# MULTIVARIATE STATISTICS FOR NURSING RESEARCH

# Multivariate Statistics for Nursing Research

**Beverly J. Volicer, M.P.H., Ph.D.**
College of Health Professions
University of Lowell
Lowell, Massachusetts

(G&S)

**Grune & Stratton, Inc.**
(Harcourt Brace Jovanovich, Publishers)
Orlando    San Diego    San Francisco    New York    London
Toronto    Montreal    Sydney    Tokyo    São Paulo

**Library of Congress Cataloging in Publication Data**

Volicer, Beverly J.
  Multivariate statistics for nursing research.

  Bibliography: p. 315
  Includes index.
  1. Nursing—Research—Statistical methods.
  2. Multivariate analysis. I. Title.
  RT81.5.Y65 1984     519.5′35′024613     83-26601
  ISBN 0-8089-1639-4


© 1984 by Grune & Stratton, Inc.

All rights reserved. No part of this publication
may be reproduced or transmitted in any form or
by any means, electronic or mechanical, including
photocopy, recording, or any information storage
and retrieval system, without permission in
writing from the publisher.

  Grune & Stratton, Inc.
  Orlando, Florida 32887

  Distribution in the United Kingdom by
  Grune & Stratton, Ltd.
  24/28 Oval Road, London NW 1

  Library of Congress Catalog Number 83-26601
  International Standard Book Number 0-8089-1639-4

**Printed in the United States of America**
84  85  86  87    10  9  8  7  6  5  4  3  2  1

To my mother, Johanna Beers

# Contents

| | | |
|---|---|---|
| Preface | | xi |
| Chapter 1 | **Introduction** | 1 |
| | Descriptive versus Inferential Statistics | 2 |
| | Inference from Samples to Populations | 3 |
| | Inference as Hypothesis Testing | 8 |
| | Inference in the Context of Research | 11 |
| Chapter 2 | **Binomial and Normal Distributions** | 19 |
| | Binomial Distribution | 19 |
| | Normal Distribution | 24 |
| | Sampling Distributions of Proportions | 28 |
| | Testing a Proportion | 31 |
| | Comparing Two Proportions | 34 |
| Chapter 3 | **$t$-Tests** | 40 |
| | Uses of $t$-tests | 40 |
| | Sampling Distributions of Means | 43 |
| | $t$ Distribution | 47 |
| | Testing a Mean | 50 |
| | Comparing Two Means | 54 |
| | Confidence Intervals | 57 |
| | Paired $t$-test | 59 |
| Chapter 4 | **Chi-Square Tests** | 66 |
| | Uses of Chi-square Tests | 66 |
| | Chi-square Distribution | 69 |
| | 2 × 2 Tables | 71 |
| | R × C Tables | 74 |
| | Partitioning of Chi-square | 77 |
| | Goodness-of-Fit Tests | 81 |
| | Categorizing Data | 83 |

| Chapter 5 | **REGRESSION ANALYSIS** | **91** |
|---|---|---|
| | Uses of Regression | 91 |
| | Determining a Regression Line | 94 |
| | Deviations from the Regression Line | 101 |
| | Testing a Regression Hypothesis | 102 |
| | Partitioning the Regression Sum of Squares | 105 |
| | The $F$ Distribution | 108 |
| | Summary | 111 |

| Chapter 6 | **CORRELATION AND PARTIAL CORRELATION** | **118** |
|---|---|---|
| | Correlation Coefficient | 118 |
| | Testing a Correlation Hypothesis | 121 |
| | Proportion of Variance Explained | 125 |
| | Association versus Causation | 126 |
| | Partial Correlation | 128 |

| Chapter 7 | **MULTIPLE REGRESSION** | **141** |
|---|---|---|
| | Multivariate Analysis | 141 |
| | Determining a Regression Equation | 143 |
| | Testing a Multiple Regression Hypothesis | 144 |
| | Stepwise Selection of Variables | 150 |
| | Stepwise Significance Tests | 155 |
| | Shrinkage in Multiple Regression | 162 |

| Chapter 8 | **MULTIPLE REGRESSION, CONTINUED** | **171** |
|---|---|---|
| | Nonlinear Relationships | 173 |
| | Interaction | 179 |
| | Dummy Coding | 182 |
| | Summary | 186 |

| Chapter 9 | **ANALYSIS OF VARIANCE AND MULTIPLE COMPARISONS** | **193** |
|---|---|---|
| | Uses of Analysis of Variance | 193 |
| | The One-Way ANOVA Model | 194 |
| | Partitioning the Sum of Squares in One-Way ANOVA | 196 |
| | Testing the One-Way ANOVA Hypothesis | 199 |

|   |   |   |
|---|---|---|
| | Multiple Comparisons | 206 |
| | Scheffé Tests | 211 |
| | Orthogonal Contrasts | 213 |
| | Trend Analysis | 218 |
| | Summary | 220 |
| **Chapter 10** | **TWO-WAY ANALYSIS OF VARIANCE** | **225** |
| | Main Effects and Interaction Effects | 226 |
| | The General Two-Way ANOVA Model | 232 |
| | Partitioning the Sum of Squares in Two-Way ANOVA | 235 |
| | Testing Two-Way ANOVA Hypotheses | 240 |
| | ANOVA with Multiple Factors | 244 |
| | Summary | 246 |
| **Chapter 11** | **ANALYSIS OF VARIANCE, CONTINUED** | **256** |
| | Fixed and Random Effects | 256 |
| | Randomized Blocks | 258 |
| | Repeated Measures | 263 |
| | Repeated Measures with Random Assignment | 265 |
| | Multivariate ANOVA | 269 |
| | Summary | 269 |
| **Chapter 12** | **ANALYSIS OF COVARIANCE** | **277** |
| | Uses of ANOCOVA | 277 |
| | The General ANOCOVA Procedure | 279 |
| | Testing an ANOCOVA Hypothesis | 285 |
| | ANOCOVA with Multiple Covariates | 287 |
| **Chapter 13** | **FACTOR ANALYSIS AND DISCRIMINANT ANALYSIS** | **293** |
| | Factor Analysis | 293 |
| | Discriminant Analysis | 297 |
| **Chapter 14** | **POWER AND SAMPLE SIZE** | **304** |
| | Cohen's Approach to Power Analysis | 305 |
| | Difference Between Two Means | 308 |
| | Multiple Correlation | 310 |

| | |
|---|---:|
| **REFERENCES** | **315** |
| **APPENDIX: STATISTICAL TABLES** | **319** |
| **ANSWERS TO SELECTED PROBLEMS** | **327** |
| **SUBJECT INDEX** | **339** |
| **AUTHOR INDEX** | **345** |

# Preface

There is presently a discrepancy between the statistical methods taught to students in health fields and related disciplines and the statistical methods commonly used in published research articles in these fields. The development of packaged computer programs has facilitated the use, in all kinds of research, of advanced statistical techniques beyond those usually taught to nonmathematicians. These canned programs have made it possible for researchers to use the most appropriate analytic techniques (instead of the easiest to calculate) while making it difficult for consumers to understand the research results. The purpose of this book, which can be used for reference or as a text, is to acquaint the reader with those advanced techniques which are now widely used in health research but not generally understood by its consumers.

Applications of the techniques discussed have been taken from the field of nursing. Graduate students in nursing are now generally required to take courses in elementary statistics and research methods. They are expected to become consumers of nursing research, and many of them will eventually do their own research. The statistical procedures commonly included in such courses are chi-square, $t$-tests, correlation, and occasionally an introduction to one-way analysis of variance. Before canned statistical computer programs became widely available, nurse researchers used these elementary methods for data analysis. However, these procedures are appropriate for investigation of bivariate relationships rather than relationships among three or more variables. Computers have made it possible for nurse researchers to use complicated multivariate methods of data analysis more appropriate to nursing research than the elementary techniques.

Nursing research generally deals with the real world, and most real-world problems are not bivariate in nature. Nursing research commonly concerns the psychological and physical effects of nursing interventions or other variations in treatments or experiences related to health. Since these effects can be influenced by many factors, there are often several independent variables to be evaluated or controlled within one study. This means that multivariate procedures usually are appropriate. These include multiple regression and various forms of analysis of variance and covariance.

There are many advanced-level statistics texts available that deal with multivariate techniques. They tend to be fairly abstract, to require sophisticated mathematical background, and to have applications which are not relevant for nursing. *Multivariate Statistics for Nursing Research* is oriented toward the nonmathematically inclined reader, and assumes no mathematical training beyond algebra. Most of the examples are taken from actual nursing research studies or are prototypes of such studies. The intent is not to describe the mechanics of data analysis, but rather to teach the reader how to reach conclusions from complicated multivariate analyses and to judge whether the appropriate analytical methods have been used in a given situation.

Chapters 1–4 of the book include a discussion of elementary methods and can be used as a review. If the book is used as a text, these four chapters are helpful in bringing students to a similar level of comprehension of basic methods, especially hypothesis testing, prior to the introduction of more complicated methods. Chapters 5–8 cover various forms of multiple regression, including stepwise multiple regression, use of dummy coding, and investigation of nonlinear relationships. Chapters 9–12 on analysis of variance cover one- and two-way classifications, randomized blocks, repeated measures, and analysis of covariance. An introduction to factor analysis and discriminant analysis is provided in Chapter 13, and Chapter 14 includes a discussion of power and sample size. Although the examples are from nursing research, the material can be easily adapted for use in any discipline in which psychological or physical characteristics of individuals are systematically studied.

*Multivariate Statistics for Nursing Research* was developed from my experience in teaching intermediate-level statistics to students in nursing at Boston University. These students need to be able to choose the appropriate statistical procedures for their dissertation research (as well as their future research), carry out the analyses, and interpret the findings. Computers can easily do the analysis, but human judgments are necessary to determine the computer input and interpret the computer output. The ability to make these judgments is rapidly becoming important for all people interested in current nursing research, and this book will assist readers in developing this ability.

The original, self-published version of this book was titled *Advanced Statistical Methods with Nursing Research Applications*. In the present version, I have expanded the explanations of the ethics of experimentation, categorization of data, coding for categorical variables, trend analysis, multiple comparison procedures, interaction, and factor analysis. Statistical tables for the normal, $t$, chi-square, and $F$ distributions have also been included. I have retained most of the mathematical formulas that appeared in the original version. It has been my experience that formulas are very useful in teaching the logic behind hypothesis testing, even when the derivation of the formulas is not understood. The best example of this

# Preface

is in teaching the effect of sample size on the power of statistical tests. Even though they may have no idea why the test statistic has the distribution it does, students can see by the location of the $n$'s in the computational formula how an increase in sample size tends to inflate the test statistic.

I am indebted to many friends and colleagues who have made the writing of this book possible. The persistent questions of doctoral students in the School of Nursing at Boston University resulted in improvements in the text material and stimulated my own self-study of advanced topics. Among the most helpful individuals were Dorrian Sweetser, Terry Malcolm, Paulette Cournoyer, and Kathryn Hegedus. The benefits of the book have been increased by the generosity of many authors and publishers in giving permission for the adaptation of their data to use as examples of the various techniques.

Throughout the original writing and recent revisions of this book, I have received continued and enthusiastic support from numerous friends. The women who have assisted me through child care, housecleaning, car pooling, and moral support are too numerous to name. The work could not have been completed without the encouragement and cooperation provided by my husband, Ladislav Volicer. Lastly, I thank my daughters, Zuzka, Mika, and Nadya, for enduring my preoccupation with this book during the many hours required for preparation.

# MULTIVARIATE STATISTICS FOR NURSING RESEARCH

ard # Chapter 1

## INTRODUCTION

The objective of this book is to describe procedures useful in the application of statistics to various kinds of data commonly encountered in nursing research. Since research in nursing includes both experimental and nonexperimental studies and also tends to deal with both psychosocial and physiological variables in relation to patient health and illness, the data nurse researchers must deal with are extremely diverse. The statistical methods to be presented in this text are intended to be applicable to this wide range in types of observation and measurement.

One intent of the presentation of analytical procedures and examples in this book is to demonstrate that there are usually several ways to approach a particular set of data. There is seldom one technique that is the only appropriate way to analyze a body of data. Part of this is due to the fact that many of the procedures (e.g., regression and analysis of variance) commonly believed to be different techniques are actually closely related. An appreciation of the similarities of the different procedures should increase the readers' options in dealing with their own data as well as provide new insights into already published studies.

It is hoped that those who read this book will become better prepared as consumers of nursing research as well as better prepared to carry out statistical analyses of their own data. A by-product should be an increased ability to understand the statistical thinking behind much information of current general interest to the public. The mathematical basis for statistics is, of course, the same, whether the application is in nursing, another health field, or any one of the numerous areas in which statistical methods are now used. An understanding of the basic logic underlying statistical treatment of data is appropriate as part of a general education for coping with the world of today.

## DESCRIPTIVE VERSUS INFERENTIAL STATISTICS

Consider the following statements, which are typical of those found in the "results" section of nursing research studies: "During the first trimester, the number of pregnancy symptoms reported by women in the study ranged from 0 to 20, averaging 8," "The mean age in a sample of 100 nursing home residents was 83.4 years," and "of 200 patients interviewed, 82% indicated that the threat of loss of function of the senses was the most stressful event associated with a hospitalization experience."

These statements are examples of what the word "statistics" is commonly understood to mean—any piece of information expressed in numerical form. Such statistics are likely to be referred to in an elementary statistics book under the major heading of *"Descriptive Statistics."* Descriptive statistics are intended to summarize information, using percentages, averages, graphs, or other devices designed to present the data in a simple form. The intent of descriptive statistics is to characterize the data in numerical form so that one can get a picture of the nature of the observations without considering them one by one.

The other major division of statistics likely to be discussed in a statistics book is called *Inferential Statistics*. The term "inferential" is derived from the fact that inferences are made, that is, conclusions are drawn, about characteristics of a large population based on a sample of observations from that population. The theory of inferential statistics provides methods for making conclusions about what is likely to be true for a large population, given the data actually observed in the sample. For example, one of the above statements refers to a study of women in the first trimester of pregnancy, who reported an average of 8 symptoms. For a large population of women similar in age and life-style to those observed in this study, we could infer, using the theory of inferential statistics, that the number of pregnancy symptoms during the first trimester is unlikely to deviate more than a given amount from the estimated value of 8. As you will see in the descriptions of procedures included in this text, statistical theory provides a very systematic procedure for making such inferences.

Another very common use of inferential statistics is in the comparison of the experiences of two or more groups. Suppose that the 5-year survival rate for 50 breast cancer patients treated with a placebo is 30% and for 50 similar patients treated with a new cytostatic agent is 35%. An investigator who obtains data of this sort is not merely interested in the particular 100 women who happen to be in the study, but in the effectiveness of the new drug in general. In this study, the patients given the placebo (the control group) represent a large population of breast cancer patients treated by placebo. Similarly, the patients given the new drug (the experimental group) represent a large population of breast cancer patients treated by

Introduction

the new drug. The theory of inferential statistics can be used to determine whether 30% versus 35% survival is likely to represent a real or trivial difference in survival rates between these two large populations of breast cancer patients. The 100 subjects actually observed during the study are the samples from which judgment about the two larger populations can be made.

By inferential statistics we mean a process of using data about a limited number of subjects (a *sample*) to make judgments about what is likely to be true for the subjects represented by that sample (a *population*). Or we may use data from two or more samples (such as a control group and an experimental group) to make a judgment about the differences between populations represented by the samples. The use of inferential statistics always presumes a specific bit of information, or data, from one or more samples, from which one would like to make some general conclusions about the populations that the samples are taken to represent.

## INFERENCE FROM SAMPLES TO POPULATIONS

The process of statistical inference involves making judgments about populations based on sample information. Any group of people, rats, mice, cities, and so on, about which we wish to make inferences, can be considered a population. Any subgroup or portion of such a population from which we actually collect data in order to make the inference about the population is called a *sample*. It is often possible to obtain data with which to make solid statistical inferences from fairly small samples of extremely large populations when study of the whole population would be either unfeasible or actually impossible.

The procedure of taking a sample for the purpose of making inferences is not limited to statistical endeavors. Everyone takes samples all the time. When you taste a gin and tonic for the first time and decide whether to drink it, you are sampling and making inferences, because you are deciding what all the rest of the sips would probably taste like, given the one or two you have taken. When you decide to see a Fellini film because you liked the ones you saw before, you are inferring that all his films are likely to be good on the basis of your sample.

Similar examples of how inferences are casually made from samples can be observed in medicine and the health sciences. Physicians who try a new sample drug on several patients with a particular medical condition and observe beneficial effects may start to prescribe the drug routinely on all patients with the same condition. The physicians are inferring from their observed samples of a few patients that the drug will be beneficial to patients in general. Nurses who observe very negative reactions from several patients when trying to explain details of a surgical procedure to them the day before surgery may discontinue the effort. The nurses are making generalizations, or inferences, that most patients do not want to hear the information they have been trying to give, or at least don't want to hear it at the time or under the circumstances they have used. In both of these examples, a small number of patients (sample) are observed, and a conclusion is made about what is likely to be true for patients in general (population).

Any procedure in which data or observations on subjects are used to make generalizations to some unobserved subjects involves sampling and inference. The difference between inferential statistics and the ordinary thinking process by which we commonly make inferences is that the statistical method provides a systematic procedure for making the inference that is based on probability. In the examples given earlier, the inference is likely to be made in a relatively intuitive, and quite subjective, manner. Statistics provides a method for making such decisions in a relatively objective way, so that different observers of the same data are likely to come to the same conclusion.

The value of information obtained from a sample submitted to statistical analysis, just as the value of information obtained and used in a more casual manner, depends to a large extent on the manner in which the sample is taken. If the sample is taken in such a way that it is likely to be *representative* of or like the population, the inferences made about the population are likely to be quite accurate. A sample that does not represent the population, or that is biased in some way, will yield inaccurate information about the population. (If you taste a gin and tonic without stirring it and if the gin has been put into the glass first, you may be quite disappointed. Your sample information will be quite different from what it would be if you stirred the drink a few times before the sample sipping.)

As an example of bias, consider the physician's judgment about the effectiveness of a new drug described previously. Suppose that the only patients who are given the new drug are students, who tend to be younger than the average patient. This might happen because the physician assumes that older patients can easily pay for the usual drugs and therefore saves the free samples for the students. Or, the physician may feel that younger people are generally healthier than older ones and therefore might be unwilling to risk the new drug on older patients. In either case, if the observed sample consists of a younger than average group, it is a biased or nonrepresentative sample; that is, it does not truly represent the population of patients treated by the physician. It may be that the new drug works well, but only for the relatively young people on whom it was tested. In this case, a generalization about the effects of the drug made to the population of all patients may be faulty.

Introduction

Clearly, the procedure by which a sample is obtained will determine whether it is likely to be representative. The best way to maximize the chances of obtaining a representative sample is to take what is known as a *random sample*. A random sample must be picked in such a way that all subjects have an equal chance of being chosen. Stated another way, the probability of being chosen should be the same for all subjects in the population. One common way to select such a sample is to assign numbers to all subjects in the population and then select numbers at random to determine who goes into the sample. This can be done, for example, using a table of random numbers.

Sometimes all the subjects already have numbers assigned to them. For example, hospital patients have identification numbers, so one could easily identify a random sample from the population of all patients of a given hospital based on the identification numbers already assigned. This could be done with a table of random numbers. The resulting sample is referred to as a *simple random sample*. An alternative procedure would be to pick a digit randomly and then include in the sample all patients whose identification numbers end in that digit. If the study requires that patients be selected at random over a period of time, as they enter a hospital or clinic, one can use what is referred to as a *systematic sample*. For this procedure, a number is picked randomly (10 for example) and then every 10th patient who comes into the system is included in the sample.

Random sampling is most commonly used in large surveys. For example, the Gallup Poll and the Harris Poll make use of random sampling procedures. Although these polls are used to describe the opinions or voting intentions of "the American public," only a small sample of people are actually interviewed to obtain the data. The people recruited for the sample are selected in such a way that representativeness can be assumed, so that generalizations about the U.S. population can be made with a high degree of accuracy. Random sampling procedures are also used in the U.S. Census for many of the items obtained by the census takers. Such large surveys often involve modifications of simple random sampling procedures, such as *stratified random samples*. Since these techniques are very unusual in nursing research, they will not be discussed in detail. The reader should consult a text such as those by Cochran[6] or Snedecor and Cochran[41] for the details of various sampling procedures.

In many studies, and often in research in health fields, it is impossible to actually take a random sample from the population for which a generalization is to be made. This is true, for example, for any test of a new treatment for a disease. It is usually desirable to use the results of such a study to treat patients at different places and times, including patients who do not even have the disease at the time the study is done. There is generally no available, existing population of all patients with the disease from which a random sample can be drawn. Researchers who wish to investigate this sort of problem must work with the available and willing patients in their own hospitals or offices during a given period of time. The generalization of the results to a larger population rests on the assumption that the patients actually observed are likely to be representative of some larger population. In this case, the sample represents a *hypothetical* rather than an actual population, since no existing population is actually identified and sampled according to a random procedure. Determination of the population to which a generalization is to be made thus involves a good deal of judgment on the investigator's part. Demographic characteristics of the sample, including age, sex, and socioeconomic status, can be tabulated to help the researcher determine the sort of population for which the study results are likely to be representative.

The problem of biased samples can also be present when several groups are compared. Consider the possibility of nonrepresentativeness in the study of breast cancer patients mentioned earlier. In this study, we assumed that 50 patients were treated by a placebo and 50 by a new cytostatic drug. Suppose the 50 patients who received the new drug were volunteers. The fact that they were volunteers may mean that they were sicker than, younger than, or in some other way different from those who received the placebo. If there were differences like these between the two groups at the outset of the study, it would be very difficult to interpret the meaning of any difference in survival rates at the end of the study. For example, suppose that the 5-year survival rate in the experimental group turned out to be higher than the 5-year survival rate in the control group, but that it also happened that the control group subjects were sicker than the experimental subjects at the time the study began. The investigator would be unable to determine whether the survival rate was higher in the experimental group because of beneficial effects of the drug or because this group was healthier than the control group to begin with.

In the case of a study involving the comparison of groups, it may be possible to avoid bias through a procedure known as *randomization*. Randomization means that, starting with a group of subjects, such as breast cancer patients, assignment to the comparison (e.g., control vs experimental) groups is made at random. Each subject has a 50-50 chance of being in either group. This could be done, for example, by assigning the first patient who enters the study to the control group, the second to the experimental group, and so on. If patients are assigned to groups in such a manner, one would expect the groups to have approximately the same number of married and unmarried subjects, the same average age, and to be similar in any other characteristics (due to the effects of chance). The purpose of such a procedure is, of course, to make the two groups alike

# Introduction

at the beginning of the study, so that any difference observed at the end can be attributed to the effects of the treatment itself.

When patients are assigned to sample groups by a randomization procedure, random sampling is seldom used, so that the samples represent hypothetical rather than actual populations. To carry out such a randomized study, the researcher cannot start by selecting a random sample, but must use only subjects who are available and willing to participate in the study. The randomization procedure in effect yields two samples. In the case of a drug study, the control group sample represents a hypothetical population of breast cancer patients treated by a placebo, and the experimental group sample represents a hypothetical population of breast cancer patients treated by the drug under study. In generalizing the results, the investigator or consumer of the research needs to be aware of the characteristics of the individuals in these samples and the conditions under which they were studied and should not claim that the results will hold for populations of individuals different from those studied. In studies not based on random sampling, that is, in most studies with which researchers in health are concerned, a large element of judgment will be involved in making generalizations about results.

Discussion of experimental studies such as the one just described always raises ethical concerns among nurse researchers. Concern for patients as individuals makes issues involved in manipulation of experimental subjects assume crucial importance in the design and execution of many nursing research studies. Even for studies involving interviews or observations rather than subject manipulation, the concern is present, although it is less important than in true experimental studies. Since randomization is the best way to establish causation, it is very important for nurse researchers to be able to deal with these concerns. There are several ethical issues in experimental studies that should be of concern to any nurse who becomes involved in such research.

One issue to be considered is whether it is ethical to withhold treatment from patients by putting them into control groups. Since an experiment should be undertaken only when the effect of the treatment is unknown, it is generally not true that a treatment known to be effective is being withheld from control group patients. If the treatment is known to be effective, there is no need for the experiment. This problem can also be viewed from the opposite angle—that is, whether it is ethical to submit a patient to an experimental treatment whose effectiveness is not known. The logical extension of this argument is that no new treatment should ever be tried, and it is doubtful that many individuals would agree with this.

A powerful argument can be made for the fairness of randomization of subjects into experimental and control groups when there are limited resources. When it is impossible for all patients to receive treatment, randomization may be the most ethical solution, rather than the personal judgment of researchers as to who most deserves to receive the treatment. In any situation where limitations of cost, space, personnel, and other factors necessitate that the treatment or intervention be implemented over an extended period of time, randomization is a good way to allocate subjects. Those who are assigned to the control group can then receive the treatment later, when more resources become available, should the treatment prove to be effective.

These issues vary greatly in importance across various types of studies, and they include the appropriateness of informed consent and its effect on the research as well as the potential risks and benefits to the subjects. For example, issues for a study of the effects of child care availability on the appointment keeping ability of clinic patients are likely to be quite different from issues for a study of alternative treatments for breast cancer. One must consider such variables as potential patient benefit, possible side effects, and effort required of experimental subjects. A detailed examination of these issues is not within the scope of this text. Refer to Smith[39] for an excellent discussion of contemporary ethical dilemmas in behavioral research and guidelines for research involving human subjects.

## INFERENCE AS HYPOTHESIS TESTING

Statistical inference is commonly used to generalize from sample data to a population or to populations by way of *hypothesis testing*. Each particular statistical technique includes a plan for hypothesis testing. The choice of a particular technique is determined by the number of groups studied and the nature and number of variables to be analyzed. Although many kinds of hypotheses can be tested by statistical procedures, the type of hypothesis most commonly tested is what is referred to as the *null hypothesis*. A null hypothesis is an assumption, for example, that two or more groups do not differ, that two variables are not correlated, or that two traits are not associated. In an experimental study, a null hypothesis is an assumption that the experimental variable has no effect.

Before going on to an example of hypothesis testing, consider the difference between a null hypothesis and what one might call a *research hypothesis*. The research hypothesis is the actual assumption or hunch in an investigator's mind that is the basis for study. A researcher who compares the effect of a new cytostatic agent with a placebo hopes and expects that survival will be higher in the experimental group than in the control group, or the study would not be undertaken at all. The researcher certainly could not get approval from a human subjects committee to subject patients

# Introduction

to a new treatment with no evidence to suggest that it might improve survival rates. Ordinarily the research hypothesis will be opposite to the null hypothesis, since most researchers are looking for differences and associations, rather than no differences and no associations.

The null hypotheses used by statistical procedures are required by the nature of the techniques themselves; in other words, hypotheses are stated in a null form to make them testable. It is a common practice in research in the social sciences, including nursing, to state in verbal form the null hypotheses to be tested in a study, rather than the research hypotheses which are those hunches actually in the investigator's mind at the outset. This is an unnecessary and confusing practice. The null hypotheses can be assumed with the given statistical techniques and do not have to be stated verbally. The research hypotheses, on the other hand, summarize and clarify the hunches of the researcher, based on the theoretical and/or empirical rationale behind the study, and should be clearly stated.

As an example of the procedure for hypothesis testing, consider the breast cancer study described earlier. In this study, the 5-year survival rates for a control group and an experimental group are to be compared. The sequence of steps used to test a null hypothesis for these two groups will be given here. Later, you will learn the details of this and other hypothesis testing procedures. At this point, a general outline will give you an idea of the process of statistical inference.

The null hypothesis used for comparing two groups states that the two groups do not differ on the criterion or dependent variable under consideration. In the example, the null hypothesis is that the 5-year survival rates with placebo and with the new drug are equivalent. This can be written as:

$$H: p_1 = p_2$$

or

$$H: p_1 - p_2 = 0$$

The value $p_1$ stands for the proportion of survivors in a hypothetical population treated by the new drug, and the value $p_2$ stands for the proportion of survivors in a hypothetical population treated by the placebo. Since we cannot actually observe $p_1$ and $p_2$, our judgment about the similarity or difference between these two values will be based on what we actually do observe in the experimental and control groups, that is, in the samples that represent these two hypothetical populations.

It is important to note that the hypothesis is made about population values rather than sample values. We will actually observe the proportion of survivors in the sample control and experimental groups and will thus know whether they are equal, without having to hypothesize or assume anything. The hypothesis or assumption is made about the two populations these samples represent—that is, two populations we will not be able to observe but which we would like to generalize about. It should be obvious at this point that our decision about the null hypothesis will involve taking some chance of error. We will not be able to say positively whether the null hypothesis is true, since we will not observe the entire populations. We will have to settle for a statement that the evidence for rejection of the null hypothesis is either strong or insufficient.

The next step in the procedure is to collect data. Assume that in this study, a sample of 100 patients are randomly assigned to two groups of 50 each and followed for 5 years. The 5-year survival rates for these two groups will be called $\hat{p}_1$ and $\hat{p}_2$. These values are sample *estimates* of $p_1$ and $p_2$. Remember that $p_1$ and $p_2$ are unknown, since they are population values. They are the proportions of survivors for all patients treated by the new drug and all patients treated by the placebo, from hypothetical but not actually observed populations.

The third step is to compare the observed data with the outcome predicted by the null hypothesis. In this case, the null hypothesis states that there is no difference in the population survival rates. If this is true, then $\hat{p}_1$ and $\hat{p}_2$ should be very close together. Close agreement between the two sample proportions will suggest that the population values $p_1$ and $p_2$ are also very similar or equal. A large difference between $\hat{p}_1$ and $\hat{p}_2$ will imply that there is a difference between the two groups, that is, between treatment and placebo. We are really asking the question, "How reasonable does the hypothesis about population values look when evaluated according to the results shown in the sample data?"

The final step is to make a decision to either *retain* or *reject* the null hypothesis. A statistical test can be used to determine whether $\hat{p}_1$ and $\hat{p}_2$ are so close together that $H: p_1 = p_2$ should be retained, or whether $\hat{p}_1$ and $\hat{p}_2$ are so far apart that $H: p_1 = p_2$ should be rejected. This test is based on the use of probability. If the null hypothesis is true, the difference between $\hat{p}_1$ and $\hat{p}_2$ is likely to be very small, since it will represent merely chance variation in the samples. If the null hypothesis is not true, the difference in these two population values will likely be represented by a substantial difference in the two sample values. Since we are making an inference that is based on incomplete information (sample data as opposed to population data), there is always a chance of making an error. Using statistics, we can make a decision that is most probably right, and can also evaluate the chance of error, that is, of rejecting the null hypothesis when it is true.

As stated earlier, it is common in research to make a null hypothesis that one hopes to be able to reject. In this study, the null hypothesis says that the survival rate for patients on the new drug will be equal to the survival rate for those on the placebo. Anyone doing such a study would very likely expect the new drug to perform better than the placebo, and the research would anticipate that $\hat{p}_1$ would thus be quite a bit greater than $\hat{p}_2$. In statistics there is a kind of backward reasoning process. A null hypothesis is assumed, and then data are collected in an effort to reject this hypothesis in favor of an *alternative hypothesis*. The alternative hypothesis in this case is that there is a difference in survival rates in the two hypothetical populations represented by the control and experimental groups.

## INFERENCE IN THE CONTEXT OF RESEARCH

Using inferential statistics, we will be able to make a judgment about what is likely to be true of a population based on a sample, or about how two or more groups compare with each other. The validity of such an inference, however, will be determined by the context of the research study itself. In evaluating the statistical results, one should consider how the sample was taken, how the comparison groups were chosen, and how the measurements were obtained or recorded. Statistics can provide an objective way of evaluating the numbers but statistical procedures make the assumption of random sampling. You will have to consider how the data were collected to determine what a statistical conclusion means for any particular research study. The way in which a sample is chosen or comparison groups established is one of the most important things to consider in interpreting a statistical result. The following two examples will illustrate the effect of sampling on inference.

Following a presidential decision, a report of the subsequent telephone calls to the White House will often be made. This was common practice in the Nixon era. "The calls are running 9–1 in favor of the president's decision," for example, may be reported. The suggested inference is that "the people" are strongly in agreement with the decision that has been made, that is, that 90% of the population is in favor of the decision. This inference is based on a statistical fact—that 90% of the sample, namely, the callers, are in favor of the president's decision. Any conclusion about what "the people" think would have to take into consideration what sort of people are represented by the sample of callers, and this would be an extremely difficult task.

Consider which people are most likely to call the White House. Perhaps it is mainly those people who support the decision who are willing to spend the money and take the effort to call. We really don't have any idea about the opinions of the people who did not call. This is an example of data that statistically appear to show a striking conclusion, but when seen in the light of the sampling procedure (i.e., the way in which the callers have selected themselves) really give no information about the opinion of "the people." In this case, the sample is quite likely to be biased and nonrepresentative of the population. A statistical test will show only what is suggested by the data but does not take into account how the data were obtained.

Another common way that errors in inference are made is by the inappropriate use of comparison groups. Suppose that a nurse wants to study the response of patients to daily stimulation in the form of 1 hour conversations with volunteers on any subject of interest to the patients. The nurse's hypothesis is that patients receiving this kind of stimulation will recover sooner than others. Volunteers are to see some patients daily and others not at all. The only restriction is that patients who are unable or unwilling to talk with volunteers are to be left alone. At the end of a month, mean length of stay for those receiving volunteer visits is compared with mean length of stay for other patients. The means are 7.3 days for the former group and 12.7 for the latter. A statistical test on these data would probably suggest a large and significant difference in length of stay. Again, the data suggest an inference—that talking with patients helps them get well faster.

The problem is, as before, with the sampling procedure. Those who are in the experimental or conversation group may be younger, healthier, or in some way different from those in the control or no-conversation group. The assignment of people to groups has not been done in such a way that the groups are likely to be similar. Differences in length of stay may be due to initial differences in the groups rather than a treatment effect. A dramatic statistical effect may be observed that has nothing to do with any treatment effect. It is important to understand that the statistical tests assume random samples, and that the statistical findings must always be put back into the context of the study methodology.

In the course of reading this book you will learn about statistical procedures, and then you will consider research studies in which the procedures have been used. In every instance you should first consider what the statistics tell you, that is, what inference the data suggest. As you make this inference, you will then want to consider the data analysis in the context of the research design, to determine whether the suggested conclusion is justifiable in terms of the manner in which the data were collected. Consult a text such as Campbell and Stanley[3] for problems

Introduction

involved in such issues, which are often referred to as problems of internal and external validity.

## PROBLEMS

1. Corey et al.[9] studied factors thought to be associated with child abuse, using data obtained from medical records. Their sample of battered children included 48 children up to 6 years of age who were hospitalized for battering at a Midwestern public children's hospital from 1965 through 1973. The hospital used for the study was selected because it was the only hospital in the state that had patients from all socioeconomic levels and all geographic areas and treated all types of medical cases. For a comparison group of nonbattered children, the investigators obtained records of a random sample of 50 nonbattered children of the same age group and admitted to the same hospital during the same time period as the sample of battered children. Answer the following questions, based on the information given above:

(a) Describe the population that you could reasonably assume is represented by the sample of battered children.
(b) Describe the population that you could reasonably assume is represented by the sample of nonbattered children.
(c) Why do you think the researchers used children hospitalized for other reasons than battering as a comparison group (e.g., instead of children in the general population)?
(d) Why do you think the investigators included all the battered children in their sample, instead of taking a random sample, as they did for the nonbattered children?
(e) Why do you think the researchers wanted to select a hospital with patients from all socioeconomic levels and all geographic areas of the state and all types of medical cases?

2. Cleland et al.[5], conducting research to identify social and psychologic influences on employment of married nurses, obtained a study sample from the list of registered nurses in Michigan in 1972. From the list, the researchers selected all nurses who were less than 60 years old, presently married and living with spouse, had at least one child 18 years of age or younger, resided in the metropolitan Detroit area, and were born between October 1 and March 31. A letter explaining the general nature of the study was sent to the 7063 nurses who met the above criteria, asking each to respond with an enclosed postcard to indicate willingness to participate in the study. Each of the 2351 nurses who agreed to participate in

the study received an unmarked (anonymous) copy of the questionnaire, with a reminder postcard, and 2100 (89%) of the questionnaires were returned, of which 1998 (85%) were usable. Answer the following questions, based on the above information.

(a) Would it be possible to use random sampling for such a study? If so, propose a procedure.
(b) Why do you think the researchers selected nurses born between October 1 and March 31? Could this selection create any bias in the sample?
(c) How does the geographic area from which subjects were chosen affect generalization of the results?
(d) How might the findings be affected by the fact that about two-thirds of the nurses who met the criteria for inclusion in the study did not agree to participate?

3. To study postmastectomy patients 4 years after surgery, Woods and Earp[47] obtained a sample of such patients through the hospitals where their surgery was performed. Of the 134 hospitals in North Carolina, 24 reported to the State Tumor Registry at the time the study was done. Of the 24 reporting hospitals, 6 were selected. In addition to requiring the cooperation of the medical administrations of each hospital, the choices were made to obtain variability in type of hospital and region of the state in which they were located. The hospitals ranged in bed size from 121 to 823 (163 is average for all 134 hospitals in the state) and included university teaching hospitals, large community hospitals, and small voluntary hospitals. The sample was chosen as follows: All women who had had a mastectomy performed in 1972 at one of these six hospitals were selected if they:

1) were known to the Registry
2) were residents of North Carolina at the time of surgery and at the time of the interview
3) had tumors in stages 1 to 3 of the disease classification at the time of surgery (i.e., free of metastasis beyond involvement of regional nodes)
4) were free of recurrent breast disease by self-report at the time of the interview.

These criteria yielded 122 women who were sent letters by their surgeons requesting their participation in the study and their consent to be interviewed. Of the 122, 21 had died but were not listed as dead with the Registry, one had moved out of state, one had a disabling illness, 4 were not able to be located, and 46 refused to be interviewed. This left 49 women who were interviewed, fewer than 10% of the 540 women who had had a mastectomy in North Carolina in 1972.

Answer the following questions, based on the above information:

(a) The sample selected for the study is not a random sample. Explain why it is not, and discuss whether there would be any way to obtain a random sample of postmastectomy patients for North Carolina.
(b) How could the results be biased by the fact that only 24 of the hospitals in the state report to the State Tumor Registry?
(c) How could the results be biased by the fact that only 6 of the 24 hospitals reporting to the State Tumor Registry were selected for the study?
(d) Why did the researchers eliminate women who were not residents of North Carolina at the time of their surgery?
(e) Why did the researchers eliminate women who were not residents of North Carolina at the time of the study itself?
(f) Why did the researchers include only women with tumors in stages 1 to 3 at the time of surgery?
(g) How might the fact that 21 of the women selected for the study had died affect representativeness of the sample?
(h) How might the fact that 46 of the women selected for the study refused to be interviewed affect representativeness of the sample?
(i) Discuss how the researchers might attempt to ascertain how representative their sample actually was. Read the article to see what they actually did.

4. In a study of morale among aged people in institutions, Chang[4] interviewed 30 residents, aged 65 to 96, in four skilled nursing facilities. The four institutions qualified as skilled nursing facilities according to Department of Health, Education and Welfare standards for certification and participation in Medicare and Medicaid programs. Two of the facilities were free-standing and the other two were geographically connected to acute-care hospitals. The capacity of the parent institutions was from 100 to 350 beds, with a range of 22 to 62 beds on the units from which study subjects came. Individuals who met the following criteria were included in the study:

1) age 65 or over
2) sufficient energy level to participate in the testing procedures (e.g., not in acute stages of chronic illness, not suffering from pain or elevated temperature, not complaining of fatigue)
3) able to read and understand English
4) oriented to person and place and able to give oral and written informed consent

5) self-rating their health as "fair" or better
6) no previous admission to the same unit in the selected skilled nursing facility
7) in the same institution on the same unit for at least 2 weeks and not more than 6 months
8) Caucasian, and had lived most of their lives in the United States

Based on the information above, answer the following questions:

(a) Describe the population that you could reasonably assume is represented by the sample used for this study.
(b) Why do you think the researcher used only subjects who rated their own health as "fair" or better?
(c) How could the researcher determine whether the facilities used were representative of skilled nursing facilities in general?
(d) Discuss how the various selection criteria simplify the study while simultaneously limiting generalization of the results.

5. Consider the following hypothetical study. A questionnaire was mailed to a random sample of 1000 recent graduates of Boston University School of Nursing to find out the types of jobs the graduates had taken. The purpose of this study was to evaluate the preparation provided by the school in relation to jobs taken by the students. Results from the 500 questionnaires that were returned were tabulated as indicated in Table 1-1.

The investigators concluded that the curriculum should go in two directions—preparation for staff nurse positions and preparation for graduate school work—since the majority of respondents indicated these two types of activity.

(a) Describe the population that you could reasonably assume is represented by the sample of 1000 graduates to whom the questionnaire was mailed.

**Table 1-1.** Number and Percent of 500 Boston University Graduates Classified by Job Type

| Type of job | N | Percent, % |
| --- | --- | --- |
| Staff nurse in hospital | 250 | 50 |
| In graduate school | 150 | 30 |
| Other nursing positions | 85 | 17 |
| President of bank | 5 | 1 |
| Lifeguard | 5 | 1 |
| Unemployed | 5 | 1 |

- (b) Describe the population that you could reasonably assume is represented by the 500 graduates who returned the questionnaire.
- (c) How might the 500 individuals who did not return the questionnaire differ from the ones who did in such a way as to make the sample nonrepresentative? Think of specific ways in which the nonrespondents might differ or not differ from the respondents.
- (d) Assume that the researchers have access to student records for the 1000 graduates to whom the questionnaire was mailed. For which of the sources of bias identified in item c would it be possible to compare the respondents and nonrespondents, to identify any differences?
- (e) Discuss the conclusion of the investigators, in the light of your answers to the above questions.

6. Suppose that you are asked to take a sample of the population of patients enrolled at a neighborhood health center to find out their opinions about whether the center is fully serving their needs. Suggest at least three procedures by which the sample could be obtained (both good and bad). For each procedure, determine:

- (a) What are the possible sources of nonrepresentativeness?
- (b) How feasible would the procedure be in terms of time, money, and likelihood of good response?

7. In a hypothetical study comparing traditional classroom teaching with a new open classroom idea, each of 200 first-grade students was randomly assigned to one of two classes. Some of the parents of children assigned to the open classroom refused to have their children "used" in an experiment, and these children were sent to the traditional classroom. The classes were maintained for a year, and intelligence testing of all the children was done at the end. The statistical analysis indicated much higher levels of intelligence in the open classroom group, according to the measurement tool used.

- (a) How does the refusal of some parents to cooperate affect the interpretation of these results?
- (b) How could the number of children who were switched to the traditional classroom affect the interpretation of the results (e.g., 2 vs 50)?
- (c) How could the procedure of assignment to groups be done to avoid the problem of switching between the groups but still make the groups comparable?

8. Discuss the feasibility of a randomized study to answer each of the following questions:

(a) Does fluoride in drinking water reduce tooth decay among children?
(b) Does smoking cause lung cancer?
(c) Does increased verbal stimulation help children learn to talk sooner?
(d) Does diabetic teaching by trained nurses increase diet compliance?

# Chapter 2

# BINOMIAL AND NORMAL DISTRIBUTIONS

## BINOMIAL DISTRIBUTIONS

The word "variable" refers to any characteristic that varies among observed cases or subjects. Age, blood pressure, sex, number of times hospitalized, and marital status are examples of variables that might be observed among a sample of hospital patients. Those variables that can take on only two values are referred to as *binomial* variables. For example, sex has the categories, "male" and "female" as its only possible values and is thus a binomial variable. Other examples are type of patient (medical or surgical) and marital status (married or not married). A tabulation of the proportion of a population in each of the two possible categories of a binomial variable is referred to as a *binomial distribution*. Examples using the binomial distribution are included in this chapter because of the simplicity with which the binomial distribution can be used to illustrate hypothesis testing. You will see in later chapters that alternative procedures are more commonly used in nursing research.

As a model for the binomial distribution, consider the outcomes of a coin tossing experiment. There are only two possible outcomes of tossing a coin—heads or tails. Therefore, the outcome of a coin tossing experiment is a binomial variable. Consider the probability of each of the two possible outcomes:

$$Pr \text{ (head)} = ? \qquad Pr \text{ (tail)} = ?$$

You know that, given a fair coin, the probability of a head is 1/2, and the probability of a tail is 1/2. This listing of the probability of each possible outcome is called a *probability distribution* and, in this case, a *binomial probability distribution*. Notice that the sum of the probabilities is 1. The sum of probabilities of all the possible outcomes of any such experiment must always equal 1.

The coin tossing experiment just described is equivalent to taking a random sample of size 1 from a population where 50% are male and 50% are female. The probability of choosing a male is 1/2, and the probability of choosing a female is 1/2. Or consider a population of hospital patients in which 50% of the patients have cancer. If one patient is chosen at random, the probability is 1/2 that one of the cancer patients will be chosen and 1/2 that one of the others will be chosen.

The idea of a probability distribution can be extended to a situation where a coin is tossed more than once. Suppose, for example, that a coin is tossed 4 times. Using binomial distribution theory and some elaborate formulas, or a binomial table in a statistics book, we can list all the possible outcomes of this experiment and determine the probability associated with each one. These are:

$$
\begin{aligned}
Pr\,(4\ \text{heads}) &= .0625 \\
Pr\,(3\ \text{heads, 1 tail}) &= .2500 \\
Pr\,(2\ \text{heads, 2 tails}) &= .3750 \\
Pr\,(1\ \text{head, 3 tails}) &= .2500 \\
Pr\,(0\ \text{heads}) &= \underline{.0625} \\
& \phantom{=}\ 1.0000
\end{aligned}
$$

The above listing is, of course, another example of a binomial probability distribution, since it gives the probability associated with each of the four possible outcomes of the experiment.

This experiment can also be regarded as a simulation of a real situation. Suppose a population exists with 50% males and 50% females. If a random sample of size 4 is taken from this population, the above probability distribution can be used to predict the probability of various outcomes. For example, the probability that the sample will consist of 4 males is .0625, the probability of 3 males and 1 female is .2500, and so forth. For any population with a given proportion in each category of a binomial variable, the theory behind the binomial distribution allows us to determine the probability of any particular outcome for a given size sample. Note that calculation of the probabilities of the various outcomes of a sample are always based on an assumption or hypothesis about what the true population is like. In the case of tossing a coin, the above distribution describes what could be expected in 4 tosses, assuming the coin is fair, that is, assuming

$$Pr\,(\text{head}) = 1/2$$

or, equivalently,

$$Pr\,(\text{tail}) = 1/2$$

# Binomial and Normal Distributions

This theoretical binomial distribution also tells us what we might expect to observe when sampling from a population assumed to contain 50% males and 50% females. According to the figures, a sample of size 4 consisting of all males is relatively unlikely to happen; that is, $Pr$ (4 males) = $Pr$ (4 heads) = .0625. Such a sample result might lead us to question the original assumption or hypothesis that the population really has equal proportions of males and females. Such an outcome would tend to suggest that the true proportion of males in the population may be larger than 50%. This example illustrates the basic way in which statistical inference operates. We first make a hypothesis about the values of some variable in the population—in this case, the proportion of males in the population—and then observe a sample. A sample result with a low probability of occurrence, given the original assumption (i.e., 50% males in the population), suggests that this assumption should be rejected.

The binomial probability distribution can also be determined for situations where the probability of each of the two outcomes is not equal to 1/2. Consider a population where 80% of the people are diseased and 20% are not. For a random sample of 5 people from this population, the theoretical probabilities for each sort of outcome are as follows:

$Pr$ (5 diseased)           = .32768
$Pr$ (4 diseased, 1 not)    = .40960
$Pr$ (3 diseased, 2 not)    = .20480
$Pr$ (2 diseased, 3 not)    = .05120
$Pr$ (1 diseased, 4 not)    = .00640
$Pr$ (none diseased)        = .00032
                              1.00000

Notice that this distribution with $p$ = 4/5 (80%) is not symmetric, as is the case for $p$ = 1/2. Here, the probability is concentrated at one end of the distribution. It is likely that the sample will contain more diseased than healthy individuals, rather than a nearly equal number of each. Using such a binomial probability distribution, we could test a hypothesis about a population proportion. Consider the example that follows.

Suppose that experience has indicated that the usual incidence of a certain infection in any unvaccinated population is about 80%. We are interested in the incidence of this infection among people treated with a new vaccine. For a small preliminary study of the effectiveness of the vaccine, a sample of 5 people are inoculated. This small sample comes from a hypothetical population, specifically, that population consisting of a large number of people inoculated with the new vaccine. The sample is not a random sample, since no actual population is identified and sampled; there is no existing population consisting of individuals inoculated with the new vaccine. In order to make any generalization about the effects of the vaccine, it is necessary to assume that the sample of 5 people represents a random sample of all people who could in the future be treated with the vaccine. If the researcher is willing to assume this, a statistical inference about the effect of the vaccine on the incidence of infection can be made.

The first step used in the procedure for statistical inference is to establish a null hypothesis. The null hypothesis in this case is the assumption that the new vaccine is ineffective. If this is true, the incidence of infection in the hypothetical population of patients treated by the vaccine should be equal to the known incidence of infection in similar but unvaccinated populations. The latter figure is known to be 80%, so the null hypothesis is

$$H: p = .80$$

where $p$ is the proportion infected in the hypothetical population. If this null hypothesis is true, and if the sample of 5 patients actually inoculated is assumed to act as a random sample from this population, then $\hat{p}$, the proportion of sample patients infected, should be about 80% or 4 out of 5.

Note that the null hypothesis can be also stated in terms of the proportion not infected, instead of the proportion infected. If the known incidence of infection in an unvaccinated population is 80%, the proportion not infected must be 20%. Therefore, the null hypothesis could be stated as

$$H: p = .20$$

In this case, the null hypothesis refers to the proportion not infected, and the analysis would compare the observed proportion not infected in the sample with the hypothesized proportion not infected. Similarly, a null hypothesis can refer to either the proportion male or the proportion female in a population. Or a null hypothesis can refer to either the proportion of surgical patients or the proportion of medical patients in a population. The results of the statistical analysis will be equivalent, so that the choice of how to phrase the null hypothesis in a binomial situation is a matter of the researcher's preference.

Collection of data is the second step in the hypothesis testing procedure. For this study a sample of 5 people are inoculated. Suppose that of these 5, 1 becomes infected and 4 do not. The incidence of infection in this sample is, therefore,

$$\hat{p} = 1/5$$

or

$$\hat{p} = .20$$

A comparison of data obtained from the sample with the outcome predicted by the null hypothesis indicates a striking difference between the sample infection rate, 20%, and the assumed rate of 80% in the hypothetical population represented by this sample. If the null hypothesis were true and the vaccine was really ineffective, we would expect a sample infection rate closer to 80% than the observed 20%. The large discrepancy between the observed value and the value expected according to the null hypothesis suggests that the null hypothesis should be questioned and perhaps rejected.

The probability distribution of outcomes for a sample of size 5 from a distribution with $p = .80$, listed above, provides an objective criterion for evaluating the large discrepancy between the observed and expected values. The probability of the observed sample outcome of 20% infected is, according to the figures given earlier, equal to .00640, on the assumption that the sample represents a population with a true infection rate of 80%. In other words, the chance of getting only 1 in 5 infected if the vaccine is ineffective is about 6.4 in 1000. The fact that this probability is so small, specifically, less than 1 in 100, suggests that the sample does not represent a population with a true infection rate of 80%. The rate of infection in the hypothetical population is probably not equal to .80, and the null hypothesis should be rejected. The outcome suggests a much lower rate of infection than .80, or, in other words, that the vaccine is effective.

It should be noted that the probability distribution does indicate that there is a chance that 1 in 5 in the sample could be infected, given a true rate of infection of .80. This chance is equal to .00640, or about 6.4 in 1000. The chance of none infected in this situation is .00032, so the probability of one or more infected is about .00672. In other words, there is a very small chance that the vaccine is not effective, but that only one of the 5 people in the sample were infected anyway. If this is true, the decision to reject the null hypothesis is an error, that is, an incorrect decision. This chance of error is so small, however, that we will reject the null hypothesis and take this very small chance that an error is being made. Since we can never actually observe the incidence of infection in the entire population, we won't ever know definitely whether an error has been made, but we do know that the chance or probability that such an error has been made is very small. This kind of error, that of rejecting the null hypothesis when it is true, is called a *Type I error*. Of course, if we wanted to be even more stringent, we could decide to reject the null hypothesis only if none of the 5 people we infected, in which case the chance of error would be .00032.

This illustration gives you an idea of how to use a probability distribution to test a null hypothesis. The known probability distribution under the null hypothesis allows you to determine the probability of error associated with rejecting the null hypothesis. We haven't yet discussed how much probability should be allowed for this small chance of error, which is referred to as the *level of significance*. Since the binomial distribution we have discussed here is not too commonly used, we will not discuss it further. Unless the sample size is extremely small, it is common to use the normal distribution as an approximation for the binomial to test hypotheses about proportions. The normal distribution and its usefulness for testing hypotheses about proportions, as well as the determination of level of significance, are the subjects of the remainder of this chapter.

## NORMAL DISTRIBUTION

Everyone over 5 years old has experienced the idea of a normal distribution, although it might not have been called by that name. In every grade school class there are a few very young students and a few older, with most of the ages clustered around some average. There are a few very short students and a few very tall ones, with most tending toward some typical height. On a test there are usually only a few very high and a few very low marks, with the majority of marks somewhere in the middle. Variables such as age, height, and grades, for a large population, tend to have the characteristic shape indicated in Figure 2-1.

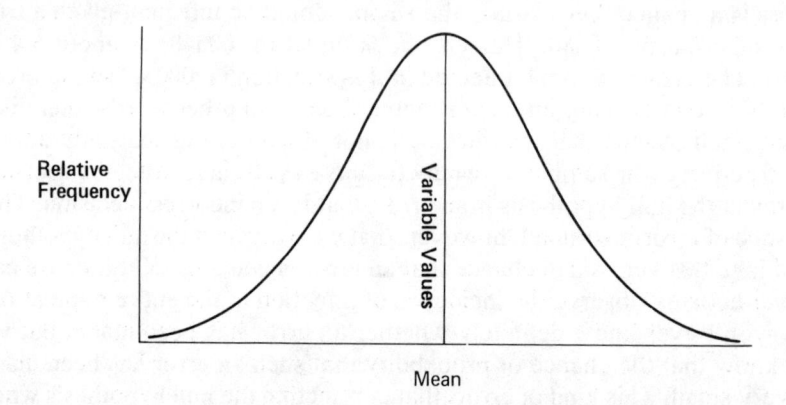

**Figure 2-1.** Normal distribution.

# Binomial and Normal Distributions

In the graph in this figure the values of the variables are plotted along the horizontal axis and relative frequency of occurrence on the vertical axis.

This shape is called the *normal distribution,* or sometimes the *Gaussian distribution* or *bell curve.* Temperature, blood pressure, and pulse are examples of variables that tend to be normally distributed in large populations. Many commonly observed variables are distributed normally, and more theoretical work in statistics has been done with this distribution than with any other probability distribution. There is consequently a great amount of theoretical knowledge about the normal distribution and about distributions of sample statistics obtained from normal populations. We will use some of these theoretical results to test hypotheses about proportions. Later, these same results will be useful for testing hypotheses about means and other population parameters.

There are two *parameters* or population characteristics that are used to describe any normal distribution. These are

$$\text{mean } \mu$$

and

$$\text{variance } \sigma^2 \text{ (or standard deviation } \sigma\text{)}$$

The mean is the value at the center of the distribution, and the variance is a measure of variation or spread of observations about the mean. Knowledge of these two parameters for any normally distributed variable in a population allows us to describe in detail the shape of the distribution of the variable and to determine the relative frequency of values that the variable takes on above, below, or between any specified values. Values of common interest are those representing the mean, and 1, 2, and 3 standard deviations above and below the mean.

The graph shown in Figure 2-2 describes any normally distributed variable. According to the graph, one can expect 68.3% of the values of a normally distributed variable to lie within 1 standard deviation of the mean, 95.5% of the values to lie within 2 standard deviations of the mean, and 99.7% of the values to lie within 3 standard deviations of the mean. Proportions of the distribution lying between any other two points on the graph can also be specified, and all these proportions will hold true for any normal distribution, regardless of the actual values of the mean and variance.

As an example of how this knowledge about the normal distributions can be useful in describing the relative frequencies of various values of a variable in a population, consider the distribution of serum cholesterol

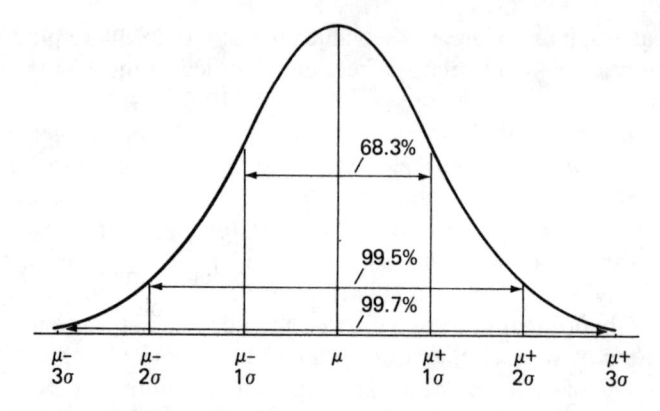

**Figure 2-2.** Normal distribution, indicating proportions within 1, 2, and 3 standard deviations of the mean.

level in a population. Suppose the serum cholesterol level is known to be normally distributed with a mean of 250 and a standard deviation of 10. The distribution of this variable is indicated in Figure 2-3.

In this population, we would expect 68.3% of the people to have serum cholesterol levels between 240 and 260, 95.5% between 230 and 270, and 99.7% between 220 and 280. A similar graph can be constructed for any normally distributed variable, provided the mean and variance are known.

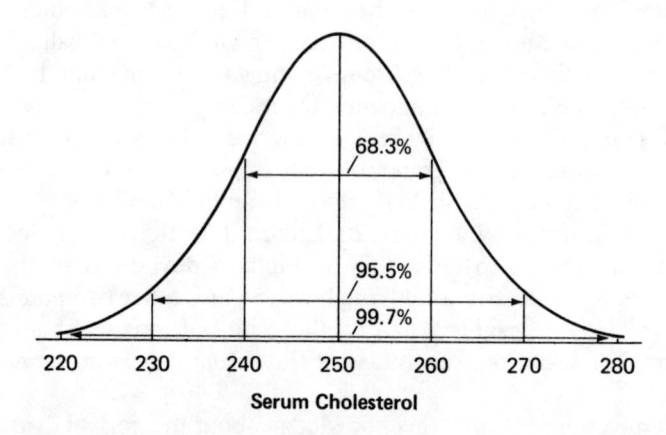

**Figure 2-3.** Normal distribution of serum cholesterol level with mean 250, standard deviation 10.

For the distribution just described, consider a simple procedure by which we can translate each serum cholesterol value into a standardized form. This is done according to the following formula:

$$z = \frac{x - \mu}{\sigma}$$

In this formula, $x$ represents any serum cholesterol value, and $z$ is the standardized score for that value. In order to determine what the $z$ value, called the $z$ score, represents, consider a serum cholesterol value of $x = 260$. The $z$ score for this value is

$$z = \frac{x - \mu}{\sigma}$$
$$= \frac{260 - 250}{10} = \frac{10}{10} = 1$$

Notice that a serum cholesterol of 260 is precisely 1 standard deviation (in this case 10 units) above the mean of 250. The $z$ score for any value turns out to represent the *number of standard deviations* by which that value deviates from the mean. If this transformation is made on all $x$ values from a normal distribution, the transformed values will have a distribution that is called the *z distribution* or the *standardized normal distribution*.

Regardless of the original values of $\mu$ and $\sigma$, that is, for any normally distributed variable, the standardized normal distribution (the distribution of the $z$ values) is normal in shape with $\mu = 0$ and $\sigma = 1$. Figure 2-4 shows the graph of the standardized normal distribution.

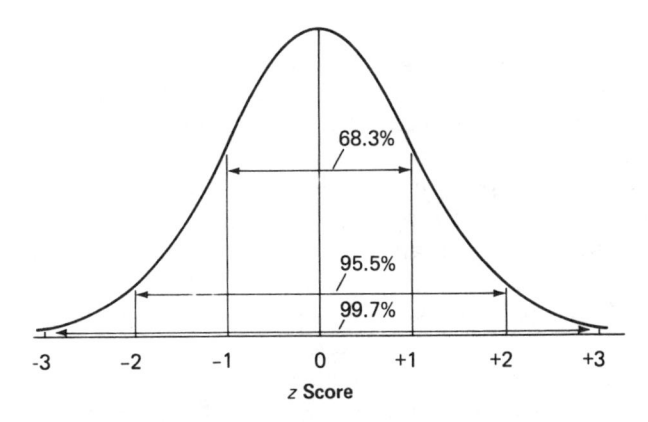

**Figure 2-4.** Standard normal distribution.

Just as for any other normal distribution, the percentages represent the proportion of observations lying in each area. Since this theoretical distribution is continuous, rather than a discrete distribution like the binomial, the probabilities are represented by areas under the curve, and the total area under the curve is equal to 1. The above graph shows that 99.7% of the distribution is within 3 standard deviations of the mean, so that, for example, 0.3% of the total area is more than 3 standard deviations away from the mean.

The fact that any variable that has a normal distribution can be transformed into the standard normal curve makes this curve useful in many situations. The graph indicates that 68% of the standard curve, for example, is within 1 standard deviation of the mean 0. This means that if we have any value, say, $v$, known to have a normal distribution, then 68% of the time we could expect

$$z = \frac{v - \mu}{\sigma}$$

to lie between $-1$ and $+1$. Using tables of the standard normal distribution, such as Table A in the Appendix, one can determine the proportion of values between any two points on the curve. In the next section, you will see how these properties of the standard normal curve allow for testing hypotheses about proportions.

## SAMPLING DISTRIBUTIONS OF PROPORTIONS

A very important fact to understand when dealing with statistical inference is that the theoretical distributions of several sample estimates of population values tend to be normally distributed. For example, consider a large population in which 60% of the people have health insurance and 40% do not. For this binomial variable, insured versus not insured, the value of $p$, the proportion insured, is $p = .60$. Suppose that a sample is taken to estimate $p$, the proportion with health insurance. The sample proportion with health insurance, $\hat{p}$, is likely to be close to $p$ (60%). If another sample of the same size is taken, it is also likely to give an estimate close to 60%. A few such sample estimates will be way too high or too low, but in general they will cluster around 60%. It turns out that the distribution of all such possible sample estimates of $p$ for a given sample size, called the *sampling distribution of p*, has the form shown in Figure 2-5.

# Binomial and Normal Distributions

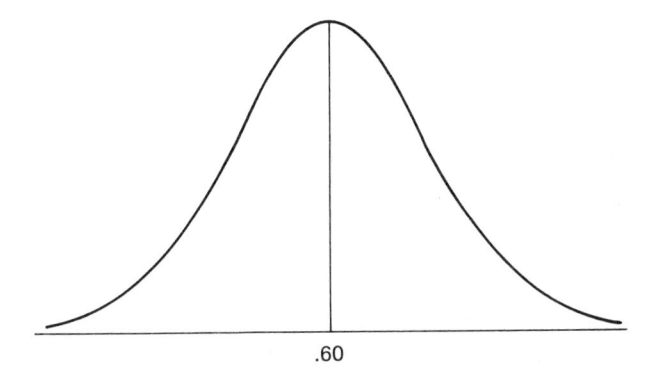

.60

**Figure 2-5.** Sampling distribution of a sample proportion for samples of size $n$ from a population with $p = .60$.

For reasonably large samples, this distribution is approximately normal. Its mean and standard deviation can be shown to be

$$\mu = p$$

and

$$\sigma = \sqrt{pq/n}$$

where $p$ is the true proportion in the population, $q = 1 - p$, and $n$ is the sample size. This means that any value from this distribution, that is, any sample proportion $\hat{p}$, can be converted to a $z$ score as follows:

$$z = \frac{v - \mu}{\sigma}$$

$$= \frac{\hat{p} - p}{\sqrt{pq/n}}$$

This approximation is generally considered adequate when $np \geq 5$ and $n(1 - p) \geq 5$. This fact makes it possible to test a hypothesis about a proportion using the normal distribution, provided the sample size is not too small. This procedure is explained in the next section of this chapter.

A similar theoretical result holds when two sample proportions are obtained to test a null hypothesis of the form

$$H: p_1 = p_2$$

or

$$H: p_1 - p_2 = 0$$

For example, suppose that $\hat{p}_1$ is a sample estimate of $p_1$, the proportion of patients who develop complications with traditional nursing care, and $\hat{p}_2$ estimates $p_2$, the proportion of patients who develop complications with primary nursing care. The difference between the two sample proportions, $\hat{p}_1 - \hat{p}_2$, is an estimate of the actual difference between $p_1$ and $p_2$ and tends to be close to the actual difference. If two more samples of the same sizes as the first two are obtained, their difference is also likely to be close to the actual difference, $p_1 - p_2$. Consider the sampling distribution of all possible values of $\hat{p}_1 - \hat{p}_2$, the estimates of the difference between $p_1$ and $p_2$. The shape of this distribution is illustrated in Figure 2-6.

This distribution is approximately normal, with the adequacy of the approximation increasing as sample size increases. Its mean and standard deviation are

$$\mu = p_1 - p_2$$

and

$$\sigma = \sqrt{pq/n_1 + pq/n_2}$$

where $p_1$ and $p_2$ are the true proportions of those with complications in the two populations and $n_1$ and $n_2$ are the two sample sizes. The quantity $p$ is a combined estimate of the proportion with complications from both samples, that is,

$$p = \frac{a_1 + a_2}{n_1 + n_2}$$

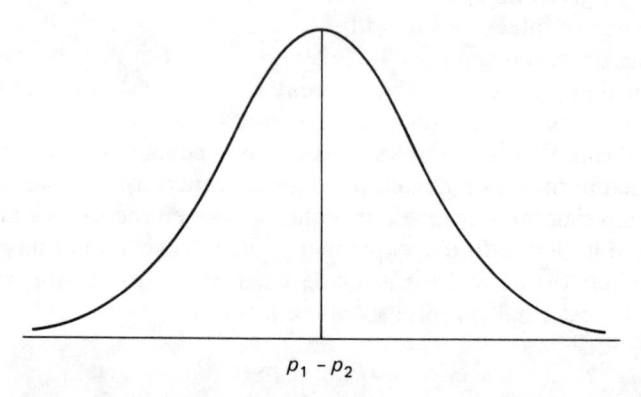

**Figure 2-6.** Sampling distribution of the difference between two sample proportions for samples of size $n_1$ and $n_2$ from populations with proportions $p_1$ and $p_2$.

Binomial and Normal Distributions

where $a_1$ and $a_2$ are the number with complications from samples 1 and 2, respectively, and $q = 1 - p$. Therefore, any value from this sampling distribution, that is, the difference between two sample proportions, $\hat{p}_1 - \hat{p}_2$, can be transformed to a z score as follows:

$$z = \frac{v - \mu}{\sigma}$$

$$= \frac{(\hat{p}_1 - \hat{p}_2) - (p_1 - p_2)}{\sqrt{pq/n_1 + pq/n_2}}$$

This result will allow us to use what we know about normally distributed variables to test hypotheses about the difference between two proportions, as you will see in a later section in this chapter.

## TESTING A PROPORTION

Earlier in this chapter we considered a hypothesis about the incidence of infection in subjects treated with a new vaccine. The null hypothesis was $H: p = .80$, where 80% represented the usual incidence of infection in an untreated population. Consider this problem again, using a sample of size 50 instead of 5, which makes it possible to use the normal approximation to test the same hypothesis. The same steps as before will be followed.

The null hypothesis $H: p = .80$ is again used as the expected incidence of infection, given no effect of the vaccine. If the vaccine has no effect, the incidence of infection should be similar to that of an untreated population. The observed sample of size 50 is assumed to be a sample from a hypothetical population of subjects treated by the new vaccine. The incidence of infection in this hypothetical population is 80%, according to the null hypothesis. That is, the hypothetical population has an infection rate equal to that normally observed, or, in other words, the vaccine is useless.

A sample of 50 people are inoculated. The incidence of infection in this sample is $\hat{p} = .20$, or, in other words, 10 people are infected. The sample infection rate of 20% is now compared with the predicted rate of 80%. The large difference between what is observed in the sample and what is hypothesized about the population suggests that, if the sample can reasonably be said to represent the population, the actual rate of infection in the population is not likely to be equal to 80%, but rather lower than 80%. The standardized normal distribution allows us to make an objective appraisal of the impression presented by the data.

The normal approximation to the binomial distribution provides a procedure for deciding whether to accept or reject the null hypothesis. According to the theory of the normal distribution, the quantity

$$z = \frac{v - \mu}{\sigma}$$

fits a standard normal curve, where $v$ is a sample value from a normal distribution, and where $\mu$ and $\sigma^2$ are the mean and variance, respectively, of the distribution of all such sample values. In the case of a sample proportion, which we have said earlier has a sampling distribution that is approximately normal for reasonably large samples,

$$z = \frac{v - \mu}{\sigma}$$

$$= \frac{\hat{p} - p}{\sqrt{pq/n}}$$

Substituting the numerical values from our example into the above formula, we have

$$z = \frac{.20 - .80}{\sqrt{(.80)(.20)/50}} = -10.7$$

when the null hypothesis $H: p = .80$ is true.

According to what we know about the standardized normal distribution, 95.5% of the distribution is between $+2$ and $-2$, which represents 2 standard deviations above or below the mean of 0. This means that if the null hypothesis $H: p = .80$ is true, then .80 is the mean of the sampling distribution of $\hat{p}$, and 95.5% of the time we would expect to observe a sample $\hat{p}$ within two standard deviations of this mean. Converting to the $z$ score, which has a mean of 0 and a standard deviation of 1, we would thus expect that 95.5% of the time the $z$ score should lie between $+2$ and $-2$. The value of $z = -10.7$ obtained in this example is appreciably more than 3 standard deviations below the mean; that is, the outcome is very unlikely to have occurred if the true population proportion is equal to .80.

We can interpret this result as follows. Since 95.5% of the time we expect a $z$ score to fall between $+2$ and $-2$ when the null hypothesis is true (and 99.7% of the time between $+3$ and $-3$), the outcome of $z = -10.7$ is very unlikely to occur when the null hypothesis is true. In this example, the sample proportion $\hat{p} = .20$ is far below the hypothesized value $p = .80$, and it has converted to a $z$ value that is far below zero. A

# Binomial and Normal Distributions

sample $\hat{p}$ very close to .80 would have resulted in a $z$ value closer to zero. It is obvious that $z$ values far away from zero occur when the observed or sample value, $\hat{p}$, is very different from the value of $p$ assumed by the null hypothesis. A large discrepancy between what is observed in the sample ($\hat{p}$) and what is hypothesized in the population ($p$) suggests that the hypothesis was wrong and should be rejected.

In making a rule for just exactly how large $z$ must be in order to reject the null hypothesis, we will adopt the conventionally used 5% *level of significance*. This rule says that whenever the $z$ value calculated from the data falls within the 95% area of the theoretical $z$ distribution around zero, the null hypothesis should be accepted and that whenever the $z$ value falls outside the 95% area, the null hypothesis should be rejected. Remember that the theoretical probability distribution of $z$ describes the probability of various outcomes under the assumption that the null hypothesis is true. The value 5% represents the allowance we make for error, that is, the probability that we will obtain a $z$ value outside the 95% area when the null hypothesis is actually true. In such a case, we will follow the rule and reject the null hypothesis and will thus be making an error 5% of the time.

The actual area of the standardized normal distribution that includes 95% of the distribution is the area lying between $z$ values of $+1.96$ and $-1.96$, as illustrated in Figure 2-7. Using the 5% level of significance as a criterion, we should accept the null hypothesis whenever the calculated $z$ value is between $\pm 1.96$ and reject the null hypothesis whenever the calculated $z$ value is outside these limits. The area between the $\pm 1.96$ limits is called the *acceptance region,* and the areas above and below $\pm 1.96$

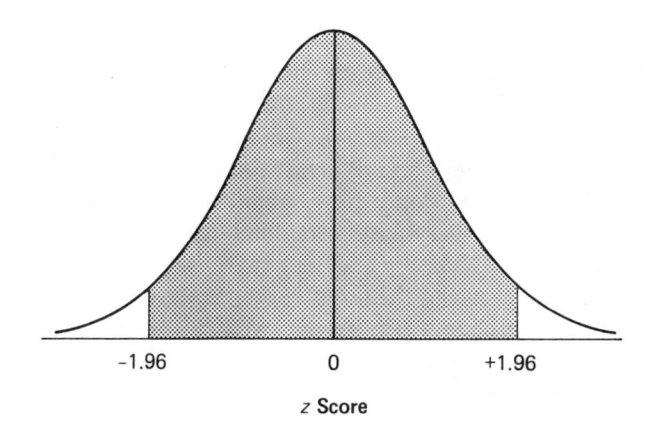

**Figure 2-7.** Area of standardized normal distribution, including 95% of the distribution.

constitute what is referred to as the *rejection region*. The above result, $z = -10.7$, is clearly in the rejection region, and the null hypothesis can be rejected by using the 5% level of significance. Our conclusion is that the incidence of infection in a population inoculated with the new vaccine will not be equal to 80%, and the sample data suggest that it may be substantially lower than 80%.

## COMPARING TWO PROPORTIONS

Suppose, instead of a sample of 50 patients treated with a new vaccine, we want to study two groups of patients. The two groups are formed by randomization and are constituted in such a way that group 1 receives concentration A of the new vaccine and group 2 receives concentration B of the new vaccine. The research problem is to determine whether the incidence of infection differs between these two groups. The same general procedure for hypothesis testing can be used as that just indicated for a hypothesis about one proportion.

The null hypothesis for this study is that there is no difference in the incidence of infection in the two hypothetical populations represented by group 1 and group 2. Symbolically, it is written as

$$H: p_1 = p_2$$

or

$$H: p_1 - p_2 = 0$$

A sample of 50 people are inoculated with concentration A of the vaccine and 50 people with concentration B. The incidence of infection in group 1 is $\hat{p}_1 = .75$ and in group 2 is $\hat{p}_2 = .71$. The observed difference between the sample proportions is $\hat{p}_1 - \hat{p}_2 = .04$. Remember that this difference between the two sample proportions is an estimate of the difference between the two actual population proportions, which we have hypothesized to be equal to zero. In this case, there is minimal difference between the two sample proportions, which suggest that there is little evidence for suspecting a difference between the population proportions. In order to carry out an objective test of this impression, we again make use of the standardized normal distribution.

We stated earlier that the value

$$z = \frac{v - \mu}{\sigma}$$

# Binomial and Normal Distributions

is distributed as a standard normal curve, where $v$ is a normal sample value and $\mu$ and $\sigma^2$ are respectively the mean and variance of the distribution from which that sample value comes. We indicated earlier that for the difference between two proportions,

$$z = \frac{v - \mu}{\sigma}$$

$$= \frac{(\hat{p}_1 - \hat{p}_2) - (p_1 - p_2)}{\sqrt{pq/n_1 + pq/n_2}}$$

where $\hat{p}_1 - \hat{p}_2$ is the difference between the sample proportions and $p_1 - p_2$ is the difference between the population proportions assumed by the null hypothesis.

Replacing the symbols by their appropriate values in this example, we have:

$$z = \frac{(\hat{p}_1 - \hat{p}_2) - (p_1 - p_2)}{\sqrt{pq/n_1 + pq/n_2}}$$

$$= \frac{.04 - 0}{\sqrt{(.73)(.27)/50 + (.73)(.27)/50}}$$

$$= 0.45$$

This value of $z$ is between $-1.96$ and $1.96$, which means that the hypothesis should be accepted, using the 5% level of significance.

In this case $z = 0.45$ corresponds to 35% of the standardized normal curve. In other words, 35% of the standardized normal curve lies between $+.45$ and $-.45$. This leaves 65% of the curve outside of the calculated $z$ value. The percentage representing the amount outside of the calculated $z$ value is often called the *p value*. These data, if presented in a research article, might be accompanied by the notation $p = .65$. Or, more likely, the notation might just say $p > .05$, which means that the $z$ value, whatever it is, is too low to be significant at the .05 level.

Inspection of the formula by which $z$ is calculated is instructive. If the null hypothesis is true and the two different concentrations of the new vaccine have the same effect, the sample values $\hat{p}_1$ and $\hat{p}_2$ are likely to be similar. This will make $\hat{p}_1 - \hat{p}_2$ quite small and tend to make $z$ close to zero. As a result, the null hypothesis is likely to be accepted. A large difference between $\hat{p}_1$ and $\hat{p}_2$ will tend to make $z$ large and thus tend to result in rejection of the null hypothesis.

All the statistical inferences used in this book will be made in a manner similar to those described in this chapter. We will make a null hypothesis, usually one we would like to reject. We will then collect data and reject the null hypothesis only if the observed data yield a test value such as $z$ (i.e., a *test statistic*) that is unlikely to occur, given the theoretical distribution of the test statistic that follows from the null hypothesis. For rejection of the null hypothesis, the test statistic must be so unusual that the chance of such an outcome occurring merely by chance is small, usually less than 5% and sometimes even less than 1%. In future chapters, we will discuss theoretical distributions other than the normal distribution, since many test statistics computed from sample data follow distributions other than the normal distribution. You should keep in mind that the procedure for inference, that is, the logic of the procedure, will remain as it has been described in this chapter.

## PROBLEMS

1. A hospital ward has 20 patients, 17 of whom are 25 years old or older and 3 of whom are under 25. One patient is selected at random for an interview about attitudes toward nurses.

   (a) What is the probability that a patient over 25 is selected?
   (b) What is the probability that a patient under 25 is selected?

2. Of 2000 cardiac patients treated at a hospital during 1969–1971, 1200 survived their first myocardial infarction.

   (a) What is the probability of patient survival of the first myocardial infarction, based on this population (i.e., the survival rate)?
   (b) What is the probability of death?
   (c) In 1972, a new intensive care unit was opened at this hospital. The first 5 patients admitted to this intensive care unit all survived the first myocardial infarction. What is the survival rate for this sample?
   (d) What is the probability that the first 5 patients in such an intensive care unit would survive the first myocardial infarction by chance, that is, if the patients are similar to the 2000 treated during 1969–1971 and if intensive care has no effect on survival? Use Table 2-1 to answer this question.
   (e) Do you think the intensive care unit has significantly improved chances of survival of the first myocardial infarction, if these patients are representative of the ones studied earlier?

3. Refer to Table A in the Appendix to answer the following questions. What is the probability of a $z$ score

# Binomial and Normal Distributions

**Table 2-1** Binomial Probability of Each Outcome for $p = .60$, $n = 5$

| | |
|---|---|
| $Pr$ (no survivors) = | .010 |
| $Pr$ (1 survivor) = | .077 |
| $Pr$ (2 survivors) = | .230 |
| $Pr$ (3 survivors) = | .346 |
| $Pr$ (4 survivors) = | .259 |
| $Pr$ (5 survivors) = | .078 |

(a) above zero?
(b) between $z = \pm 1.96$?
(c) above $z = 1.96$?
(d) to the left of $z = 0.4$?
(e) above $z = 0.1$ and below $z = 1.2$?
(f) below $z = -0.05$?
(g) between $z = \pm 2.58$?

4. Refer to Table A in the Appendix to answer the following questions. What $z$ score(s)

(a) has 50% of the standard normal curve above it?
(b) has 25% of the standard normal curve above it?
(c) has 2.5% of the standard normal curve above it?
(d) include 90% of the standard normal curve?
(e) include 80% of the standard normal curve?
(f) include 95% of the standard normal curve?
(g) include 99% of the standard normal curve?

5. In a study examining the effect of orientation on the practice of basic preventive health measures and changes in the practice of breast self-examination in response to the October 1974 mass media coverage of Mrs. Betty Ford's mastectomy, Turnbull[43] questioned 160 women enrolled in masters' degree programs. Based on their answers to questions about physical health behaviors such as dental care, nutrition, exercise, and so on, the respondents were classified into two groups, health-oriented and non-health-oriented. The practice of breast self-examination at least every 3 months prior to Mrs. Ford's surgery was reported as more frequent among the health-oriented group than among the non-health-oriented group. Subjects were asked whether Mrs. Ford's mastectomy led to any change in their practice of breast self-examination, and the responses were tabulated as shown in Table 2-2.

(a) What null hypothesis can be tested by the figures shown in the table?

**Table 2-2.** Change in Practice of Breast Self-Examination After Mrs. Ford's Surgery, by Health Status of Orientation ($n = 160$)

| Respondents | After Mrs. Ford's Surgery More Practice | No Change in Practice | Total |
|---|---|---|---|
| Health-oriented | 16 | 74 | 90 |
| Non-health-oriented | 27 | 43 | 70 |
| Total | 43 | 117 | 160 |

(b) Calculate $\hat{p}_1$ and state verbally what it represents.
(c) Calculate $\hat{p}_2$ and state verbally what it represents.
(d) Calculate $p$, the combined estimate of the population proportion of interest.
(e) Calculate the $z$ score.
(f) Test the null hypothesis, using the calculated score, at the .01 level of significance.
(g) State the $p$ value.
(h) How would you explain the results?
(i) How would you determine whether Mrs. Ford's surgery had any long-term effects on the practice of breast self-examination?

6. In the study by Corey et al.[9] described in Problem 1 of Chapter 1, data were obtained from medical records for 48 battered and 50 non-battered children for several demographic characteristics and medical history items. The researchers wished to look for differences on these variables between the battered children and the nonbattered children, and the items chosen for analysis were binomial in form. Tables 2-3 and 2-4 show the frequencies of battered and nonbattered children in various categories of the demographic characteristics and medical history items.

**Table 2-3.** Frequency of Demographic Characteristics of Battered and Nonbattered Children

| Group | Sex Male | Female | Siblings No | Yes | Battered Sibling No | Yes | Mother Married No | Yes |
|---|---|---|---|---|---|---|---|---|
| Battered | 25 | 23 | 14 | 32 | 17 | 15 | 9 | 38 |
| Nonbattered | 27 | 23 | 9 | 34 | 34 | 0 | 6 | 44 |

# Binomial and Normal Distributions

**Table 2-4.** Frequency of Medical History Characteristics of Battered and Nonbattered Children

| Group | Delivery Full-Term | Delivery Premature | Postnatal Hospitalization Normal | Postnatal Hospitalization Extended | Home Care Normal | Home Care Special |
|---|---|---|---|---|---|---|
| Battered | 28 | 6 | 26 | 8 | 26 | 8 |
| Nonbattered | 43 | 7 | 35 | 14 | 37 | 13 |

(a) Why do you suppose the total numbers of battered and nonbattered children are not 48 and 50, respectively, for all of these frequency tabulations?

(b) What null hypothesis can be tested by the figures on the delivery variable?

(c) Calculate $\hat{p}_1$. State verbally what it represents.

(d) Calculate $\hat{p}_2$. State verbally what it represents.

(e) Calculate $p$, the combined estimate of the population proportion of interest.

(f) Calculate the $z$ score.

(g) Test the null hypothesis, using the calculated $z$ score, at the .05 level of significance.

(h) State the $p$ value.

(i) State your conclusion in substantive terms.

(j) Repeat questions b through i for the other variables for which data are given in the above tables.

(k) Write a general statement about what this study indicates with respect to the differences between battered and nonbattered children.

# Chapter 3

# *t* TESTS

## USES OF *t* TESTS

We have already discussed binomially distributed variables such as sex, survival, type of patient, and so on, where each person is classified into one of two categories. Using such binomially distributed variables, we have also studied ways of testing hypotheses about the proportion of subjects in a population who possess some characteristic, as well as hypotheses about the difference between two proportions. In this chapter we turn to the study of variables that take on other types of distributions. We refer to many such variables as *continuous,* because they take values along a continuum. Although such variables are recorded as discrete values, they cannot be measured exactly. Examples are age, height, weight, blood pressure, and temperature. For these variables, means rather than proportions are most useful to describe sample data. We might take a sample of patients of size 50 and describe them as having a mean age of 43.2, for example. For the investigation of hypotheses about the mean value of a continuous variable in a population, or hypotheses about the difference between means of two populations, the most commonly used statistical procedures are referred to as *t tests*.

One way that such tests can be used is in the comparison of an observed mean or average value in a sample with some value hypothesized for the population. This corresponds to the procedure described in Chapter 2 for testing a sample proportion against a hypothesized value for the population from which the sample was drawn. For the cases to be described in this chapter, however, the variable to be analyzed is continuous, so that the analysis will be carried out in terms of means instead of proportions.

Consider a situation where a *t* test would be appropriate. Suppose that we want to know whether the average age in the population of all undergraduate nurses is equal to the average age of U.S. college students in general. Assume that we know that the average age of all college students is 19.8 years. We could make a null hypothesis that the average age of undergraduate nurses is equal to 19.8. This is written:

$$H: \mu = 19.8$$

According to this null hypothesis, we are assuming that the mean age for the population consisting of all nursing students is no different from that for the population consisting of all U.S. college students.

A sample of nurses would provide a sample mean age that could be tested against this hypothesized population value. In this chapter we will discuss a procedure for using a $t$ test to compare a sample mean with a hypothesized population mean. In this example, the procedure would allow us to determine whether it is reasonable to accept the null hypothesis that the mean age of nursing students is no different from the mean age of all college students. If the mean age in the sample of nurses were far away from 19.8, and if the sample was collected in such a way that we could assume it represented all nursing students, we would decide to reject the null hypothesis and would conclude that nursing students are not similar in mean age to other students. The procedure, of course, determines how "far away" the sample mean should be from 19.8 in order for the null hypothesis to be rejected.

The use of a $t$ test in the situation just described, where a hypothesis is made about one population mean, is relatively unusual in nursing research. $t$ Tests are much more commonly used to test hypotheses about the difference between means of two populations. Such tests are analogous to the comparison of two proportions, with mean values being compared instead of proportions. The selection of a $t$ test procedure versus the $z$ score from the normal distribution depends on the nature of the data to be analyzed. If we want to compare the proportion of women over age 30 among patients seeking abortions in comparison to those not seeking abortions, we can use the normal approximation to the binomial. If, on the other hand, we want to see whether there is a difference in mean age between these two groups, the $t$ test is appropriate. Any statistical technique is designed to handle data collected in a specific form, and the way in which the data have been collected and summarized will determine the kind of analysis that is appropriate.

One very common situation in which a $t$ test is used to compare two means is an experimental study with a control group and an experimental group. In Chapter 1 we discussed a study of the effect of the use of volunteers on length of stay in the hospital. The data resulting from this study would be in the form of a sample mean or average length of stay for each of the two groups of patients, those receiving a volunteer visit and those not receiving volunteer visits. A $t$ test would be used to determine whether the difference between these two means is sufficient to suggest a real difference between the means of the hypothetical populations corresponding to the two samples, that is, whether the difference is *significant*. To say that a result is significant is another way of saying the null hypothesis is rejected.

Another very common use of *t* tests is in the analysis of survey data. A survey usually involves the collection of data on many variables from each of the individuals in the sample. Some of the variables will be of the qualitative or categorical form, such as male–female, yes–no answers to questions, married–single, and Republican–Democrat. Others will be quantitative or continuous, such as age, income, number of children, and number of years in school. The relationship between one qualitative variable and one quantitative variable can be investigated by use of a *t* test. For example, a researcher might want to know whether the mean age of Republicans differs from the mean age of Democrats, or whether the mean number of years in school differs for males versus females. Each of these examples requires a comparison of two groups, as in a controlled study, except that these groups are not "treatment" groups and are not formed by randomization.

There are circumstances other than controlled studies and surveys in which one may wish to compare the means of two groups. Many such situations occur in nursing where a comparison is to be made between people with a particular characteristic or experience and people without. For example, national board scores for a sample of nurses from a traditional program could be compared with scores for a sample of nurses from a new, innovative program, to determine whether there is any difference in mean scores between the two populations. Or mean scores on a test of knowledge about diabetes could be compared for a sample of diabetic patients receiving nursing education about the disease with a sample of similar patients not receiving this education. For such situations, a *t* test would be appropriate for testing the null hypothesis of no difference between the two populations.

It is clear from the above examples that the *t* test for the difference between two means can be used in a great variety of situations. The procedure for using this test is independent of the type of situation from which the data were obtained and is appropriate when means from two samples are to be compared. The statistical test, however, will only determine whether the difference between the sample means is large enough to suggest a true difference between the population means. You will have to refer to the details of the specific study in question in order to interpret the substantive meaning of the results indicated by the statistical test. In particular, a significant difference between experimental and control group means does not in itself demonstrate causality.

# t Tests

Yet another type of *t* test, which should not be confused with the two just described, is referred to as the *paired t test*. The paired *t* test is appropriate for situations in which before–after measures have been taken on the same subjects or in which subjects have been paired prior to randomization into experimental and control groups. In these cases, the two sets of measures are correlated; they should not, therefore, be analyzed as if they are based on two independent samples. The paired *t* test, which is used for data of this type, provides a more powerful test than the *t* test for independent samples because it takes the correlation between pairs of observations into account.

## SAMPLING DISTRIBUTIONS OF MEANS

Since *t* tests make use of knowledge about the sampling distributions of means, the relevant sampling distributions should be discussed prior to describing the *t* distribution. You will recall that when the variable *v* has a normal distribution, the quantity

$$z = \frac{v - \mu}{\sigma}$$

has a standard normal distribution, where $\mu$ and $\sigma^2$ are respectively the mean and variance of the original distribution. Two values that have approximately normal distributions when sample sizes are reasonably large are a sample proportion and the difference between two sample proportions. Recall that this statement means that the sampling distribution, that is the distribution of all possible sample proportions of a given size or of all possible differences between two proportions for given sample sizes, tends to be normally distributed. We have already discussed procedures for substituting the appropriate values for $\mu$ and $\sigma$ into the *z* formula to carry out hypothesis tests about proportions.

Now, consider the situation where we have a continuous variable that is normally distributed in a population, from which we select a random sample and calculate the sample mean, which we will denote by the symbol $\bar{x}$. For example, consider an infinite population with a normal distribution of age, a mean age of $\mu = 40$, and a standard deviation of $\sigma = 10$. Suppose that a sample of size 4 is taken from this population in order to estimate $\mu$. The value of the sample mean age, $\bar{x}$, is likely to be fairly close to the true value of 40, assuming that $\bar{x}$ is the distribution of all the sample means of size 4 that could theoretically be chosen from this same population. Some of these estimates will be far under 40 and some far over 40, but they will generally cluster around 40. It turns out that the sampling distribution of all such possible samples is normal in shape, as shown in Figure 3-1.

The mean of this sample distribution is 40, the same as the mean of the distribution of the original variable in the population. However, the standard deviation of the sampling distribution turns out to be smaller than the standard deviation of the original distribution, since the means will tend to be more centrally located than the original values of the variable. If the original standard deviation is denoted by the value $\sigma$, it turns out that the standard deviation of the sampling distribution of means is

$$\sigma_{\bar{x}} = \frac{\sigma}{\sqrt{n}}$$

where $n$ is the sample size. In this case, for example, since $\sigma = 10$ and $n = 4$,

$$\sigma_{\bar{x}} = \frac{\sigma}{\sqrt{n}} = \frac{10}{\sqrt{4}} = \frac{10}{2} = 5.$$

The value

$$\sigma_{\bar{x}} = \frac{\sigma}{\sqrt{n}}$$

is referred to as the *standard error of the mean*. In general, then, the sampling distribution of a sample mean for a sample of size $n$, from a

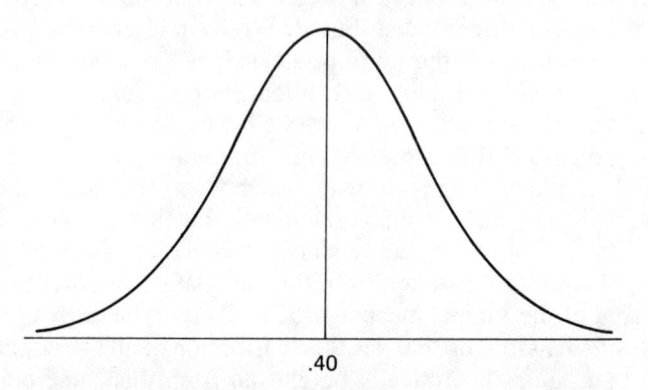

**Figure 3-1.** Sampling distribution of a sample mean for samples of size $n$ from a population with $\mu = 40$.

normal distribution with mean $\mu$ and standard deviation $\sigma$, is normal with mean $\mu$ and standard deviation $\sigma_{\bar{x}} = \dfrac{\sigma}{\sqrt{n}}$.

The theoretical derivation of the results just given requires the assumption that the underlying or original distribution from which the sample is obtained is normally distributed. Strict adherence to this assumption would limit the use of the above results to testing hypotheses about sample means only when one knows that the distribution of the variable in the population is normal in shape. It has been demonstrated that such a strict assumption is not necessary, however, provided sample sizes are not too small. It can be shown that the sampling distribution of a sample mean is approximately normally distributed with mean and variance as described above, regardless of the shape of the original distribution, and that the adequacy of this approximation improves as sample size increases. This result, called the *central limit theorem,* allows us to assume a normal sampling distribution of the sample mean for virtually any situation where the sample size is reasonably large.

The Central Limit Theorem is important for testing hypotheses about means. According to this theorem, $\bar{x}$, a sample mean, is a quantity that is approximately normally distributed, with mean $\mu$ and standard deviation

$$\sigma_{\bar{x}} = \frac{\sigma}{\sqrt{n}},$$

where $\mu$ and $\sigma$ represent the mean and standard deviation in the original distribution, respectively. Therefore, the quantity

$$z = \frac{\bar{x} - \mu}{\sigma_{\bar{x}}} = \frac{\bar{x} - \mu}{\sigma/\sqrt{n}}$$

can be used to test a hypothesis about a population mean $\mu$, given a sample mean $\bar{x}$.

You will recall that in the case of sampling distributions for proportions, in addition to the fact that a sample proportion tends to be normally distributed, the difference between two sample proportions also tends to be normally distributed. A similar result holds for the difference between two independent sample means; that is, the sampling distribution of the difference between two sample means $(\bar{x}_1 - \bar{x}_2)$ tends to approximate a normal distribution. The mean of this sampling distribution is

$$\mu = (\mu_1 - \mu_2)$$

the difference between the means of the two populations from which the samples were taken. Further, the standard deviation of this distribution is

$$\sigma_{\bar{x}_1 - \bar{x}_2} = \sqrt{\sigma_1^2/n_1 + \sigma_2^2/n_2}$$

where $\sigma_1^2$ and $\sigma_2^2$ are the variances of the two populations and $n_1$ and $n_2$ are the two sample sizes. The value $\sigma_{\bar{x}_1 - \bar{x}_2}$ is referred to as the *standard error of the difference between means*. Using the usual procedure for obtaining a standard score,

$$z = \frac{v - \mu}{\sigma}$$

we obtain in this case

$$z = \frac{(\bar{x}_1 - \bar{x}_2) - (\mu_1 - \mu_2)}{\sqrt{\sigma^2/n_1 + \sigma^2/n_2}}$$

The above value is a $z$ score that can be used to test a hypothesis of the form

$$H: \mu_1 = \mu_2$$

We have now derived formulas for converting either a sample mean or the difference between two sample means into $z$ scores that can be used to carry out hypothesis tests about means. Calculation of these $z$ scores requires that the values for $\mu$ (or $\mu_1 - \mu_2$) and $\sigma$ (or $\sigma_1$ and $\sigma_2$) be *known*. The typical null hypothesis to be tested in the one sample case would be $H: \mu = k$, where $k$ is a constant, and $k$ would be used as a value for $\mu$ in the test statistic. For two samples, one would generally test the null hypothesis

$$H: \mu_1 = \mu_2$$

that is

$$H: \mu_1 - \mu_2 = 0$$

so that zero would be used as a value for $\mu_1 - \mu_2$. However, $z$-test statistics can rarely be actually computed, since the population variances $\sigma^2$ (or $\sigma_1^2$ and $\sigma_2^2$) are seldom known. The next section describes how the $t$ distribution can be used to solve this problem.

# *t* DISTRIBUTION

Suppose that we want to test a hypothesis about mean length of hospital stay for surgical patients. We would obtain a sample mean, $\bar{x}$, based on a sample of size $n$. The population mean and variance, $\mu$ and $\sigma^2$, would not be known, and thus it would be impossible to compute the test value

$$z = \frac{\bar{x} - \mu}{\sigma/\sqrt{n}}$$

In such cases the null hypothesis gives a value to use in the formula for $\mu$, but it is necessary to estimate $\sigma^2$ from the sample data. The value

$$s^2 = \frac{\sum_{i=1}^{n}(x_i - \bar{x})^2}{n - 1}$$

which is called the *sample variance,* is calculated and used as an estimate of $\sigma^2$. Then $\sigma_{\bar{x}}$, the standard error of the mean, is estimated by $s_{\bar{x}} = s/\sqrt{n}$.

In the case of two samples, each sample provides an estimate of variance, and the two sample variances are calculated as follows:

$$s_1^2 = \frac{\sum_{i=1}^{n}(x_i - \bar{x}_1)^2}{n_1 - 1}$$

and

$$s_2^2 = \frac{\sum_{i=1}^{n}(x_i - \bar{x}_2)^2}{n_1 - 1}$$

Then $\sigma_{\bar{x}_1 - \bar{x}_2}$, the standard error of the difference, can be estimated by

$$s_{\bar{x}_1 - \bar{x}_2} = \sqrt{s_1^2/(n_1 - 1) + s_2^2/(n_2 - 1)}$$

This formula is a biased estimate, which approaches the unbiased estimate as the sample size increases. The unbiased estimate, which assumes that the population variances are equal, is based on a *pooled estimate of variance*,

$$s_p^2 = \frac{(n_1 - 1) s_1^2 + (n_2 - 1) s_2^2}{n_1 + n_2 - 2}$$

which is a weighted average of $s_1^2$ and $s_2^2$. The unbiased estimate of the standard error of the difference then becomes

$$s_{\bar{x}_1 - \bar{x}_2} = \sqrt{s_p^2/n_1 + s_p^2/n_2}$$

If the values in one sample are much more spread out than those in the other, the pooled estimate of variance may be inappropriate. See Snedecor and Cochran (41) for further discussion of this issue.

The values

$$z = \frac{\bar{x} - \mu}{\sigma_{\bar{x}}} = \frac{\bar{x} - \mu}{\sigma/\sqrt{n}}$$

and

$$z = \frac{(\bar{x}_1 - \bar{x}_2) - (\mu_1 - \mu_2)}{\sigma_{\bar{x}_1 - \bar{x}_2}} = \frac{(\bar{x}_1 - \bar{x}_2) - (\mu_1 - \mu_2)}{\sqrt{\sigma^2/n_1 + \sigma^2/n_2}}$$

were given earlier as the standard $z$ scores for testing hypotheses about means. When sample values, $s^2$ for one sample and $s_p^2$ for two samples, are used as variance estimates in these formulas, the two quantities are no longer distributed according to the standard normal distribution. Instead, they have what is called the *t distribution* and can be denoted as

$$t = \frac{\bar{x} - \mu}{s_{\bar{x}}} = \frac{\bar{x} - \mu}{s/\sqrt{n}}$$

and

$$t = \frac{(\bar{x}_1 - \bar{x}_2) - (\mu_1 - \mu_2)}{s_{\bar{x}_1 - \bar{x}_2}} = \frac{(\bar{x}_1 - \bar{x}_2) - (\mu_1 - \mu_2)}{\sqrt{s_p^2/n_1 + s_p^2/n_2}}$$

In order to test hypotheses about means when only sample variances are available, we must use the probabilities under the curve that correspond to the theoretical distribution of $t$ rather than $z$.

# t Tests

The *t* distribution is very similar in shape to the standard normal distribution, except that it is more spread out. For small samples, a comparison of the two distributions might appear as indicated in Figure 3-2.

The *t* distribution is actually not just one distribution, but a family of distributions. It has no fixed shape, as does the *z* distribution, but rather changes shape, according to the sample size used in each situation. With a very small sample, the *t* distribution is more spread out than the *z* distribution, as indicated in Figure 3-2. As the sample size increases, the *t* distribution concentrates toward the center and approaches exactly the same shape as the *z* or normal distribution.

The fact that the *t* distribution changes according to the sample size means that there is no "standard" *t* distribution, as there is a "standard" normal distribution. The proportion under a part of the curve between two fixed *t* values depends on the sample size. The parameter related to sample size, which determines the shape, is called *degrees of freedom;* examples of this will be given in the following applications of the *t* distribution. Table B in the Appendix indicates probabilities for various *t* distributions, based on the degrees of freedom.

*t* Tests are commonly described as appropriate when sample sizes are small (e.g., < 30). If you consider the shape of the *t* distribution in relation to the standard normal distribution, as shown in Figure 3-2, you will see why this is so. Consider the implications of the difference between the two distributions in terms of determining a 95% area under the curve in each case. You may recall that 95% of the *z* distribution lies between $z = \pm 1.96$. Since the *t* distribution for small samples is more spread out than the *z* distribution, the area between $t = \pm 1.96$ includes *less than* 95% of the entire *t* distribution. This means that if we test hypotheses about means

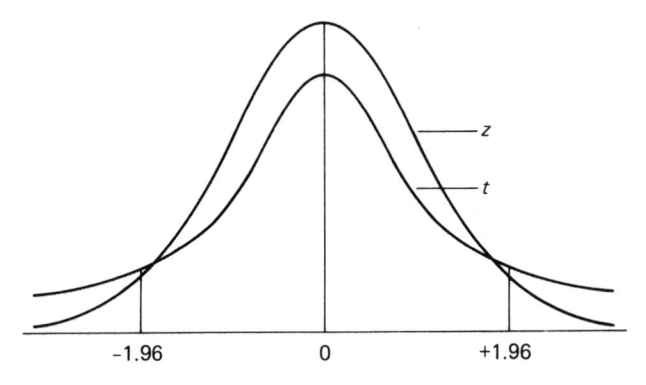

**Figure 3-2.** Comparison of standardized normal *(z)* distribution with *t* distribution *(t)* for small samples.

using the $t$ distribution and the 5% level of significance, a larger $t$ value than 1.96 will be required to reject the null hypothesis.

For a large sample, the $t$ value required to reject a null hypothesis at the 5% level will be very close to 1.96, since the $t$ distribution for large samples is close to the standard normal distribution. Thus for a large sample we could calculate the test statistic and refer to the standard normal distribution rather than the $t$ distribution. The distinction is important when small samples are used, which is frequently the case in experimental nursing research or any other similar research on human subjects. In the next section we will consider some examples in which the $t$ tests described in this section would be useful.

## TESTING A MEAN

Suppose that we want to determine the average number of days lost from work per year for individuals taking large doses of vitamin C. A random sample of 25 employees is selected from a large company, and all 25 people are supplied with large quantities of vitamin C that they are asked to take daily for a year. The analysis of these data takes the form of a $t$ test.

The average number of days lost from work for the company's employees as a whole for the study year is 10.3 days. Therefore, the null hypothesis

$$H: \mu = 10.3$$

makes the assumption that the use of vitamin C makes no difference in days lost from work. Here $\mu$ stands for the mean lost days from work in a hypothetical population of people taking vitamin C, that is, people corresponding to those in the sample. If vitamin C has no beneficial effects, loss of work in this hypothetical population should be the same as for the whole company, on the average.

Results at the end of the year show an average of 7.3 days lost from work in the sample, with a sample variance of 1.2. In terms of the notation given earlier, this can be written as

$$\bar{x} = 7.3$$

and

$$s^2 = 1.2 \ (s = 1.095)$$

# t Tests

The mean number of days lost in the sample group is 7.3, compared with the expected value according to the null hypothesis of 10.3. Loss of days is lower in the sample than predicted by the null hypothesis, suggesting that vitamin C may have some effect. The $t$ test will be used to determine whether this difference is in fact statistically significant.

According to the theory of the $t$ distribution, if $\bar{x}$ is a sample mean, $s^2$ is an estimate of the population variance $\sigma^2$, and $n$ is the sample size, then

$$t = \frac{\bar{x} - \mu}{s/\sqrt{n}}$$

has a $t$ distribution with $n - 1$ degrees of freedom, *when the null hypothesis is true.*

In this case, substitution of the sample values in the formula for $t$ yields

$$\begin{aligned} t &= \frac{\bar{x} - \mu}{s/\sqrt{n}} \\ &= \frac{7.3 - 10.3}{1.095/\sqrt{25}} \\ &= \frac{-3}{1.095/5} \\ &= -13.5 \end{aligned}$$

For a $t$ distribution with $n - 1 = 24$ degrees of freedom, the distribution is as indicated in Figure 3-3.

According to the graph in Figure 3-3, if the null hypothesis is true, the computed $t$ value should be between $-2.064$ and $+2.064$ 95% of the time. The $t$ value of $-13.5$ is well outside this range, and the null hypothesis should thus be rejected at the .05 level of significance. This result could appear in a research article accompanied by the notation "$p < .05$." As a matter of fact, the computed $t$ value lies outside the range $-2.797$ to $+2.797$, which includes 99% of the distribution, so that the result would probably appear as "$p < .01$." Rejection of the null hypothesis in this example means that the researcher concludes that the mean days lost from work would be significantly different for employees taking vitamin C than for a similar population not taking vitamin C. Comparison of the sample mean, 7.3 days, with the hypothesized population mean, 10.3 days, shows that the mean days lost from work is lower than expected.

The formula for $t$ illustrates the logic of the hypothesis testing. Consider first the numerator of $t$. Values of $\bar{x}$ close to $\mu$, the value assumed

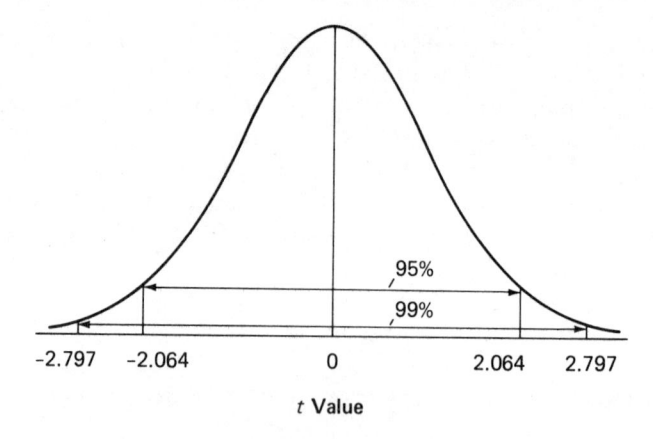

[Figure: bell curve with cutoffs at −2.797, −2.064, 0, 2.064, 2.797 on the t Value axis, showing 95% and 99% regions]

**Figure 3-3.** Cutoff points for 95% and 99% of the *t* distribution with 24 degrees of freedom.

by the null hypothesis, will tend to make *t* small. A small value of *t* (a *t* value close to 0) will lead to acceptance of the null hypothesis that vitamin C has no effect on mean days lost from work due to colds. If vitamin C does have an effect, the true $\mu$ in the hypothetical population is lower than 10.3, and the sample $\bar{x}$ is likely to be lower than 10.3, which will tend to make *t* large and lead to rejection of the null hypothesis.

The *t* value is affected by the denominator of the test statistic as well as the numerator. The denominator in this sort of test, which in this case is

$$\frac{s}{\sqrt{n}}$$

estimates the standard error of the mean. It is affected by the size of both *s* and *n*. Large variation in the sample values, which is expressed by a large value of $s^2$, will tend to reduce *t* and make it harder to obtain a statistically significant result. A large sample, that is, large *n,* will tend to increase *t* and make it easier to obtain a statistically significant result. Thus in situations where the variation of the variable under study is known to be substantially large, it will be necessary to obtain a fairly large sample to increase the likelihood of rejecting the null hypothesis. A smaller difference between $\bar{x}$ and $\mu$ is necessary to reject the null hypothesis when the sample size is large than when it is small. The effect of sample size on likelihood of rejecting the null hypothesis will be discussed further in Chapter 14.

# *t* Tests

At this point, we have only discussed what are known as *2-tailed tests*. Rejection of the null hypothesis is indicated by extreme values on either end of the distribution. In the type of study reported here, this does not really make sense in terms of the theoretical framework of the research. The employees who receive large doses of vitamin C are not expected to have *more* days of absence than usual. If vitamin C has an effect, it is expected that the effect will be in the direction of reducing the number of days lost from work.

Sometimes, when the investigator expects results to be in one direction only, a *one-tailed test* is used. In this case, this would be done by making the total rejection area of 5% completely at the lower end of the *t* distribution, since *t* is expected to be negative. The *t* table values for 24 degrees of freedom are shown in Figure 3-4.

In this case, the *t* value of −13.5 is significant at the .01 level as well as the .05 level, so that the null hypothesis would be rejected in either case. Note that the use of a one-tailed test makes it *easier* to reject the null hypothesis, since a smaller *t* value is required. For the case of 24 degrees of freedom, −1.711 is sufficient to reject the null hypothesis for a one-tailed test, whereas −2.064 was shown earlier to be necessary for a two-tailed test. A value of *t* between −1.711 and −2.064 would be significant with the use of a one-tailed test, but not significant with the use of a two-tailed test. In cases where the rationale for the study indicates a prediction of an effect in a specific direction, the researcher can increase the chances of obtaining significant results, and is justified in doing so, by using a one-tailed test rather than a two-tailed test.

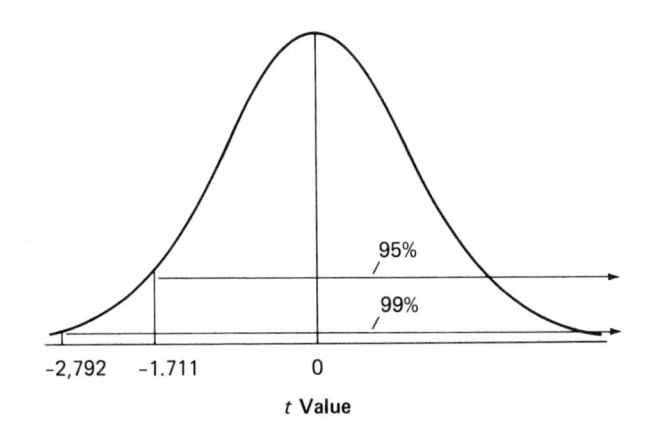

**Figure 3-4.** Cutoff points for 95% and 99% of the lower end of the *t* distribution with 24 degrees of freedom.

The study described in this section is a good example of one in which the researcher would want to be careful to put the results of the statistical analysis in perspective, by looking at the methodology of the study in detail. One could hypothesize that selection for inclusion in the study had a psychological effect on participants (Hawthorne effect), which either reduced their tendency to get colds or made them appear at work anyway. It would also be difficult to determine whether the subjects actually took the vitamin C daily, or whether other employees heard about the study and started to self-medicate themselves with vitamin C. This hypothetical study is poorly designed for the purpose of showing a causal effect, but the statistical handling of the data is perfectly adequate. Watch for highly significant results, statistically speaking, that don't indicate much in terms of scientific knowledge. The next section illustrates how a study of the effects of vitamin C could be done by a somewhat different approach.

## COMPARING TWO MEANS

A study of the effect of vitamin C on days lost from work could be done in a different way from that described above, so that a comparison of two means would be involved. Assume that 50 employees are selected at random to participate in the study. They are randomized into two groups. Each subject in group 1 receives a vitamin C placebo, and each subject in group 2 receives real daily vitamin C supplements. The analysis of the data takes the form of a $t$ test for the difference between two means.

Symbolically, the null hypothesis can be expressed as

$$H: \mu_1 = \mu_2$$

According to this hypothesis, the mean number of days lost from work is the same for people on vitamin C as for people on the placebo, that is, for people in the two hypothetical populations represented by the two samples. The two groups are followed for a year; assume that the results are as follows:

| Group 1 (Placebo) | Group 2 (Vitamin C) |
|---|---|
| $\bar{x}_1 = 9.3$ | $\bar{x}_2 = 8.3$ |
| $s_1 = 2.1$ | $s_2 = 1.9$ |
| $n_1 = 25.0$ | $n_2 = 25.0$ |

The difference between the sample means is

$$\bar{x}_1 - \bar{x}_2 = 9.3 - 8.3 = 1.0$$

that is, people in the experimental group lost on the average one less day from work than people in the control group. The statistical test provides for a comparison of this difference between the sample means with the difference of zero assumed by the null hypothesis.

According to the theory of the $t$ distribution, if $(\bar{x}_1 - \bar{x}_2)$ is the difference between the two sample means of sizes $n_1$ and $n_2$, and $s_p^2$ is a pooled estimate of variance from the two samples, then

$$t = \frac{(\bar{x}_1 - \bar{x}_2) - (\mu_1 - \mu_2)}{\sqrt{s_p^2/n_1 + s_p^2/n_2}}$$

has a $t$ distribution with $n_1 + n_2 - 2$ degrees of freedom, *when the null hypothesis is true*.

The pooled estimate of variance is obtained by simply substituting the corresponding sample values into the formula for $s_p^2$, as follows:

$$\begin{aligned} s_p^2 &= \frac{(n_1 - 1) s_1^2 + (n_2 - 1) s_2^2}{n_1 + n_2 - 2} \\ &= \frac{(25 - 1)(2.1)^2 + (25 - 1)(1.9)^2}{25 + 25 - 2} \\ &= 4.01 \end{aligned}$$

Then the $t$ value is calculated as follows:

$$\begin{aligned} t &= \frac{(\bar{x}_1 - \bar{x}_2) - (\mu_1 - \mu_2)}{\sqrt{s_p^2/n_1 + s_p^2/n_2}} \\ &= \frac{(9.3 - 8.3) - 0}{\sqrt{4.01/25 + 4.01/25}} \\ &= 1.75. \end{aligned}$$

The test statistic, that is, the computed value $t = 1.75$, is then tested against the distribution of $t$ with

$$n_1 + n_2 - 2 = 25 + 25 - 2 = 48$$

degrees of freedom.

Since the vitamin C group is really expected to do better than the control group, a one-tailed test would be justified in this case. The usual $t$ table does not have 48 degrees of freedom, but jumps from 40 to 60. To be on the conservative side, we will use the value required for rejection with 40 degrees of freedom. The $t$ table indicates a 95% value as shown in Figure 3-5. The computed $t$ value is 1.75, and so the null hypothesis is rejected. The results could be stated as "significant at the $p < .05$ level." Since the $t$ value is not large enough to make the results significant at the .01 level, an alternative description of the $p$ value could be ".01 $< p <$ .05." A significant result in this example means that we conclude that mean days lost from work is significantly lower for people on vitamin C than for those not on vitamin C.

From the formula for the $t$ value, it is clear that a large difference between $\bar{x}_1$ and $\bar{x}_2$ will tend to make $t$ large and thus tend to lead to rejection of the null hypothesis. This is what the researcher hopes will happen if vitamin C really does lower the mean days lost from work. If the null hypothesis is true, $\bar{x}_1$ and $\bar{x}_2$ should in most cases be close together and should result in a $t$ value too small to reject. The denominator of the test,

$$\sqrt{s_p^2/n_1 + s_p^2/n_2}$$

is an estimate of the standard error of the difference. As in the one sample case, the denominator is affected by both variation and sample size. If very small samples are used, or if variation is large, a large difference between the sample means will be necessary to obtain a large enough $t$ value to result in rejection of the null hypothesis. In Chapter 14 we will return to this issue of sample size and rejection of the null hypothesis.

You might compare the methodology for this study with the one sample design described in the previous section. The two-sample study

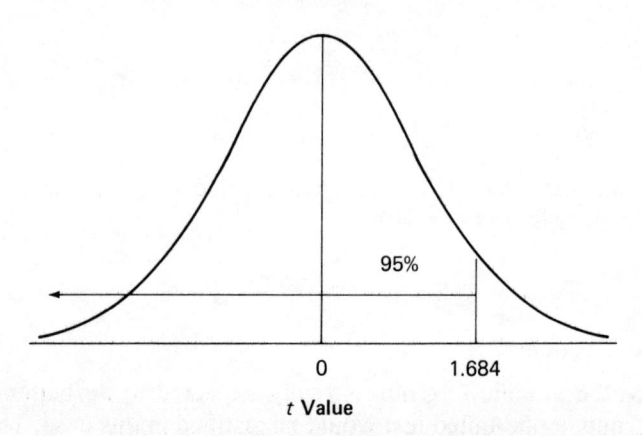

**Figure 3-5.** Cutoff point for 95% of the upper end of the $t$ distribution with 40 degrees of freedom.

provides a much stronger case for a claim that use of vitamin C reduces days lost from work. Since the control group in this design takes a placebo, there is no reason to think that one of the two groups should be consciously affected differently from the other. The second study is stronger evidence for causality, even though the test results were more highly significant (lower $p$ value) in the first study. Be sure to put the statistical results together with the study methodology when you attempt to evaluate the conclusions of any research project.

## CONFIDENCE INTERVALS

The theoretical distribution of $t$ tells us that for a $t$ value calculated to test a hypothesis about a population mean, we can expect that 95% of the time the calculated $t$ value will lie within the specific values of $t$ that include 95% of the probability distribution, *when the null hypothesis is true*. This fact is sometimes written as a probability statement:

$$Pr(-t_{.05} < \frac{\bar{x} - \mu}{s/\sqrt{n}} < t_{.05}) = .95$$

In this equation $t_{.05}$ refers to the critical value of $t$ needed to reject at the .05 level, which depends, of course, on the degrees of freedom, and thus on the sample size.

By algebraically manipulating this equation, we can arrive at a probability statement about $\mu$, the unknown mean, as follows:

$$.95 = Pr(-t_{.05} < \frac{\bar{x} - \mu}{s/\sqrt{n}} < t_{.05})$$

$$= Pr(-t_{.05} \frac{s}{\sqrt{n}} < \bar{x} - \mu < t_{.05} \frac{s}{\sqrt{n}})$$

$$= Pr(-t_{.05} \frac{s}{\sqrt{n}} < \mu - \bar{x} < t_{.05} \frac{s}{\sqrt{n}})$$

$$= Pr(\bar{x} - t_{.05} \frac{s}{\sqrt{n}} < \mu < \bar{x} + t_{.05} \frac{s}{\sqrt{n}})$$

This result means that 95% of the time (in identical experiments) we expect the true value of $\mu$ to lie between $\bar{x} - t_{.05} s/\sqrt{n}$ and $\bar{x} + t_{.05} s/\sqrt{n}$. The interval between these two values is called a *95% confidence interval for* $\mu$, and the two values are called the *confidence limits*.

Since with most studies of reasonably large sample size the required value of $t$ approaches as a limit the $z$ score 1.96, which is close to 2, the 95% confidence interval is often approximated as $\bar{x}$ plus or minus 2 standard errors ($s/\sqrt{n}$ is 1 standard error). Also, of course, confidence intervals for 90%, 99%, and so on, can be constructed by choosing the appropriate $t$ values from the table. Obviously, a large sample, that is, a large $n$, tends to produce a small standard error and thus tends to make the confidence interval narrower than for a small sample. In addition, the confidence interval also tends to be narrower when the standard deviation $s$ is small than when it is large.

A confidence interval can also be constructed for the difference between two means. In this case the original probability statement is

$$Pr(- t_{.05} < \frac{(\bar{x}_1 - \bar{x}_2) - (\mu_1 - \mu_2)}{\sqrt{s_p^2/n_1 + s_p^2/n_2}} < t_{.05}) = .95$$

Again by algebra, this becomes

$$.95 = Pr\{(\bar{x}_1 - \bar{x}_2) - t_{.05}\sqrt{s_p^2/n_1 + s_p^2/n_2} < \mu_1 - \mu_2$$
$$< (\bar{x}_2 - \bar{x}_2) + t_{.05}\sqrt{s_p^2/n_1 + s_p^2/n_2}\}$$

This equation defines a 95% confidence interval for $\mu_1 - \mu_2$, the true but unknown difference between the population means.

In both cases the interval defined by the confidence limits corresponds with the result of the test of the null hypothesis. In the case of a test of one mean, $H: \mu = k$, where $k$ is some constant, stating that this null hypothesis is rejected at the .05 level is equivalent to stating that the 95% confidence interval for $\mu$ does not include $k$. In testing the hypothesis for the difference between two means, $H: \mu_1 - \mu_2 = 0$, a statement that this null hypothesis is rejected at the .05 level is equivalent to stating that the 95% confidence interval for $\mu_1 - \mu_2$ does not include zero. If the null hypothesis $H: \mu = k$ is accepted by the statistical test, the corresponding confidence interval for $\mu$ will include $k$. Similarly, if the null hypothesis $H: \mu_1 - \mu_2 = 0$ is accepted by the statistical test, the corresponding confidence interval for $\mu_1 - \mu_2$ will include 0.

Confidence intervals are often included in research reports to give the reader an eyeball idea about the precision with which an estimate has been made. For example, if one has estimated the mean age for a sample of patients with myocardial infarction as 58.7 with a standard error of 4, the confidence interval would be expressed as

$$58 \pm 8$$

# PAIRED t TEST

The two sample *t* tests we have already discussed in this chapter are made with the assumption that the two samples are independent, that is, that individual observations in one sample are not matched or paired with corresponding observations in the other sample. If the observations have been paired, so that each subject in the second sample has been purposefully matched or identified with a subject in the second sample, then the *t* test we have described is not an appropriate procedure for analysis of the data.

Pairing is sometimes done prior to randomization to ensure that the experimental groups are equivalent at the beginning of a study. For example, litter-mates in laboratory studies might be assigned one to each study group. In this case each group includes one animal from each litter. Or in a nursing study of the effects of patient teaching on psychological well-being of patients following mastectomy, patients might be first paired in terms of age and length of time since surgery. In other words, the researcher would identify pairs of subjects similar on these two variables, and then randomly assign one of each pair to the experimental group and one to the control group.

The pairing procedure just described, which is also referred to as *matching,* is made on the basis of a variable known to be correlated with the *criterion* or *dependent* variable, that is, the variable hypothesized to be affected by the treatment. The paired *t* test takes into account the correlation between the paired observations, with the effect that the error (denominator) term in the test statistic is lower and thus the test is likely to be more powerful (more sensitive) than the one used for two independent samples.

Paired data also occur when repeated measurements or observations are made on the same subjects. For example, in the above nursing study, a measure of psychological well-being might be made on each subject before and after patient teaching, with no use of a control group and an experimental group. Similarly, observations of blood pressure are sometimes made on the same subjects at two different times. In such instances, the sets of observations consist of measurements on the same subjects at two different time points, rather than measurements on two different independent groups. Generally, the two sets of observations will be correlated, since each individual will be relatively consistent, and the paired $t$ test will take account of this correlation.

The easiest way to do the paired $t$ test is to first compute the difference between the measurements for each pair. Suppose, for example, that a study of the effect of vitamin C is done by first tabulating days lost from work in a sample of size 20 for 6 months. Then the sample subjects are given vitamin C for 6 months, and days lost from work are again tabulated. By taking the difference between days lost from work for each subyect,

(Days lost months 1–6) minus (days lost months 7–12)

we define a new variable for each of the 20 pairs of observations. Some subjects will lose more days on vitamin C and some less, but if vitamin C has no effect, the average of the differences will be about 0. If vitamin C has an effect, the average of the differences will be higher than 0.

A one-sample $t$ test is done in this case. The null hypothesis is $H: \mu_d = 0$, where $\mu_d$ is the mean change in number of days lost from work. The sample mean, $d$, is the mean difference in number of days lost from work for the 20 subjects in the sample, and $s_d$ is just the sample standard deviation of the differences. The calculated $t$ is

$$t = \frac{\bar{d} - \mu_d}{s_d/\sqrt{n}}$$

which is the same as the one sample $t$ test discussed earlier, except that the variable studied is the difference between two values rather than one value alone. The degrees of freedom are $n - 1$, since $n$ differences are being considered, and significance is determined in the same way as for the ordinary one sample $t$ test.

Once again, the methodology suggested by this study of the effects of vitamin C should be compared with the methodologies described earlier. This design is appealing because we are actually measuring a change in the subjects. However, there would be numerous problems in attributing a significant decrease in days lost from work to the effect of vitamin C. Consider the possibility of the Hawthorne effect again, or the possibility that the second 6 months of the study occurred during a season of the year when there is a low incidence of colds, or the possibility that the sick leave policy of the company changed during the course of the study. You can doubtless think of additional problems in interpretation of such data. Consult Campbell and Stanley[3] for a more systematic discussion of before–after studies and associated problems in interpretation of data.

# PROBLEMS

1. Refer to Table B in the Appendix to answer the following questions. For a two-tailed test, what $t$ value is required to reject the null hypothesis at the

   (a) .05 level, for a sample of size 10?
   (b) .01 level, for a sample of size 10?
   (c) .05 level, for a sample of size 20?
   (d) .01 level, for a sample of size 20?
   (e) .05 level, for two independent samples of size 10 each?
   (f) .01 level, for two independent samples of size 10 each?
   (g) .05 level, for two independent samples of size 20 each?
   (h) .01 level, for two independent samples of size 20 each?

2. Answer questions a through h for one-tailed $t$ tests.

3. Explain why the $t$ value required for rejection of the null hypothesis is always higher for the .01 level than for the .05 level, for a given number of degrees of freedom.

4. In this chapter, three different research designs were suggested for investigating the effectiveness of vitamin C on reducing the number of days lost from work. Consider the implications of the different procedures.

   (a) How do the differences in design affect the implications that can be derived from the results in each case?
   (b) Which design is the best and which is the most practical?

5. In a hospital where early discharge planning has been instituted, the average length of stay for a random sample of 61 patients is 5, and the standard error of the mean is 1. Assume that the mean length of stay prior to early discharge planning was 7.2 days.

   (a) If early discharge planning has no effect on length of stay, what would be the null hypothesized value for length of stay for patients with early discharge planning?
   (b) Calculate the $t$ value required to test the null hypothesis stated in question a.
   (c) Test the null hypothesis, using the .05 level of significance. State whether you used a one- or two-tailed test and explain your choice.
   (d) State your conclusion in substantive terms.

6. It is commonly assumed that giving information to patients will have the effect of reducing anxiety and thereby reduce pain. Kim[27] investigated this assumption by providing preparatory information about sensation to surgical patients on the evening prior to surgery and comparing their reported pain the day after surgery with that of control patients not receiving preparatory information. To test her contingency model, she also classified patients as either high or low on physical-danger trait anxiety, according to their scores on an inventory of trait anxiousness. She hypothesized that preparatory information would reduce pain for subjects low on physical-danger trait anxiety and would increase pain for subjects high on physical-danger trait anxiety. The study, therefore, included four groups, two experimental groups and two control groups, with one experimental group high on anxiety and one low, and one control group high on anxiety and one low. The data included the analysis of pain scores (pain scored so that a higher score represents higher pain than a lower score) shown in Table 3-1.

(a) What null hypothesis, stated in your own words, can be tested by the data from both groups for those high on physical-danger trait anxiety?
(b) Calculate the pooled estimate of variance necessary to carry out the test of the null hypothesis mentioned in question a.
(c) Would you be justified in using a one-tailed test in this situation? Discuss.
(d) Calculate the $t$ test statistic and test the null hypothesis, using the .01 level of significance.
(e) Calculate a 99% confidence interval for $\mu_1 - \mu_2$ and explain how it corresponds to the results of the hypothesis test.
(f) Answer questions a through e with reference to patients low on physical-danger trait anxiety.

**Table 3-1.** Comparison of Pain Scores Between Experimental and Control Groups of Patients with High and Low Physical-Danger Trait Anxiety

| Physical-Danger Trait Anxiety | Experimental Group $\bar{x}$ | $s$ | Control Group $\bar{x}$ | $s$ | $t$ Value |
|---|---|---|---|---|---|
| High ($N = 42$) | 0.750 ($N = 22$) | 1.054 | −0.036 ($N = 20$) | 0.259 | |
| Low ($N = 23$) | −1.353 ($N = 10$) | 0.750 | −0.173 ($N = 13$) | 0.519 | |

(g) How well do the results of the analysis support the hypotheses put forward by the researcher?
(h) For each of the two tests, does it make any difference whether the critical value is taken from the $t$ distribution or the $z$ distribution? Discuss.

7. In Chapter 1, Problem 2, a study of social and psychological influences on employment of married nurses was described. In this study, Cleland et al.[5] analyzed responses to 145 questions to identify factors related to employment status on which all the respondents could be scored. Four of the factors identified in the analysis were:

(1) career desirability—a high score indicates the individual feels that having a career is highly desirable
(2) economic value of work—a high score indicates that financial rewards of working are very important to the individual
(3) satisfaction with nursing—a high score indicates a high level of satisfaction with one's job and with nursing as a profession
(4) conducive home situation—a high score indicates a home in which the tasks are shared by husband and wife

As part of the analysis, the researchers calculated and compared mean scores on these factors for nurses classified according to their level of position. Mean scores are given in Table 3-2.

(a) State in substantive terms the null hypothesis that can be tested by the data for both groups on career desirability
(b) Calculate the pooled estimate of variance required to test the null hypothesis stated in item a.
(c) Calculate the $t$ test statistic and test the null hypothesis, using the .05 level of significance.
(d) State your conclusion in substantive terms.

Table 3-2. Mean Scores of Employment Status Factors by Level of Position ($N = 1767$)

| Factors | Staff Level ($N = 1168$) $\bar{x}$ | $s$ | Head Nurse ($N = 599$) $\bar{x}$ | $s$ | $t$ Value |
|---|---|---|---|---|---|
| Career desirability | 8.56 | 5.7 | 10.52 | 6.1 | |
| Economic value of work | 9.84 | 2.4 | 9.95 | 2.3 | |
| Satisfaction with nursing | 51.38 | 7.6 | 52.05 | 8.1 | |
| Conducive home situation | 39.36 | 16.8 | 41.95 | 19.2 | |

(e) Calculate a 95% confidence interval for $\mu_1 - \mu_2$ and explain how it corresponds to the results of the hypothesis test.
(f) Answer questions a through e for the factors of economic value of work, satisfaction with nursing, and conducive home situation.
(g) For each test carried out above, does it make any difference whether the critical value is taken from the $t$ distribution or the $z$ distribution? Discuss.

8. Dittmar and Dulski[12] carried out a study to examine the effects on hospitalized elderly patients of receiving sleep medications at earlier than traditional times. They hypothesized that sleep medication takes effect at a later time in older patients than younger, because of slow absorption and that, therefore, the effects might be extended later into the morning hours. This could adversely affect aged patients' ability to care for themselves and thus might result in longer than necessary hospital

Table 3-3. Patient Scores on Activities of Daily Living Before and After Change in Time of Sleep Medication ($n = 21$)

| Patient | Before | After | Difference |
|---|---|---|---|
| 1 | 81 | 85 | +4 |
| 2 | 176 | 180 | +4 |
| 3 | 94 | 98 | +4 |
| 4 | 114 | 126 | +12 |
| 5 | 201 | 210 | +9 |
| 6 | 190 | 190 | 0 |
| 7 | 163 | 166 | +3 |
| 8 | 204 | 219 | +15 |
| 9 | 155 | 158 | +3 |
| 10 | 125 | 129 | +4 |
| 11 | 100 | 125 | +25 |
| 12 | 143 | 165 | +22 |
| 13 | 164 | 180 | +16 |
| 14 | 93 | 118 | +25 |
| 15 | 102 | 116 | +14 |
| 16 | 160 | 183 | +23 |
| 17 | 135 | 124 | −11 |
| 18 | 103 | 99 | −4 |
| 19 | 112 | 141 | +29 |
| 20 | 204 | 204 | 0 |
| 21 | 165 | 166 | +1 |

Activities of Daily Living (ADL)

stay. Patients included in the study ($n = 21$) were given sleep medication at 8:00 P.M. for three consecutive evenings, instead of the traditional time of 9:30 to 10:00 P.M. They were observed and rated by the investigators on activities of daily living both before and after the change in time of sleep medication. The activities included dressing, mobility in bed, ambulation, use of wheelchair, toileting and feeding, and scoring was done in such a way that a high score indicates greater independence than a low score. Scores for the patients, as reported in the article, are given in Table 3-3.

(a) What null hypothesis can be tested by the data?
(b) Calculate $\bar{d}$, the mean change in ADL scores.
(c) Calculate $s_d$, the standard deviation of the differences.
(d) Calculate the test statistic and test the null hypothesis, using the .05 level of significance.
(e) What should be concluded, substantively, according to the statistical analysis?
(f) How might the fact that the investigators themselves observed and scored the ADL affect interpretation of the findings of the study?
(g) How could the problem mentioned in question f be avoided?
(h) How could you design a new study to investigate changes in ADL associated with time of administration in sleep medications, using randomization into control and experimental groups?

# Chapter 4

# CHI-SQUARE TESTS

## USES OF CHI-SQUARE TESTS

The normal approximation to the binomial was discussed in Chapter 2 as a procedure for testing a hypothesis about the difference between two proportions. In an example comparing two proportions, we described a randomized study of patients treated with two different concentrations of a new vaccine. A $z$ score was calculated to test the null hypothesis of no difference in the proportion infected between the two populations corresponding to the samples.

An alternative and more commonly used procedure for testing a null hypothesis of no difference between two proportions is called a *chi-square test*. Although this test gives the same results as the normal approximation using the $z$ score, it is conceptualized in a slightly different way. Individuals in the sample are classified according to their scores for each of the two dichotomous variables, and the analysis is carried out in terms of frequencies rather than proportions.

Application of the chi-square test to the example of patients treated with two different concentrations of a new vaccine would require that each patient be classified two ways, according to the two variables involved, that is, concentration of vaccine received and presence or absence of infection. These data would be presented as a cross-classification or "2 × 2" table like the following:

|  |  | Infection Yes | No |  |
|---|---|---|---|---|
| Concentration | A | 38 | 12 | 50 |
|  | B | 36 | 14 | 50 |
|  |  | 74 | 26 | 100 |

# Chi-Square Tests

In this table, the numbers represent frequencies or counts of individual subjects in each category. For example, 38 people received concentration A and became infected, while 12 received concentration A and did not become infected. The values outside the table represent marginal totals; for instance, 74 people became infected and 26 did not.

A chi-square test on such data could be used to determine whether the two variables are associated, that is, whether an individual in group A is more or less likely to become infected than one in group B. Stating this in terms of proportions, the chi-square test would determine whether the proportion who became infected in group A is equal to the proportion infected in group B. The results would be essentially equivalent to the results obtained earlier, using the normal approximation to the binomial distribution. In this case the chi-square would give nonsignificant results, as did the normal approximation to the binomial. The analysis of 2 × 2 tables using chi-square is one of the most commonly used statistical techniques and is appropriate when the association between two binomial-type variables is to be studied.

Chi-square analysis has an advantage over the normal approximation to the binomial because the procedure can be extended to the comparison of more than two proportions. Thus chi-square analysis is much more widely applicable than the $z$-score procedure and so is more commonly seen in research reports. For example, suppose that the study of a new vaccine involved the comparison of four instead of two different concentrations of the new drug. The resulting data would be described in the form of what is called a 4 × 2 table:

|  | Infection Yes | Infection No |
|---|---|---|
| A |  |  |
| B |  |  |
| C |  |  |
| D |  |  |

Concentration

The research question would be the same as before, namely, whether presence or absence of infection is associated with being in one group rather than another. The null hypothesis in this case would be that the proportion infected is the same in all four groups.

Chi-square analysis is also useful in situations other than randomized experiments. For example, suppose that an investigator wants to know whether blood type is associated with presence of a certain disease, that is, whether blood type distribution differs between infected and noninfected people. In order to answer this question, data would be organized in the form of a 2 × 4 table:

|  |  | Blood Type |  |  |  |
|---|---|---|---|---|---|
|  |  | 0 | A | B | AB |
| Disease | Present |  |  |  |  |
|  | Absent |  |  |  |  |

Chi-square analysis of such data would determine whether individuals classified by disease state differ according to blood type. If there were no difference between the two distributions, we would say that the disease occurs "independently" of blood type. The examples so far described are commonly referred to as chi-square *tests of association*.

Another type of situation where chi-square is used is in *goodness-of-fit* tests. This test is a way of comparing the distribution of observations into several categories with what is expected according to a specific research hypothesis. Consider a study of seasonal variation in births in a hospital. If there is no seasonal variation, the number of births should be about the same each month, with a slight adjustment for differences in the number of days in each month. A chi-square analysis would be used to compare the number of births observed in each month with the number expected according to the hypothesis of no seasonal variation, to determine whether there is significant variation by months.

Any chi-square problem can be considered in terms of a table with one or more rows and one or more columns. In each case the values of frequencies of observations in the cells of the table are compared with what is expected according to the null hypothesis. The null hypothesis for chi-square tests of association is always that of no association, or, alternatively stated, that the row variable varies independently of the column variable. The null hypothesis for chi-square goodness-of-fit tests is that the observations are distributed into categories according to a specified pattern.

One point of clarification should be made before we proceed to discuss the chi-square distribution and its use in testing hypotheses about proportions. Chi-square analysis is based on frequency data tabulated in a series of rows and columns and makes the assumption that all the observations are independent. This means that each frequency entry in the chi-square table represents a different individual in the study. The table must be structured and labeled so that each individual in the study is counted once and only once in the table, and therefore the total number of observations in the table is equal to the sample size. Occasionally, in nursing research as well as other research, chi-square analysis is inappropriately applied to tables that do not meet the requirements just described. This error is most commonly seen in cases where repeated observations on the same individuals are combined into one table for chi-square analysis. Such data do not meet the assumption of independent observations required by chi-square analysis, and in these cases the procedures to be discussed in this chapter are not valid.

## CHI-SQUARE DISTRIBUTION

You may recall that the $t$ distribution has a parameter called *degrees of freedom,* which varies with the sample size, and that the shape of the $t$ distribution varies as the degrees of freedom vary. The chi-square distribution also has degrees of freedom associated with it, and in this case the shape of the distribution is even more drastically affected by changes in degrees of freedom than the $t$ distribution. In addition, the chi-square distribution does not extend from $-\infty$ to $+\infty$, as do the normal and $t$ distributions, but has only nonnegative values. Some examples of the shape of the chi-square distribution are given in Figure 4-1.

The degrees of freedom for a specific problem determine the specific theoretical chi-square distribution to be used for testing the null hypothesis, just as for the $t$ distribution. You will remember that degrees of freedom for the $t$ distribution are determined by the sample sizes. For the chi-square distribution, the degrees of freedom depend on the number of

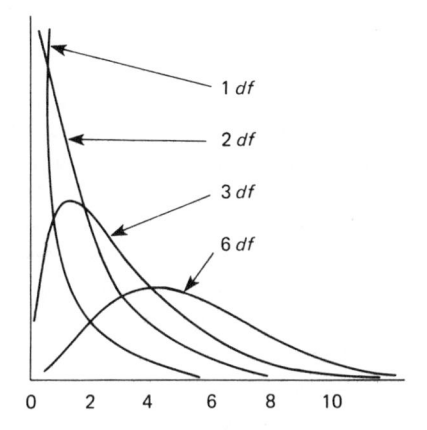

**Figure 4-1.** Chi-square distributions with 1, 2, 3, and 6 degrees of freedom.

rows and columns in the table to be analyzed, as you see in the examples that follow.

The following formula is used to compute a chi-square test statistic from sample data:

$$\chi^2 = \sum_{\text{all cells}} \frac{(O - E)^2}{E}$$

Here, $O$ stands for the observed value in each cell of the table and $E$ stands for the expected value in each cell of the table. The difference between these is squared and divided by the expected value, and this quantity is computed and summed over all cells of the table to determine the chi-square value.

The null hypothesis for tests of association is always that the row and column variable are not associated. The expected values for the chi-square formula are computed under the assumption of no association. Therefore, if the null hypothesis is true, the observed values will be close to the expected values, and the $\chi^2$ will be relatively small. If the null hypothesis is false, the observed values will vary from the expected ones substantially, and the $\chi^2$ will be relatively large. In other words, a very small calculated chi-square suggests that the null hypothesis should be accepted, while a large chi-square value suggests it should be rejected. This means that chi-square is always a one-tailed test. The chi-square is handled like the $t$ test in that extreme values lead to rejection of the null hypothesis. The difference is that all extreme chi-square values are at one end of the distribution. Chi-square is always positive, since it is always the sum of squared, that is, positive numbers. A large discrepancy between observed and expected values makes the chi-square large (and positive) and provides evidence for rejection of the null hypothesis.

The tabled chi-square distribution, as given in Table C of the Appendix, is based on the assumption of no association. If there is no association, the only difference between the observed and expected values is due to sampling error. As with the $z$ test and $t$ test, the values of .05 and .01 are customarily used as the allowance for error due to chance. Thus the calculated chi-square value will be compared with the tabled value, and the null hypothesis will be rejected when the calculated chi-square is larger than the tabled value for the specified level of significance.

Note that the theoretical chi-square distribution gives the approximate rather than exact distribution of the sample chi-square statistic and that the adequacy of the approximation improves as the sample size increases. A traditional rule of thumb is that the chi-square analysis is adequate when no expected values are less than 1 and not more than 20% of the expected values are less than 5. This means that in a 2 × 2 table, for example, none

# Chi-Square Tests

of the expected values should be less than 5. In some situations, small cell frequencies can be handled by collapsing categories together to increase the expected values. Other possibilities are to use what is called "Yates's correction for continuity," or, in the case of 2 × 2 tables, "Fisher's exact test." See Ferguson (14) for further discussion of the problem of small cell frequencies and description of the procedures just mentioned.

## 2 × 2 TABLES

Any data in which people, or any units of observation, can be classified according to two variables, and in which each of these variables has two categories, can be analyzed by use of the chi-square. Such data may be from an experimental study, where one of the variables is the classification into experimental or control group and the outcome variable is dichotomous. Or, it may be data on two of many variables from a survey, or comparison of any two groups on a binomial variable. The question is always the same: is classification on one variable independent of classification on the other variable?

Consider a study involving a sample survey of American Nursing Association members. One question to be answered is whether nurse practitioners earn more or less money than other nurses. The questionnaire asks respondents to check their income as either under or over $10,000. Assume that for 300 nurses of similar age and experience, respondents are classified according to type of job and salary. The results of the survey, that is, the *observed values,* are as follows:

|  | Salary > $10,000 | Salary < $10,000 |  |
|---|---|---|---|
| Nurse practitioner | 25 | 25 | 50 |
| Other nurses | 100 | 150 | 250 |
|  | 125 | 175 | 300 |

Using chi-square and the ordinary hypothesis testing procedure, we can determine whether there is a significant difference in salary for these two groups of nurses.

The null hypothesis for chi-square can just be written as

$$H: \text{no association}$$

or

$$H: p_1 = p_2$$

This means literally that the proportion of nurse practitioners who earn over $10,000 is equal to the proportion of other nurses earning over $10,000, in the populations corresponding to the two samples. This is the same hypothesis as $H: p_1 = p_2$ for two proportions, except that in this case the testing will be explained in terms of observed and expected frequencies rather than proportions in the two groups.

The data observed in the study are presented above. The entries in the cells of the table are called *cell frequencies*. They are not proportions, but rather numbers of people observed to lie in each of the four categories of classification. According to the null hypothesis, there is no difference in salary for these two groups. The following calculations will allow us to determine whether this null hypothesis is reasonable in light of the observed data.

To perform the chi-square analysis, we must determine the proportion among all respondents who meet the criterion of interest. In this case, the criterion of interest is that of earning over $10,000 salary. According to the observed data, the proportion who earn over $10,000 among all the sample respondents is

$$\frac{125}{300} = 41.67\%$$

If the null hypothesis is true, then approximately 41.67% of the nurse practitioners should earn over $10,000 and approximately 41.67% of the other nurses should earn over $10,000. Now, 41.67% of the nurse practitioners is

$$0.4167 \times 50 = 20.8$$

This is the number we would expect to observe in the upper left cell of the table, if the null hypothesis is true, that is the number of nurse practitioners we expect to be earning over $10,000 or the *expected value*. Similarly,

$$0.4167 \times 250 + 104.2$$

is the expected number of other nurses who earn over $10,000.

The expected values for the other two cells can be obtained by subtraction of the two quantities just obtained from the corresponding marginal totals. The following table gives the expected values for each cell in parentheses, for comparison with the values actually observed:

# Chi-Square Tests

**Salary**

|  | > $10,000 | < $10,000 |  |
|---|---|---|---|
| Nurse practitioner | 25 (20.8) | 25 (29.2) | 50 |
| Other nurses | 100 (104.2) | 150 (145.8) | 250 |
|  | 125 | 175 | 300 |

According to this table, the number of nurse practitioners earning over $10,000 is greater than expected (25 observed vs 20.8 expected), and the number of other nurses earning over $10,000 is fewer than expected (100 observed vs 104.2 expected). Use of chi-square will determine whether this difference between observed and expected values is likely to be due to chance variation in the samples or to some real difference in income between these two types of nurse.

The observed and expected values are used to calculate a chi-square value:

$$\chi^2 = \sum \frac{(O - E)^2}{E}$$

$$= \frac{(25 - 20.8)^2}{20.8} + \frac{(25 - 29.2)^2}{29.2} + \frac{(100 - 104.2)^2}{104.2} + \frac{(150 - 145.8)^2}{145.8}$$

$$= 1.74$$

Next, this value is located on the appropriate chi-square distribution, which is determined by the degree of freedom associated with the problem. In this case, if just one of the four expected values is determined, the others can be calculated, since the totals for each row and column are fixed. This means that only one value is free to vary, and all the others depend on that value. The degrees of freedom is therefore equal to 1.

The tabled values for the chi-square distribution with one degree of freedom are given in Figure 4-2.

Since the observed value of 1.74 is less than 3.84, the null hypothesis cannot be rejected at the .05 level of significance (i.e., $p > .05$). The difference in salaries observed between nurse practitioners and other nurses may be due to chance variation in the samples rather than a real difference between the two populations.

There is a mathematical connection between the chi-square distribution with 1 degree of freedom and the normal distribution. Each value on this chi-square distribution is the square of a value of the normal distribution. The chi-square distribution is like the normal distribution folded

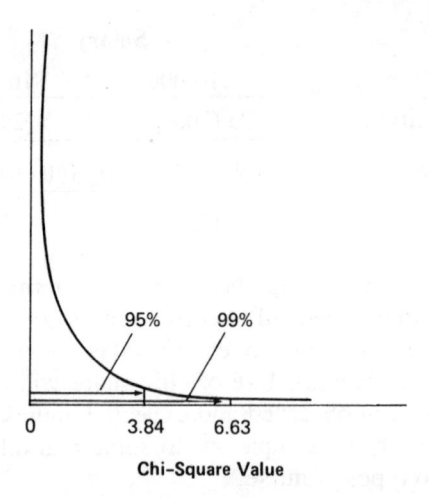

**Figure 4-2.** Cutoff points for 95% and 99% of the chi-square distribution with 1 degree of freedom.

in half in the middle. The correspondence can be seen by a comparison of figures in Tables A and C of the Appendix. The values of chi-square above 3.84 (5% of the distribution), for example, correspond to the values above $\sqrt{3.84} = 1.96$ (2.5%) and below $\sqrt{3.84} = -1.96$ (2.5%) on the normal distribution. Similarly, values of chi-square above 6.63 (1% of the distribution) correspond to the values above $\sqrt{6.63} = 2.58$ (.5%) and below $\sqrt{6.63} = -2.58$ (5%) on the normal distribution. This correspondence demonstrates the equivalence of the chi-square test for a 2 × 2 table and the $z$ score to compare two proportions. For any such problem, if you compute the $z$ score and square it, the result will be equal to the value for $\chi^2$ that you would obtain by chi-square analysis of the same data. In other words, any data that produced a $z$ score greater than 1.96 or less than −1.96 would also produce a chi-square larger than 3.84, leading to rejection of the null hypothesis in either case.

## R × C TABLES

The chi-square distribution, as we have stated earlier, applies to tables with more than 2 rows or more than 2 columns. The analysis for such tables is very similar to that described for a 2 × 2 table. The only major difference is that the degrees of freedom is not equal to 1, but rather depends on the number of rows and columns in which the data are arranged.

# Chi-Square Tests

Thus the size of the table determines the specific theoretical chi-square distribution with which the calculated value must be compared. The following example will provide an illustration.

Suppose that in the study described above, data were collected for three different kinds of nurses. Assume that nurse teachers as well as practicing nurses were surveyed, so that a comparison between three occupations could be made. Assume that the data are as follows, in the form of a 3 × 2 table:

|  | **Salary** > $10,000 | < $10,000 |  |
|---|---|---|---|
| Nurse practitioner | 25 | 25 | 50 |
| Other nurses | 100 | 150 | 250 |
| Nurse teachers | 20 | 80 | 100 |
|  | 145 | 255 | 400 |

This is the same information as presented earlier, with data on teachers now included.

The null hypothesis is again

$$H: \text{no association}$$

This null hypothesis is, of course, equivalent to the statement that the proportion making over $10,000 is the same in all three groups, or

$$H: p_1 = p_2 = p_3$$

As with chi-square analysis for 2 × 2 tables, this analysis will be carried out by a comparison of observed and expected frequencies, rather than actual calculations of the proportions.

According to the data, the proportion of all nurses in the survey who earn more than $10,000 is

$$\frac{145}{400} = 36.25\%$$

If the null hypothesis of no association between type of nurse and salary is true, 36.25% of the nurses in each of the three groups could be expected to earn over $10,000. Application of this percentage to the total number of nurses in each of the three groups determines the expected values noted in parentheses in the following table:

|  | Salary > $10,000 | Salary < $10,000 |  |
|---|---|---|---|
| Nurse practitioner | 25 (18.1) | 25 (31.9) | 50 |
| Other nurses | 100 (90.6) | 150 (159.4) | 250 |
| Nurse teachers | 20 (36.3) | 80 (63.7) | 100 |
|  | 145 | 255 | 400 |

The observed values in the > $10,000 category for the nurse practitioner and other nurse groups are higher than the expected values (25 observed vs 18.1 expected and 100 observed vs 90.6 expected), while the observed value for the teacher group is lower (20 observed vs 36.3 expected). Thus the nurse practitioners and other nurses do better than expected in this sample, while teachers do relatively worse, in terms of salary. The chi-square test can be used to determine whether the difference is significant.

A chi-square value is calculated as follows:

$$\chi^2 = \sum \frac{(O - E)^2}{E}$$

$$= \frac{(25 - 18.1)^2}{18.1} + \frac{(25 - 31.9)^2}{31.9} + \frac{(100 - 90.6)^2}{90.6} + \frac{(150 - 159.4)^2}{159.4}$$

$$+ \frac{(20 - 36.3)^2}{36.3} + \frac{(80 - 63.7)^2}{63.7}$$

$$= 17.14$$

To locate this chi-square value on the proper chi-square distribution, it is necessary to determine the degrees of freedom. One can see from the table that if two of the expected values are determined, the others are fixed by subtraction from the marginal totals. Two values are free to vary, and thus the chi-square has 2 degrees of freedom. For any chi-square with $R$ rows and $C$ columns, the degrees of freedom will turn out to be

$$(R - 1) \times (C - 1)$$

The critical values for the hypothesis test in this case are as indicated in Figure 4-3. Since the observed chi-square value of 17.14 is greater than 9.21, the null hypothesis can be rejected at the .01 level of significance ($p$

# Chi-Square Tests

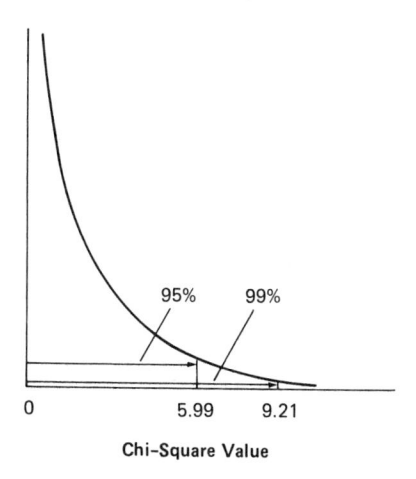

**Figure 4-3.** Cutoff points for 95% and 99% of the chi-square distribution with 2 degrees of freedom.

< .01). The conclusion is that there is a significant association between type of nurse and salary, and the chance that this conclusion is in error is less than 1%.

## PARTITIONING OF CHI-SQUARE

When a chi-square analysis is done on a table that has more than two rows and two columns, the researcher may be interested in a detailed study of differences between certain sample subgroups. In the example of the $R \times C$ table described previously, the chi-square is significant, indicating an association between type of nurse and salary. One cannot conclude from the significant result that all three groups differ, just that they are not all the same. In such a case, we can do what is called a *partitioning* of chi-square. The chi-square test for this example has 2 degrees of freedom. This means that instead of the overall chi-square test with 2 degrees of freedom, two independent chi-square tests can be made, with 1 degree of freedom each, and two hypotheses can be tested. The two computed chi-square values will account for the 2 degrees of freedom and will add to a value nearly equal to that calculated for the overall chi-square test.

The chi-square of 17.14 that was calculated for these data indicated evidence of an association between type of nurse and salary. Inspection of the observed data indicates that more nurse practitioners and other nurses earned over $10,000 than expected, while fewer teachers earned over $10,000 than expected, under the null hypothesis of no association between type of nurse and salary. At this point, we might want to compare only the two groups who earn more than expected, to see whether they differ.

This can be done by a 2 × 2 chi-square analysis, with the data for teachers omitted. This is in fact the original 2 × 2 chi-square table discussed earlier in this chapter, and the resulting chi-square is 1.74 with 1 degree of freedom, a nonsignificant result. Since the analysis indicated no difference between nurse practitioners and other nurses, we might combine the data for these two types of nurse and compare the combined group with teachers to get a second independent chi-square value with 1 degree of freedom, as follows:

|  | **Salary** | | |
|---|---|---|---|
|  | > $10,000 | < $10,000 | |
| Nurse practitioners and other nurses | 125 (108.75) | 175 (191.25) | 300 |
| Nurse teachers | 20 (36.25) | 80 (63.75) | 100 |
|  | 145 | 255 | 400 |

The above data now take the form of a 2 × 2 table, and the analysis is thus like that described earlier for tables with 2 rows and 2 columns. The proportion with salary over $10,000 is calculated as

$$\frac{145}{400} = 36.25\%$$

and expected values for each of the four cells are calculated as before, treating the combined nurse practitioners and other nurses as one group. The null hypothesis is that there is no difference in the proportion earning over $10,000 for teachers compared with the other two nurse groups combined.

The resulting chi-square is 15.23 with 1 degree of freedom, significant at the .01 level. The chi-square of 15.23 and the chi-square of 1.74 for nurse practitioners versus other nurses represent two independent sources of variation in the data relating salary to type of nurse. Each of these chi-square values has 1 degree of freedom, so that the total degrees of freedom is 2, and the two chi-square values can be summed as follows:

$$15.23 + 1.74 = 16.97$$

# Chi-Square Tests

The value of 16.97 is very close to the original overall chi-square of 17.14 with 2 degrees of freedom, and the chi-square values of 15.23 and 1.74 represent a partition or division of the overall chi-square into two independent parts. This partition indicates that the significant association between type of nurse and salary indicated by the overall chi-square of 17.14 is explained by, or results from, a difference between teachers and other nurses. The partitioning of the chi-square has yielded more information about the nature of differences in salary than did the original chi-square analysis on the three nurse groups.

Any chi-square resulting from a contingency table with more than two rows and two columns has more than 1 degree of freedom, and partitioning of the overall chi-square and the degrees of freedom into several tests can be done to study the data in detail. The number of tests that can be performed is equal to the number of degrees of freedom for the overall chi-square for the table, although fewer can be done if desired. The main restriction on the comparisons to be made is that they should be independent. This means that overlapping cells in the table cannot be used for different chi-squares. In the above data, a comparison between salaries of nurse practitioners and other nurses has 1 degree of freedom, and a comparison between salaries of other nurses and teachers has 1 degree of freedom. However, these two chi-square tables are not independent, but rather overlapping, and would not be a proper partition of the overall chi-square for the table.

As an example of a fairly complicated set of data where partitioning of chi-square might be useful, consider a study of the use of drugs among college students. Suppose that the data are tabulated as follows:

|  |  | Class |  |  |  |
|---|---|---|---|---|---|
|  |  | Freshman | Sophomore | Junior | Senior |
|  | None |  |  |  |  |
|  | Marijuana only |  |  |  |  |
| Use of illegal drugs | Marijuana and narcotics |  |  |  |  |
|  | Marijuana and LSD |  |  |  |  |
|  | Marijuana, narcotics, and LSD |  |  |  |  |

A significant chi-square for this $5 \times 4$ table, with $(R - 1) \times (C - 1)$ or $4 \times 3 = 12$ degrees of freedom, would indicate some association between class standing and use of illegal drugs but would not explain the nature of the association very adequately. We might want to study this relationship in further detail but would probably not want to examine 12 different chi-squares, even though 12 could theoretically be computed for this table, since 12 degrees of freedom are available for partitioning.

There are many ways in which these data might be partitioned into several independent chi-square tests. One follows:

A. (3 degrees of freedom)

|  | | F | So | J | Se |
|---|---|---|---|---|---|
| Use of illegal drugs | None | | | | |
|  | Any | | | | |

B. (3 degrees of freedom)

|  | | F | So | J | Se |
|---|---|---|---|---|---|
| Use of illegal drugs | Marijuana only | | | | |
|  | Marijuana and others | | | | |

C. (6 degrees of freedom)

|  | | F | So | J | Se |
|---|---|---|---|---|---|
| Use of illegal drugs | Marijuana & narcotics | | | | |
|  | Marijuana & LSD | | | | |
|  | Marijuana, narcotics, & LSD | | | | |

The first chi-square could answer the question, "Are there class differences in the proportion of students who use any illegal drugs?" The second would provide an answer to the question, "For illegal drug users, are there class differences in the proportion who use marijuana only, as compared with the use of hard drugs as well as marijuana?" The third

# Chi-Square Tests

would answer the question, "For those students who use hard drugs in addition to marijuana, are there class differences in the pattern of drugs used?" These three chi-square statistics are independent, since no comparisons are made that involve overlapping of cells in the table. Going from A to C, you can see that each subsequent data set is contained in one combined group of cells in the previous table.

Since each of the chi-square statistics in this partition has more than 1 degree of freedom, it would be possible to break each of these down further to obtain more detailed comparisons. Two independent comparisons from A, for example, are:

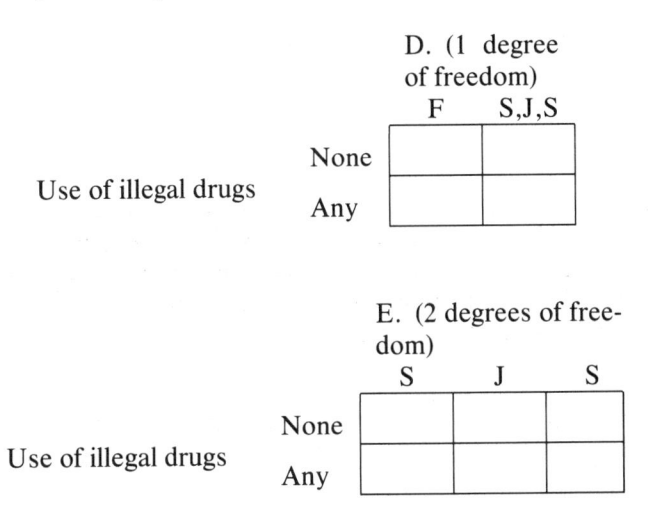

D. (1 degree of freedom)

|  | F | S,J,S |
|---|---|---|
| None |  |  |
| Any |  |  |

Use of illegal drugs

E. (2 degrees of freedom)

|  | S | J | S |
|---|---|---|---|
| None |  |  |  |
| Any |  |  |  |

Use of illegal drugs

The researcher must choose the partition to be made in a specific situation, since several alternatives are available. The choice is often made by identifying groups within the table that do not appear to differ, testing by chi-square, and then combining such groups when the results indicate no significant difference. In this way, it is possible to clarify the nature of a significant difference indicated by an overall chi-square for the entire table. Refer to Bishop et al. (1) for further discussion of analysis of cross-classified data.

## GOODNESS-OF-FIT TESTS

Suppose that an investigator suspects that people with certain blood types are more susceptible to a disease than others. In order to ascertain this, the blood types of 100 patients with the disease are tabulated as follows:

|    | N  | %  |
|----|----|----|
| O  | 35 | 35 |
| A  | 30 | 30 |
| B  | 15 | 15 |
| AB | 20 | 20 |

Total 100

These data will be analyzed using a chi-square goodness-of-fit test.
The null hypothesis is

$$H: \text{no association}$$

that is, the disease is not associated with blood type. If the null hypothesis is true, the distribution of blood types for these 100 patients should be similar to the known distribution of blood types in the normal population. The normal values for people of similar age to this sample can be used to determine the expected value for each cell of the table:

|    | % in normal population | Number expected in sample (from total of 100) | Number observed in this sample |
|----|------------------------|-----------------------------------------------|--------------------------------|
| O  | 47%                    | 47                                            | 35                             |
| A  | 39%                    | 39                                            | 30                             |
| B  | 9%                     | 9                                             | 15                             |
| AB | 5%                     | 5                                             | 20                             |

According to these expected values, there is an excess of people in the study sample with types B and AB blood (15 observed vs 9 expected and 20 observed vs 5 expected) and fewer than expected with O and A types (35 observed vs 47 expected and 30 observed vs 39 expected). Note that the data in this table are different in nature from data presented in earlier examples in this chapter. Although normal values are used to obtain expected values for the sample of diseased individuals, no sample of normal individuals is actually obtained for comparison. The fact that the expected values are obtained on a theoretical basis, that is, what is expected according to the null hypothesis, rather than by pooling values for two or more comparison groups, is what distinguishes this chi-square goodness-of-fit test from the chi-square test for association.

# Chi-Square Tests

The chi-square value is computed as before:

$$\chi^2 = \sum \frac{(O-E)^2}{E}$$

$$= \frac{(35-47)^2}{47} + \frac{(30-39)^2}{39} + \frac{(15-9)^2}{9} + \frac{(20-5)^2}{5}$$

$$= 54.14$$

For this type of test, the degrees of freedom is $k - 1$, where $k$ is the number of categories. This is due to the fact that all of the expected values can be chosen independently except the last, which can then be determined by subtraction from the total. In this case the chi-square has 3 degrees of freedom, and the tabled values are shown in Figure 4-4.

The computed value of 54.14 is significant at the .01 level. The null hypothesis is thus rejected, and the researcher can conclude that people with the disease in question probably do differ in distribution by blood type from the normal population.

## CATEGORIZING DATA

In this chapter you have seen several applications of chi-square analysis to the study of categorical data. Chi-square procedures can be used

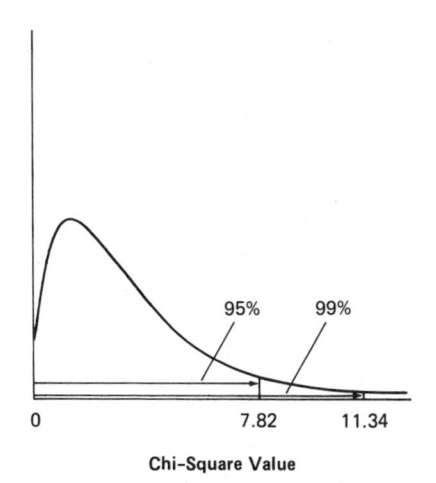

**Figure 4-4.** Cutoff points for 95% and 99% of the chi-square distribution with 3 degrees of freedom.

to test for association between two variables, each with two or more possible values, as well as for testing the goodness of fit of counted data to a theoretical distribution. Partitioning of the chi-square provides for an extension of the analysis into a more detailed examination of differences within one table. All these procedures are based on a chi-square test statistic that allows for a comparison of what is observed in the data with what would be expected on the basis of the null hypothesis.

The logic behind the chi-square test statistic is the same as that for the $t$ test. Rejection of the null hypothesis in either case is based on the degree of deviation of the observed data from what was predicted by the null hypothesis. In the case of the $t$ test, one is comparing the deviation of an observed sample mean or difference between sample means from the value, or difference between values, predicted by the null hypothesis. The only logical difference between the $t$ test and the chi-square test is that the chi-square test statistic compares observed with predicted frequencies instead of observed with predicted means. The choice between these two procedures, then, is made simply on the basis of the nature of the variables to be studied, in terms of whether they are appropriately treated as qualitative or quantitative.

Earlier in this chapter, there was an example in which chi-square analysis was used to test a null hypothesis of no relationship between type of occupation and salary. In this example, the variable type of occupation was dichotomized as nurse practitioner versus other, and the variable salary was dichotomized as over $10,000 versus under $10,000. The data were described as resulting from a self-administered questionnaire in which nurses were asked to indicate their salary as being in either the category over $10,000 or the category under $10,000. If the nurses had been asked to list their actual salaries, one could have calculated the mean salary among nurse practitioners and the mean salary among other nurses, and these two could have been compared by use of a $t$ test. It was simply the form in which the data were obtained (qualitative) that led to use of a chi-square test instead of a $t$ test.

In survey questions like the one just described, researchers often ask for personal data such as income and age in the form of categories instead of actual values. It is assumed that respondents will be more willing to give such data by indicating a range or category than they would be to write down their actual income or age. In such cases, chi-square analysis is appropriate. On the other hand, if you have actual numerical data, for example, because you asked respondents for actual age or income or because you have data from records instead of survey responses, you will not gain anything by categorizing the subjects as high, medium, and low, or under 40 versus over 40. When you convert continuous data into categorical data in this manner, you are in effect losing information about

Chi-Square Tests

variability among the subjects. The result is that the test will be less sensitive, that is, the chances of finding significant results are less than if the data are left in the original form. In a given situation, a judgment must be made as to whether the loss of variability in the data that will result from a categorical response format is more acceptable than possible refusals to answer questions that require the respondent to divulge very personal information.

## PROBLEMS

1. Refer to Table C in the Appendix to answer the following questions. Which of the following situations would lead to rejection of the null hypothesis tested with a chi-square test of association?

(a) $\chi^2 = 3.00$, for a 2 × 2 table, at the .05 level.
(b) $\chi^2 = 6.60$, for a 2 × 2 table, at the .01 level.
(c) $\chi^2 = 12.00$, for a 2 × 6 table, at the .05 level.
(d) $\chi^2 = 12.00$, for a 2 × 6 table, at the .01 level.
(e) $\chi^2 = 15.00$, for a 4 × 4 table, at the .10 level.
(f) $\chi^2 = 15.00$, for a 4 × 4 table, at the .05 level.

2. How do you know that any chi-square test statistic that is significant at the .05 level is also significant at the .01 level?

3. The data given in Table 4-1 would be problematical for chi-square analysis because some of the expected values would be too small. Suggest how categories could be combined so as to circumvent this problem.

4. In Problem 5, Chapter 2, a study of changes in the practice of breast self-examination in response to the media coverage in October 1974

**Table 4-1.** Prior Hospitalization Experience by Age ($N = 110$)

|       | Ever Hospitalized |     |       |
|-------|-------------------|-----|-------|
| Age   | Yes               | No  | Total |
| 21–30 | 2                 | 28  | 30    |
| 31–40 | 5                 | 35  | 40    |
| 41–50 | 10                | 20  | 30    |
| 51–60 | 4                 | 2   | 6     |
| 61–70 | 3                 | 1   | 4     |
| Total | 24                | 86  | 110   |

for Mrs. Betty Ford's mastectomy was described. Subjects in this study were classified as either health-oriented or non-health-oriented, based on their answers to questions about physical health behaviors. Subjects were asked whether Mrs. Ford's mastectomy had led to any change in their practice of breast self-examination, and the frequencies of respondents indicating more practice were tabulated separately for the health-oriented and non-health-oriented groups. These figures are given in the table accompanying Problem 5 in Chapter 2. Use these figures to answer the following questions.

    (a) What null hypothesis can be tested by the data?
    (b) What percentage of the respondents were health-oriented?
    (c) What percentage of the respondents reported increased practice of breast self-examination following Mrs. Ford's surgery?
    (d) What percentage of the health-oriented group would you expect to report increased practice of breast self-examination, if the null hypothesis were true?
    (e) What percentage of the non-health-oriented group would you expect to report increased practice of breast self-examination, if the null hypothesis were true?
    (f) From your answers to questions d and e, determine all the expected values for the cells of the table.
    (g) Calculate the $\chi^2$ test statistic.
    (h) Test the null hypothesis, using the .01 level of significance.
    (i) Explain the correspondence between the results of this chi-square analysis and the results of the analysis using the normal approximation to the binomial, as described in Chapter 2, Problem 5.

    5. Data from a survey of 10 nursing and 20 nonnursing students are given in Table 4-2.

    (a) Construct a 2 × 2 frequency table from the above data.
    (b) What null hypothesis can be tested using these data?
    (c) What proportion of the respondents use alcohol?
    (d) What proportion of the nurses use alcohol?
    (e) What proportion of the nonnurses use alcohol?
    (f) Use your answers to questions d and e to calculate the expected value for each cell.
    (g) Calculate the chi-square test statistic.
    (h) Test the null hypothesis, using the .05 level of significance.
    (i) State your conclusion in substantive terms.

    6. Keith and Castles[25] administered a questionnaire to staff nurses and nursing students in two community health agencies to investigate types

# Chi-Square Tests

**Table 4-2.** Type of Student (Nurse vs Nonnurse) and Use of Alcohol (Yes vs No) for 30 Boston University Students

| Student ID | Nurse | Use alcohol |
|---|---|---|
| 1  | Yes | Yes |
| 2  | Yes | Yes |
| 3  | No  | No  |
| 4  | No  | Yes |
| 5  | No  | Yes |
| 6  | No  | Yes |
| 7  | No  | No  |
| 8  | Yes | Yes |
| 9  | No  | No  |
| 10 | Yes | Yes |
| 11 | No  | No  |
| 12 | Yes | Yes |
| 13 | No  | No  |
| 14 | Yes | Yes |
| 15 | No  | No  |
| 16 | No  | No  |
| 17 | No  | No  |
| 18 | Yes | No  |
| 19 | No  | No  |
| 20 | Yes | Yes |
| 21 | Yes | No  |
| 22 | No  | No  |
| 23 | No  | Yes |
| 24 | No  | No  |
| 25 | No  | Yes |
| 26 | No  | No  |
| 27 | No  | No  |
| 28 | Yes | Yes |
| 29 | No  | Yes |
| 30 | No  | Yes |

of protection that might be acceptable to nurses making home visits in areas where they would be unwilling to go alone. Respondents were asked to say, for four alternative systems of protection, whether they would be

(1) willing to go into a community with protection where they would refuse to go alone.
(2) comfortable carrying out their nursing duties in the presence of the protector.

For four different systems of protection, the subjects (53 nursing students and 106 staff nurses) responded as shown in Table 4-3.

**Table 4-3.** Acceptance and Comfort with 4 Types of Protection System, by Type of Nurse ($N = 159$)

| Type of Protector | Number Who Would Go with Protection | | | Number Who Would Feel Comfortable Working in Presence of Protector | | |
|---|---|---|---|---|---|---|
| | Student ($N = 53$) | Staff ($N = 106$) | $\chi^2$ | Student ($N = 53$) | Staff ($N = 106$) | $\chi^2$ |
| Driver waits for you outside in car | 31 (58%) | 28 (26%) | | — | — | |
| Nurse goes with you and stays during visit | 24 (45%) | 67 (63%) | | 32 (60%) | 83 (78%) | |
| Community member goes with you and stays during visit | 25 (47%) | 61 (58%) | | 26 (49%) | 65 (61%) | |
| Hired bodyguard goes with you and stays during visit | 10 (19%) | 51 (48%) | | 5 (9%) | 45 (42%) | |

Answer the following questions, using data from the Table 4-3.

(a) Construct a 2 × 2 table to show the frequencies for those who would and would not go with protection, if accompanied by a nurse who goes along and stays during the home visit, by type of respondent. That is, fill in the cell and marginal frequencies for the following table.

|  |  | Type of Respondent | | |
|---|---|---|---|---|
|  |  | Student | Staff | Total |
| Nurse goes with you and stays during home visit | Yes |  |  |  |
|  | No |  |  |  |
|  | Total |  |  |  |

(b) What proportion of respondents in this study would accept a nurse who goes along as a protector?

# Chi-Square Tests

(c) What proportion of the nursing students would accept a nurse who goes along as a protector?
(d) What proportion of the staff nurses would accept a nurse who goes along as a protector?
(e) According to your answers to questions c and d, which type of respondent is more likely to accept this form of protection?
(f) What null hypothesis can be tested by these data?
(g) Calculate a chi-square test statistic and test the null hypothesis, using the .01 level of significance.
(h) What can you conclude in substantive terms, based on the statistical analysis?
(i) Repeat the analysis in questions a through h for each of the other three systems of protection. Then do the same analysis for differences between staff and students in proportion who would feel comfortable working in the presence of the protector, for the three relevant systems of protection.
(j) What substantive recommendations would you make from the figures shown in Table 4-3 and from your analysis?

7. In Problem 3 at the end of Chapter 1, a procedure for sample selection was described for a study of postmastectomy patients 4 years after surgery. As explained in this description, 49 women were actually interviewed for the study. Data included the number of complications occurring with the surgical procedure and symptoms of depression (4 years later). To determine whether these factors were associated, the researchers analyzed the data given in Table 4-4 (for the 43 of those interviewed who said they were at present free of all illnesses related to their breast operation).

(a) What null hypothesis can be tested by these data?
(b) What proportion of the 43 respondents fell into the low category on symptoms of depression?

**Table 4-4.** Symptoms of Depression by Number of Surgical Complications ($N = 43$)

| Surgical Complications | Symptoms of Depression Low | Symptoms of Depression High | Total |
|---|---|---|---|
| None | 14 | 4 | 18 |
| One | 7 | 1 | 8 |
| Two or more | 6 | 11 | 17 |
| Total | 27 | 16 | 43 |

(c) Based on your answer to question b, what are the expected values for all 6 cells of the table?
(d) Calculate the chi-square test statistic.
(e) Test the null hypothesis at the .05 level of significance.
(f) State your conclusion in substantive terms.

8. For Problem 7, there are 3 degrees of freedom for the chi-square analysis. Suggest a partition into either two or three independent chi-square statistics and carry out the analysis.

# Chapter 5

## REGRESSION ANALYSIS

### USES OF REGRESSION

We have already discussed the $t$-test procedure for testing a null hypothesis of no difference in means between two groups. When a $t$ test is used, the variable for which means are computed is ordinarily a continuous or quantitative variable, and the variable that defines group membership is a qualitative or categorical variable. A chi-square analysis is used to test the null hypothesis of no association between two variables when both are defined in terms of categories. Investigation of relationships between two continuous variables cannot be handled by either of these procedures unless recoding into categories is used. Regression and the closely related technique of correlation are procedures for testing a null hypothesis that two continuous variables are not related.

Regression analysis is often done for the purpose of using information about one variable to predict the value of another variable. For example, in making decisions about who should be admitted to graduate school, college faculty know from previous experience that students who have high GRE scores tend to do better in graduate school than those who score poorly. Regression provides a method for describing the relationship between GRE scores and grades received in graduate school and for predicting grades on the basis of GRE scores.

In the health field, regression analysis is useful for predicting future experience on the basis of measurements taken on individuals in the present. For example, life expectancy is sometimes predicted from weight, blood pressure, age, cholesterol level, and other parameters. The procedure is also useful for describing how two continuous variables are related. For example, it is known that blood pressure tends to increase with age. Regression analysis provides a way of graphically describing this relationship, showing normal or average blood pressures for different age levels. Growth charts based on regression techniques are also used to portray expected increases in height and weight as age increases. These sorts of pictures of normal change expected for one variable in relation to another over the course of time are useful for judging when changes in blood pressure, weight, and other variables are suggestive of disease or abnormalities in growth.

In a wider sense regression analysis allows for a systematic investigation of the relationships among variables. A researcher may be interested in testing a psychological theory that implies that the degree of patient anxiety about upcoming surgery may be associated with certain personality differences. One may be interested also in determining how health beliefs are related to smoking behavior or the use of drugs. The investigator may be more interested in explanation of the nature of the relationships among such variables than in using the results of a regression analysis in a specific clinical situation. Regression analysis provides a very powerful tool that is useful for both explanation and prediction, regardless of whether the study results are immediately applicable in a practice setting.

Because regression analysis is most commonly used for examining relationships among continuous variables, it is most appropriate for data that can be plotted on a graph, using distances on the horizontal and vertical axes to represent values of the variables. The data are usually plotted so that the *x* axis or horizontal axis represents the *independent* or *predictor* variable and the *y* axis or vertical axis represents the *dependent* or *predicted* variable.

Consider as an example the predictions of sons' heights from those of their fathers, with hypothetical data as shown in Figure 5-1.

On this graph, each dot ($x_i$, $y_i$) represents a pair of values for one father-son combination. For pair 1, for example, the father's height is 54 inches and the son's height is 53 inches, and so forth. The fact that the points tend to approximate a line with a positive slope suggests that there

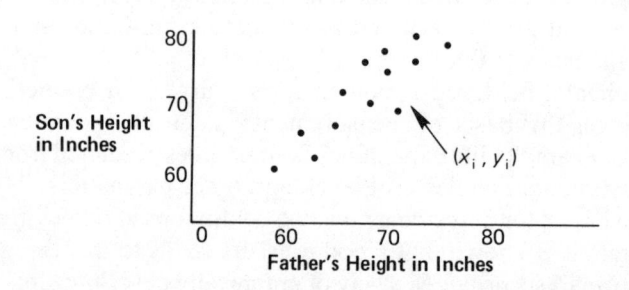

**Figure 5-1.** Scatter diagram of son's height ($y_i$) by father's height ($x_i$).

# Regression Analysis

is a direct or positive relationship between the father's and son's heights. The taller a man is, the taller his son is likely to be. Although there appears to be an upward trend, the points do not lie precisely on a straight line. Regression analysis is a procedure for calculating a formula for a straight line that approximates this upward trend in the observed data (or downward trend, if the two variables are inversely related).

Consider another example in which the relationship between two continuous variables is of interest. Suppose we would like to use weight as a predictor of IQ. Observations on weight and IQ for a sample of individuals might be plotted on a graph such as that in Figure 5-2. In this case, there is no apparent relationship between the variables; that is, IQ does not tend to either increase or decrease as weight increases. Such data can be approximated by a straight line, but the resulting line will be horizontal, with zero slope, indicating that weight is not a good predictor of IQ.

As a third example of the relationship between two continuous variables, suppose that one wants to predict income from age for a population of adults. Data on income and age might be plotted as in Figure 5-3.

These data show a relationship between age and income, but it is not a linear relationship. It would not be possible to find a straight line with a nonzero slope that would illustrate the relationship between these two variables. Regression analysis can be used to investigate nonlinear as well as linear relationships, as will be illustrated in a later chapter.

Regression and correlation procedures are most commonly used for estimation and testing for linear relationships only. Many textbooks present regression analysis methods for constructing linear models only, without even mentioning that the general procedure of regression analysis can be extended to the study of nonlinear relationships. It is very unusual in nursing research as well as other applied disciplines to see any consider-

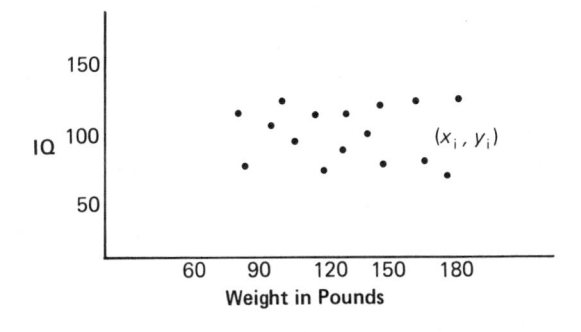

**Figure 5-2.** Scatter diagram of IQ ($y_i$) by weight ($x_i$).

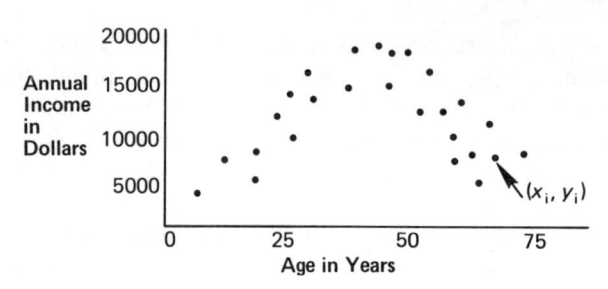

**Figure 5-3.** Scatter diagram of income ($y_i$) by age ($x_i$).

ation of nonlinear relationships. For these reasons, the following discussion is focused on the development and testing of linear relationships. A brief discussion of a technique for testing nonlinear relationships is given in Chapter 8. The reader should note that failure to find any significant linear relationship between variables does not rule out the possibility of a relationship that is nonlinear.

## DETERMINING A REGRESSION LINE

Before we consider how a regression line is determined, we will briefly review the algebra of an equation for a straight line. Readers who are familiar with this subject should skip down to the regression analysis model.

You may recall that

$$y = a + bx$$

is the equation for any straight line, plotted as in Figure 5-4.

The value $a$ is called the *y-intercept*, or the point where the line crosses the y axis. In other words, it is the value of $y$ that corresponds to $x = 0$. The value of $a$ is positive when the line crosses the y axis above the x axis and negative when the line crosses the y axis below the x axis. The value $b$, called the *slope*, is the amount that $y$ changes for every change of 1 in the value of $x$. When the value of $b$ is positive, $y$ increases when $x$ increases; and when it is negative, $y$ decreases when $x$ increases. If $b = 0$, $y$ is not a function of $x$, and the line is horizontal.

Examples of lines with equations of the form $y = a + bx$ are indicated in Figure 5-5. Note that lines 1 and 2 both have slope or coefficient of $x$ equal to 2 and are thus parallel. They differ only in the y intercept (1 versus

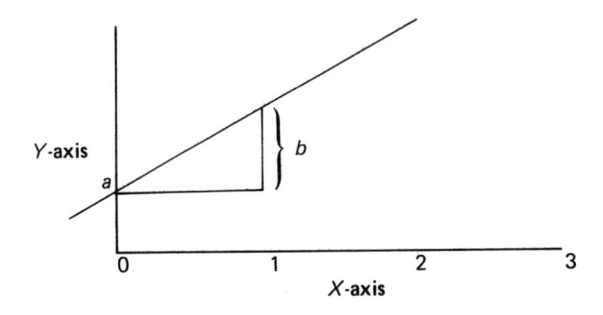

**Figure 5-4.** Graph of a straight line for the equation $y = a + bx$.

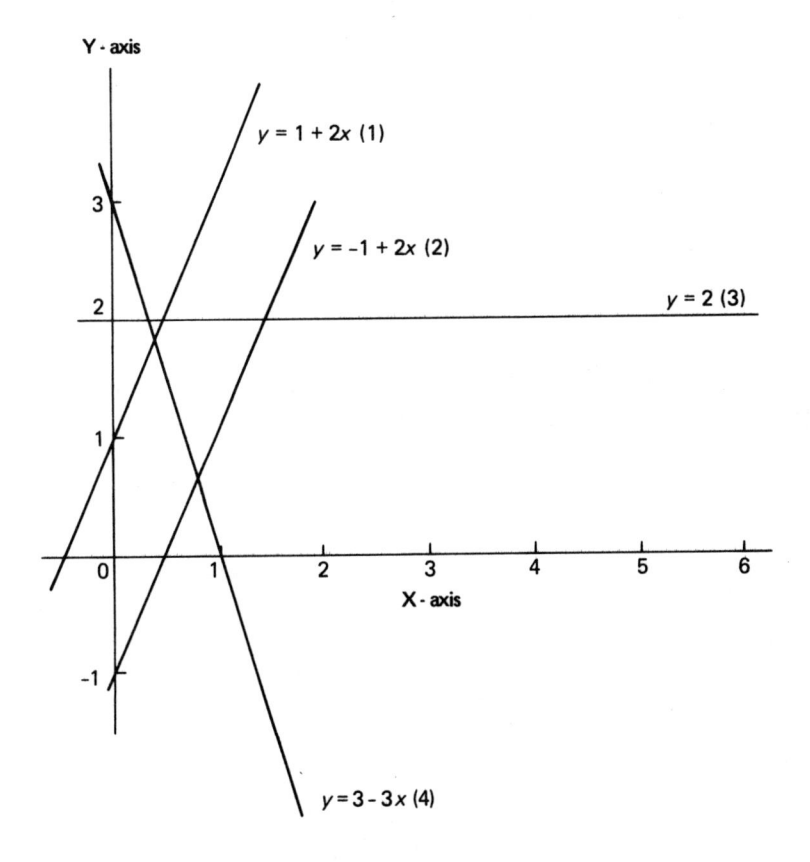

**Figure 5-5.** Graph of straight lines with equations of the form $y = a + bx$.

−1). Line 3 has 0 slope; thus the coefficient of $x$ is 0. In this case, $x$ cannot be used to predict $y$ since $y$ does not vary when $x$ does. In line 4, the slope is negative (−3), which indicates that $y$ decreases as $x$ increases.

The simplest regression analysis model assumes that the dependent or $y$ variable is a linear function of the independent variable $x$. The model for a regression equation is written:

$$y = \alpha + \beta x + e$$

In this equation $\alpha$ stands for the $y$ intercept, $\beta$ stands for the slope, and $e$ represents the variation of observations around the straight line. It is assumed by this model that for each value of $x$, there is a normal distribution of $y$ values around a mean $y$ value and that all the mean $y$ values fall on a straight line (See Figure 5-6).

The slope of this line, $\beta$, describes the increase in the mean or average value of the $y$ distribution for each increase of 1 on the $x$ distribution.

When the regression model is applied to real data, one uses a sample of $x$ and $y$ values, as opposed to the population values represented in the model. The sample of $(x,y)$ pairs is used to estimate where the true regression line is likely to be. For example, if the intent of the study is to determine the relationship between age and blood pressure, one would determine age and blood pressure for a sample of individuals. Age could be referred to as the independent or $x$ variable and blood pressure as the dependent or $y$ variable, so that the data would be in the form of a set of pairs of $(x,y)$ values.

Suppose that data are collected on a sample of size $n$. Subscripts are used for $x$ and $y$ to denote individual values, as follows:

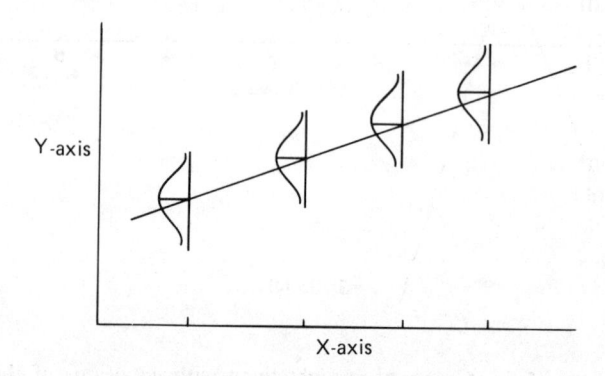

**Figure 5-6.** Model for linear regression.

# Regression Analysis

|  Variable 1<br>(e.g., Age) | Variable 2<br>(e.g., Blood Pressure) |
|---|---|
| $x_1$ | $y_1$ |
| $x_2$ | $y_2$ |
| $x_3$ | $y_3$ |
| . | . |
| . | . |
| $x_n$ | $y_n$ |

In this example, $x_3$ denotes the age of the third individual, $y_i$ denotes the blood pressure of the $i$th person, and so on. The mean age in the sample is

$$\sum_{i=1}^{n} \frac{x_i}{n} = \bar{x}$$

and the mean blood pressure is

$$\sum_{i=1}^{n} \frac{y_i}{n} = \bar{y}$$

The regression procedure determines estimates for $\alpha$ and $\beta$ from the $x$ and $y$ values observed in the sample, so that a sample or estimated regression equation can be made. For notation, the sample estimate for $\alpha$ is called $a$ or $a_{y \cdot x}$, and the sample estimate for $\beta$ is called $b$ or $b_{y \cdot x}$. The sample prediction equation used to predict $y$ from $x$ is thus written as

$$y' = a_{y \cdot x} + b_{y \cdot x} \, x$$

Just as with any other estimates of population values based on sample data, there will be sampling error in $a$ and $b$. The allowance for sampling error must be taken into account in testing hypotheses about the true but unknown population parameters $\alpha$ and $\beta$.

Since the sample points are usually scattered around and do not lie on a straight line, thee are many different straight lines that might be used to represent a trend in the data. There is a standard procedure for choosing the best line. Since the object of regression analysis is prediction of the dependent variable, it is logical that the "best" line is the one that offers the highest degree of prediction. In other words, the values of $y$ predicted by the regression equation should be as close as possible to the actually observed values of $y$.

Consider the sample data in Figure 5-7, where each point represents a sample observation on $x$ and $y$. The dotted lines in the graph in Figure

[Figure: Fitted sample regression line with equation $y' = a_{y \cdot x} + b_{y \cdot x} x$, Y-axis and X-axis labeled]

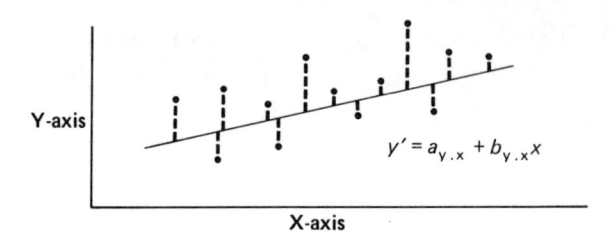

**Figure 5-7.** Fitted sample regression line showing vertical distance (deviation) from each sample point (observed $y_i$) to the line (predicted $y'_i$).

5-7 represent deviations of the observed values of y from those predicted by the regression equation (i.e., from the line). The sum of squares of all these deviations is used as an indicator of how well the regression line fits the data. A regression line for which the sum of squared deviations is small is said to "fit" the data better than a regression line for which the sum of squared deviations is large.

The formulas for calculation of a and b, the sample estimates of $\alpha$ and $\beta$, have been derived in such a way as to mathematically minimize the sum of squared deviations of the observed from the predicted values. Another way to state this is to say that if any line other than the one calculated by the formulas, to be given below, is used to describe the relationship between x and y, the sum of squared deviation of observed from predicted values will be larger than if the line is determined according to these formulas. This procedure is referred to, appropriately, as the *method of least squares*.

The formulas for a and b determined by the method of least squares are:

$$b_{y \cdot x} = \frac{\sum_{i=1}^{n} (x_i y_i) - \left\{ \sum_{i=1}^{n} x_i \sum_{i=1}^{n} y_i \right\}/n}{\sum_{i=1}^{n} x_i^2 - \left( \sum_{i=1}^{n} x_i \right)^2 / n}$$

and

$$a_{y \cdot x} = \bar{y} - b_{y \cdot x} \bar{x}$$

Regression Analysis

In the formula for $b_{y \cdot x}$

$$\sum_{i=1}^{n} x_i y_i = x_1 y_1 + x_2 y_2 + \cdots + x_n y_n$$

$$\sum_{i=1}^{n} x_i \sum_{i=1}^{n} y_i = (x_1 + x_2 + \cdots + x_n)(y_1 + y_2 + \cdots + y_n)$$

$$\sum_{i=1}^{n} x_i^2 = x_1^2 + x_2^2 + \cdots + x_n^2$$

and

$$\left(\sum_{i=1}^{n} x_i\right)^2 = (x_1 + x_2 + \cdots + x_n)^2$$

The value of $b_{y \cdot x}$ is calculated according to these formulas, and then $a_{y \cdot x}$ is obtained using the value for $b_{y \cdot x}$ and the two sample means, $\bar{y}$ and $\bar{x}$.

There is an alternative way to write the formula for $b_{y \cdot x}$. Recall that the formula for sample variance $s^2$ for a variable $x$ is

$$s_x^2 = \frac{\sum_{i=1}^{n}(x_i - \bar{x})^2}{n - 1}$$

This formula can be simplified to

$$s_x^2 = \frac{\sum_{i=1}^{n} x_i^2 - \left(\sum_{i=1}^{n} x_i\right)^2 / n}{n - 1}$$

Thus the denominator of $b_{y \cdot x}$, as shown above, can be expressed

$$\frac{\sum_{i=1}^{n} x_i^2 - \left(\sum_{i=1}^{n} x_i\right)^2 / n}{n} = (n - 1) s_x^2$$

so that an alternative way to express the value of $b_{y \cdot x}$ is

$$b_{y \cdot x} = \frac{\sum_{i=1}^{n} x_i y_i - \left\{ \sum_{i=1}^{n} x_i \sum_{i=1}^{n} y_i \right\}/n}{(n - 1)s_x^2}$$

This formula is referred to again in Chapter 6.

After $a_{y \cdot x}$ and $b_{y \cdot x}$ are calculated, the sample regression line can be written as

$$y' = a_{y \cdot x} + b_{y \cdot x} x$$

According to this equation, the variable $y$ is a function of the variable $x$. The value $a_{y \cdot x}$ is the $y$ intercept, and the value $b_{y \cdot x}$ is the slope. In statistical jargon, $b_{y \cdot x}$ is referred to as the *sample regression coefficient*. For any $x_i$, the predicted $y$ value is calculated as

$$y_i' = a_{y \cdot x} + b_{y \cdot x} x_i$$

For example, if a sample of age and blood pressure measures on $n$ individuals results in estimates of

$$a_{y \cdot x} = 74 \quad \text{and} \quad b_{y \cdot x} = 1.4$$

the equation becomes

$$y_i' = 74 + 1.4 x_i$$

Thus, the predicted blood pressure for a subject whose age is 30, for example, is

$$\begin{aligned} y_i' &= 74 + 1.40(30) \\ &= 74 + 42 \\ &= 116 \end{aligned}$$

Comparison of all such predicted values with those actually observed can then be used to determine how well the regression line fits the data.

# Regression Analysis

## DEVIATIONS FROM THE REGRESSION LINE

Following estimation of parameters of the regression line by the method of least squares, an investigator usually wants to determine how useful the line is in describing the data. Consider the two illustrations of regression lines fitted to sample data shown in Figures 5-8 and 5-9. In both situations, a fitted regression line has been determined. However, the "fit" of the line to the points is much better for Figure 5-9 than for Figure 5-8, since in Figure 5-9 the points are much closer to the line than in Figure 5-8.

The amount of error in prediction is measured by considering deviations (actually squared deviations) of the observed points from the fitted line. Since the $i$th observed $y$ is denoted by $y_i$ and the predicted value for $y_i$ according to the regression is denoted by $y'_i$, the quantity

$$(y_i - y'_i)$$

represents how far the observed $y$ value for the $i$th individual deviates from the value predicted by the regression line. In order to obtain an overall measure of the amount of deviation of all points from the fitted regression line, we simply add up the squares of deviations of all points from the line.

The total is:

$$\sum_{i=1}^{n} (y_i - y'_i)^2$$

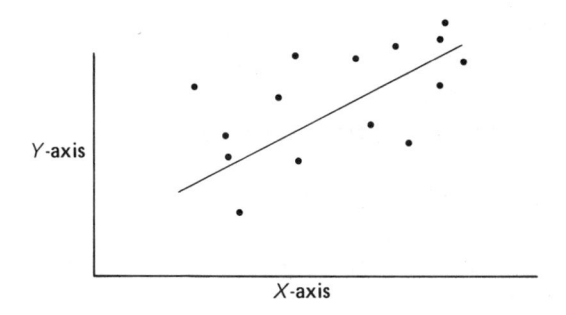

**Figure 5-8.** First example of fitted regression line.

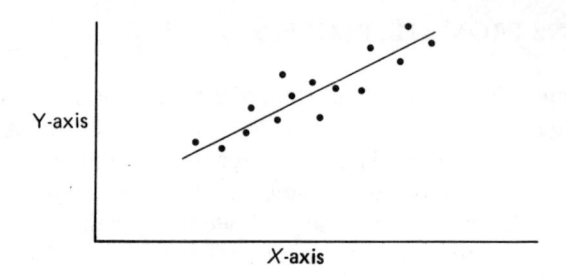

**Figure 5-9.** Second example of fitted regression line.

The total sum of squared deviations from the regression line is then used to compute the quantity

$$s_{y \cdot x}^2 = \frac{\sum_{i=1}^{n}(y_i - y_i')^2}{n - 2}$$

This variance measure, called the *mean square deviation from regression,* is used as a measure of how good the fit of the regression line is. If the line

$$y = a_{y \cdot x} + b_{y \cdot x} x$$

has a "good fit" with the data, then $s_{y \cdot x}^2$ will be relatively small. If the observed values jump around a lot and do not approximate a straight line very well, then $s_{y \cdot x}^2$ will be relatively large. In the examples shown in Figures 5-8 and 5-9, we would expect $s_{y \cdot x}^2$ to be quite a bit larger for Figure 5-8 than for Figure 5-9. The quantity $s_{y \cdot x}^2$ is used as an error term to form a test statistic for β, the unknown population regression coefficient.

## TESTING A REGRESSION HYPOTHESIS

Consider an investigation of the relationship between age and blood pressure. Suppose that a researcher hypothesizes that blood pressure increases with age and has collected data on both of these variables and plotted the data points on a scattergram, as shown in Figure 5-10. In this example, age, the independent variable, is plotted on the horizontal axis, and systolic blood pressure, the dependent variable, is plotted on the vertical axis.

# Regression Analysis

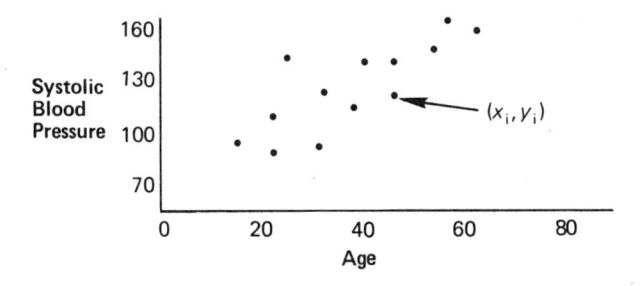

```
                   160  |                    •  •
                        |                 •  • •
    Systolic       130  |              •     •
    Blood                |                  •     •  ←── (xᵢ, yᵢ)
    Pressure       100  |           •     •
                        |        •     •
                    70  |_____
                        0      20       40       60      80
                                       Age
```

**Figure 5-10.** Scatter diagram of systolic blood pressure ($y_i$) by age ($x_i$).

The null hypothesis most commonly tested in regression analysis is

$$H: \beta = 0$$

According to this null hypothesis, the slope of the population regression line is zero. This means that $y$ is *not* a function of $x$ or, in other words, that there is no linear relationship between $x$ and $y$. If the null hypothesis is true, the fitted regression line will be horizontal (with zero slope), with minor deviation due to sampling error. Thus $b_{y \cdot x}$, the sample regression coefficient, which is the sample estimate of $\beta$, will be close to zero. If there *is* a linear relationship between $x$ and $y$, the value of $b_{y \cdot x}$ will deviate from zero as a reflection of that relationship. The significance test, to be described shortly, will indicate whether $b_{y \cdot x}$ is far enough away from zero to suggest the existence of a linear relationship between the variables.

In the example given earlier, a regression line for predicting blood pressure from age was determined to be

$$y' = 74 + 1.4x$$

The positive slope $b_{y \cdot x} = 1.4$ suggests a positive relationship between age and blood pressure, in other words, that blood pressure tends to increase with age. For every increase in age of 1 year, the blood pressure increases by 1.4 units on the average. The next step is to determine whether this apparent relationship is statistically significant, that is, likely to be a real one, or whether it just represents deviation from zero slope due to sampling error.

To test a null hypothesis about a population value, we need to know the nature of the sampling distribution of the sample estimate of the unknown population value. In this instance the sampling distribution of

$b_{y \cdot x}$, the estimator of $\beta$ is required. It can be shown mathematically that $b_{y \cdot x}$ has a sampling distribution such that

$$t = \frac{b_{y \cdot x} - \beta}{\sqrt{s^2_{y \cdot x}/(n-1) \, s^2_x}}$$

has a $t$ distribution with $n - 2$ degrees of freedom, when the null hypothesis is true. In this formuls $s^2_{y \cdot x}$ is the mean squared deviation from regression discussed in the previous section and $s^2_x$ is the sample variance of the variable $x$.

The fact that the sampling distribution of $b_{y \cdot x}$ is a $t$ distribution makes a test of the null hypothesis $H: \beta = 0$ straightforward. The test statistic is calculated by substituting zero for $\beta$ and sample values for the other quantities in the above expression. The null hypothesis is then rejected when the test statistic exceeds the critical value from the $t$ table (Table B in the Appendix), for a given significance level.

Suppose, for example, that this significance test is to be made for an association between age and blood pressure, using the data described earlier in this chapter. Recall that the sample regression equation was calculated as $y' = 74 + 1.4x$ and assume that

$$n = 42, \quad s^2_{y \cdot x} = 30, \quad \text{and } s^2_x = 20$$

Then the calculated test statistic is

$$t = \frac{1.4}{\sqrt{30/(42)(20)}}$$
$$= 7.41$$

Since the critical value for rejecting $H: \beta = 0$ at the .05 level of significance with 40 degrees of freedom is read from the $t$ table as 2.02, the null hypothesis is rejected at the .05 level. There is a significant relationship between age and blood pressure, according to the data.

The formula for $t$ shows that the further $b_{y \cdot x}$ is from zero, the larger $t$ tends to be. Thus large value of $b_{y \cdot x}$ tends to provide evidence to reject $H: \beta = 0$. The value of $b_{y \cdot x}$ cannot be evaluated without taking deviation from regression into account, however. A large sum of squared deviations from regression tends to decrease the test statistic and can make the $t$ value too small to reject, even when $b_{y \cdot x}$ is large. A small sample size also tends to reduce the size of $t$, as one can see by inspection of the formula. Computation of the $t$ value allows one to evaluate the simultaneous effects of all these parameters in determining whether the null hypothesis should be rejected.

# Regression Analysis

There is one issue that might be confusing to the reader at this point. The term "$t$ test" is commonly used to refer to a $t$ test for the difference between means from two independent samples, as described in Chapter 3. But we have just described a test for the significance of a regression coefficient that also utilizes the $t$ distribution. There are in fact several other sample estimates whose sampling distributions follow the $t$ distribution and for which hypothesis tests can thus be made by using tables of the $t$ distribution. Conventionally, these are not usually called "$t$ tests," but in actuality they make use of the $t$ distribution in the same way as the test for the difference between two means does.

Prior to the conclusion of this introduction to regression analysis, a somewhat different, although statistically equivalent, approach to the analysis will be described. Regression analysis is really analysis of variation in the dependent variable to determine what part of that variation is associated with variation in the independent variable. In other words, regression is analysis of variance. To demonstrate this, it is necessary to introduce the notion of partitioning the variation in the dependent variable into pieces that can then be combined to form a significance test. Description of these procedures constitutes the final two sections of this chapter.

## PARTITIONING THE REGRESSION SUM OF SQUARES

Several symbols have been used in this chapter to stand for different quantities of interest in a regression problem. These include $y_i$ (the actual observed value of the dependent variable for the $i$th individual), $y_i'$ (the value of the dependent variable predicted for the $i$th individual according to the regression equation), and $\bar{y}$ (the mean of all the observed values of the dependent variable).

The graph shown in Figure 5-11 illustrates the relationships between these values. The vertical distance from the horizontal axis to the value $y_i$ is the magnitude of the observed value $y_i$. As indicated by the arrows on the graph, the observed $y_i$ score for the $i$th individual can be partitioned into three segments, each representing an identifiable quantity.

The first quantity, $\bar{y}$, is just the mean of all the y values. The second quantity, $(y_i' - \bar{y})$, is the deviation of the predicted value $y_i'$ from the mean $\bar{y}$. In other words, $(y_i' - \bar{y})$ represents the effect of regression of y on the independent variable $x$. If $y$ is unrelated to $x$, the slope will be 0, the regression line will be $y = \bar{y}$, and this second quantity will be equal to zero. The third quantity, $(y_i - y_i')$, is the deviation of the observed value $y_i$ from the value $y_i'$ predicted by the regression equation. It is the third piece of this partition that is used to evaluate how adequate the fitted

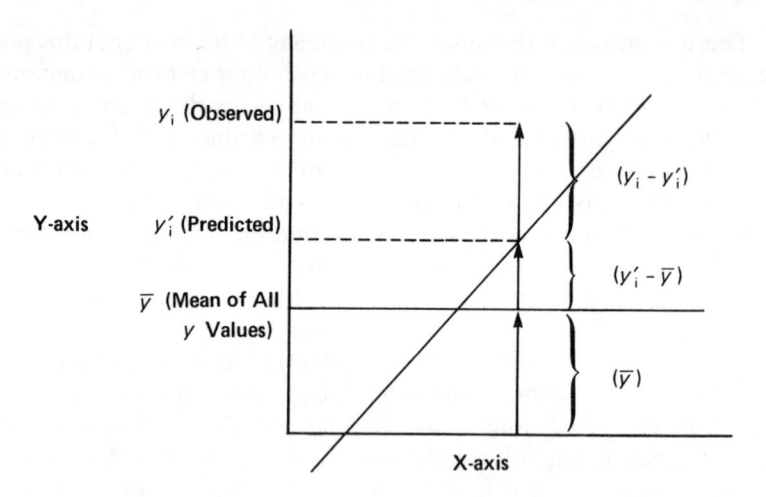

**Figure 5-11.** Partition of the regression sum of squares.

regression line is. When the fit is good, observed values will tend to be close to those predicted by the regression, and $(y_i - y_i')$ deviations will be small. When the fit is not good, that is, when observed values deviate considerably from predicted values $(y_i - y_i')$, deviations will tend to be large.

Since it is apparent from the graph that the observed $y_i$ value is the sum of the three quantities just described, one can write $y_i$ in the form

$$y_i = \bar{y} + (y_i' - \bar{y}) + (y_i - y_i')$$

Subtraction of $\bar{y}$ from both sides of this equation yields

$$(y - \bar{y}) = \bar{y} + (y_i' - \bar{y}) + (y_i - y_i') - \bar{y}$$

or

$$(y_i - \bar{y}) = (y_i' - \bar{y}) + (y_i - y_i')$$

In other words, the deviation of each observed value $y_i$ from the mean of all the $y$ observations, $\bar{y}$, can be written as the sum of two parts. You can verify that the equation just derived algebraically is true by looking back at the graph. The distance from the mean $\bar{y}$ to the observed value $y_i$ is clearly the sum of the two parts represented in the equation.

# Regression Analysis

These two parts of the difference between each observed value $y_i$ and the mean $\bar{y}$ represent two kinds of deviation, or variation, as mentioned earlier. The first part, $(y'_i - \bar{y})$, is deviation due to the regression effect, and the second part, $(y - y'_i)$, is deviation of the observed value from that predicted by the regression. Now consider what happens when these deviations are measured for all the $y_i$ values in a sample.

Recall at this point that the total variation of any set of observations around the mean is calculated as

$$s^2 = \frac{\sum_{i=1}^{n}(y - \bar{y})^2}{n - 1}$$

The numerator of $s^2$,

$$\sum_{i=1}^{n}(y_i - \bar{y})^2$$

is the total sum of squared deviations of observations in a sample from the mean of all the observations. In the regression case, the numerator is the total sum of squared deviations of observations on the dependent variable from the mean of that variable. But it was shown earlier that any one of these deviations of an observation $y_i$ from the mean could be written as

$$(y_i - \bar{y}) = (y'_i - \bar{y}) + (y_i - y'_i)$$

Thus the numerator of $s^2$ can be written as

$$\sum_{i=1}^{n}(y_i - \bar{y})^2 = \sum_{i=1}^{n}[(y'_i - \bar{y}) + (y_i - y'_i)]^2$$

$$= \sum_{i=1}^{n}(y'_i - \bar{y})^2 + 2\sum_{i=1}^{n}(y'_i - \bar{y})(y_i - y'_i)$$

$$+ \sum_{i=1}^{n}(y_i - y'_i)^2$$

It can be shown algebraically that the middle tern on the right is equal to zero, so that

$$\sum_{i=1}^{n}(y_i - \bar{y})^2 = \sum_{i=1}^{n}(y'_i - \bar{y})^2 + \sum_{i=1}^{n}(y_i - y'_i)^2$$

This last equation is called a *partition of the total sum of squares,* and each part represents a unique source of variance among the observations.
The quantity

$$\sum_{i=1}^{n} (y'_i - \bar{y})^2$$

is called the *regression sum of squares* and is a measure of the amount of prediction in the regression equation. The quantity

$$\sum_{i=1}^{n} (y_i - y'_i)^2$$

is called the *deviations sum of squares* and is a measure of the amount of deviation of observed values from the fitted regression line. The next section shows how these two quantities can be used to form a test statistic for $H$: $\beta = 0$ that is equivalent to the $t$ test for this hypothesis described earlier.

## THE *F* DISTRIBUTION

The partition of the total variation of a set of observations around the mean is referred to as *analysis of variance.* For a regression problem, the total sum of squared deviations from the mean, or the total sum of squares, is partitioned into the two parts described above. Each part represents a sum of squared values, and each has degrees of freedom associated with it. Just as the total sum of squares is divided into two parts, the total degrees of freedom ($n - 1$, from the total variance estimate $s^2$) is divided into two parts. In addition, for each part, the sum of squares can be divided by the appropriate degrees of freedom to obtain what is referred to as a *mean square.*

The partition of the total sum of squares is presented in research reports in what is called an *analysis of variance* (ANOVA) table. Table 5-1 is an example of such a table, with formulas inserted to show how each entry in the table would be calculated.

The quantity

$$\frac{\sum_{i=1}^{n} (y'_i - \bar{y})^2}{1}$$

# Regression Analysis

is called the *mean-square regression*, and the quantity

$$\frac{\sum_{i=1}^{n}(y_i - y_i')^2}{(n-2)}$$

is called the *mean-square deviation from regression*. Note that this second mean square is the quantity $s_{y \cdot x}^2$ used earlier in the denominator of the $t$ test for $H: \beta = 0$. Note also that the *total mean square*

$$\frac{\sum_{i=1}^{n}(y_i - \bar{y})^2}{(n-1)}$$

is $s^2$, the ordinary sample variance. In addition, the sums of squares and degrees of freedom columns of Table 5-1 add to the total, but the mean-square column does not.

This table provides a useful summary of the variation in observations, and we will return in future chapters to other kinds of detailed analyses of variance using this sort of table. For regression analysis, comparison of the mean-square regression with the mean-square deviation from regression allows us to evaluate the fit of the $y$ values predicted by the regression equation to the observed values. The null hypothesis to be tested (that there is no deviation due to regression) is equivalent to $H: \beta = 0$.

A test statistic is formed from the ratio of the two mean squares as follows:

$$F = \frac{\text{Mean-square regression}}{\text{Mean-square deviation from regression}}$$

or, symbolically,

$$F = \frac{\sum_{i=1}^{n}(y_i' - \bar{y})^2/1}{\sum_{i=1}^{n}(y_i - y_i')^2/(n-2)}$$

This quantity, which is sometimes called a *variance ratio*, has what is known as an $F$ distribution, when the null hypothesis is true.

The $F$ distribution, actually a family of distributions, is like the chi-square distribution in that it assumes only nonnegative values. You can see this by noting that the numerator and denominator are both sums of

**Table 5-1** Regression ANOVA

| Source of Variation | Sum of Squares | Degrees of Freedom | Mean Square |
|---|---|---|---|
| Regressions | $\sum_{i=1}^{n}(y_i' - \bar{y})^2$ | 1 | $\sum_{i=1}^{n}(y_i' - \bar{y})^2/1$ |
| Deviations | $\sum_{i=1}^{n}(y_i - y_i')^2$ | $n - 2$ | $\sum_{i=1}^{n}(y_i - y_i')^2/(n - 2)$ |
| Total | $\sum_{i=1}^{n}(y_i - \bar{y})^2$ | $n - 1$ | $\sum_{i=1}^{n}(y_i - \bar{y})^2/(n - 1)$ |

squares and thus either zero or positive. The actual formula for the distribution of $F$ is quite complex. It requires that both the degrees of freedom represented in the numerator (1) and in the denominator $(n - 2)$ be taken into account. After calculating the $F$ statistic according to the above formula, one can refer to a table of the $F$ distribution (such as Table D in the Appendix) to determine whether to reject the null hypothesis at any chosen level of significance. The null hypothesis should be rejected when there is significant prediction, which is suggested by a large $F$ ratio. Therefore, one rejects the null hypothesis when the calculated $F$ statistic exceeds the tabled value.

The specific $F$ distribution just described is only one example of a large family of $F$ distributions. There are other situations that will be described in later chapters, in which the numerator and denominator degrees of freedom take on values other than 1 and $(n - 2)$, and different $F$ distributions are defined. The usual tables for the $F$ distribution give critical values for the .05 and .01 levels of significance for various combinations of numerator and denominator degrees of freedom. The $F$ distribution discussed in this secion, that is with 1 degree of freedom in the numerator, corresponds to the $t$ distribution in such way that any given $F$ value is the square of a $t$ value associated with the same probability. You can check on this by comparing the figures in Table D (in the Appendix) for the column representing one degree of freedom in the numerator, with squared values of the figures in Table B, for the same level of significance. This means that the $F$ test given above is equivalent to the $t$ test for $H$: $\beta = 0$ given earlier.

In later chapters the topics of multiple regression and other forms of analysis of variance will be described. For most of these situations, some form of the $F$ test described in this section will be used to test null hypotheses about various relationships among variables. Although the degrees of freedom will be different, all the tests are basically in the same form, that of the ratio of one variance measure to another. Before going on to these more complicated topics, we will spend one chapter on the nature and use of correlation and partial correlation.

## SUMMARY

This chapter introduced the use of simple linear regression analysis for examining the relationship between two variables. Regression analysis provides a technique for fitting a straight line to a set of points, where each point represents scores or values for a subject on two variables, such as age and blood pressure, height and weight, and so on. The procedure also allows for a statistical test that can be used to determine whether there is a significant relationship between the two variables, based on the degree of departure of the estimated regression coefficient, $b_{y \cdot x}$, from zero. The conclusion that there is a significant relationship between the two variables means that, knowing the value on the independent variable, we can predict the value on the dependent variable more accurately than we could by just guessing the value on the dependent variable.

The next chapter will describe correlation and its relationship to regression analysis. A final point to be made is that the results of any regression analysis (or any other statistical analysis, for that matter) are dependent on the range of values for the variables that have been included in the study. A generalization that two variables are or are not statistically associated should be made with respect to the range in type of subjects for which data were collected. For example, results of a regression analysis might indicate a significant negative relationship between age and heart rate. If the study subjects ranged in age from 2 to 20, the researcher might be able to extrapolate the results to similar individuals between the ages of 2 and 20. It would not be legitimate to claim that the relationship holds for individuals of all ages, or for individuals over the age of 20, since these individuals fall out of the range of age studied. One simply would not know whether the relationship would hold for individuals over the age of 20.

Conversely, if there were no significant relationship, one could not conclude that there is no relationship for individuals of any age over 20. Nowhere is it written that two variables must be related in the same way over the entire range of values for each variable. If height and weight had the same relationship across the entire range of possible ages, we would all be in serious trouble. Many of the variables of interest to nurse researchers do not have simple linear relationships, which means that the nature of the relationship between two variables may vary dramatically over different ranges of the independent variable. Variables for which this concern is relevant include those such as age, socioeconomic level, anxiety level, stress level, and so on. If your data yield results that appear to be in conflict with findings from other studies, it is possible that results from both studies are valid, but that different ranges on the same variable were studied. This issue and its effects on various analytic procedures is discussed in later chapters.

Regression analysis is sometimes used to investigate the possibility that one variable "causes" another. For example, high anxiety may cause high blood pressure, and a regression analysis would probably indicate a positive relationship between these two variables. You should keep in mind that the demonstration of causality requires more evidence than a statistical relationship. There would be a high negative association between annual consumption of alcohol and number of cases of tuberculosis in the United States over the past 50 years, but you probably would hesitate to conclude that use of alcohol prevents TB. The contribution of statistical analysis to the study of causality is discussed later in this book.

## **PROBLEMS**

1. Plot each of the following lines on a graph:

    (a) $y = 3x$
    (b) $y = 2 + 3x$
    (c) $y = 2 + 1.5x$
    (d) $y = 2 + x$
    (e) $y = 10 - 2x$
    (f) $y = 8 - 2x$
    (g) $y = 8 - 4x$
    (h) $y = 7$
    (i) $y = -2$

2. Explain the difference between lines a and b and between lines e and f in Problem 1.

3. Explain the differences among lines b, c, and d and between lines f and g in Problem 1.

4. Explain the relationship between $x$ and $y$ indicated by lines h and i in Problem 1.

5. Johnson[23] investigated relationships between nursing aptitude, general aptitude, personality, and interest variables and academic achievement in 53 fulltime students in a school of practical nursing. As measures

# Regression Analysis

of various nursing aptitudes, the subjects were tested and scored on several subscales of the NLN Preadmission and Classification Examination (PACE). Johnson reported that previous investigators had demonstrated that the PACE is a significant predictor of success in nursing school. Nursing achievement was measured by numerical course grades for 10 individual courses and for the overall average. For each of the 10 course grades and for the overall average, Johnson selected the PACE subscale that best predicted that grade or overall average, and calculated a regression equation to show the relationship. The resulting equations are shown in Table 5-2.

(a) For the first regression equation listed in Table 5-2,

$$y = 74.54 + .35x$$

what does the symbol $x$ represent?

(b) What does the symbol $y$ represent?
(c) What is the regression coefficient?
(d) What is the direction of the relationship between $x$ and $y$ suggested by the regression equation?
(e) Answer questions a through d for the other regression equations shown in Table 5-2.
(f) Consider a student with the following subscale scores on PACE:

$$\begin{aligned} \text{Science and health} &= 60 \\ \text{Reading} &= 36 \\ \text{Vocabulary} &= 38 \\ \text{General information} &= 40 \end{aligned}$$

Determine the predicted individual course and overall grades for this student, using the regression equations given in Table 5-2.

(g) Consider a student with the following subscale scores on PACE:

$$\begin{aligned} \text{Science and health} &= 50 \\ \text{Reading} &= 30 \\ \text{Vocabulary} &= 30 \\ \text{General information} &= 30 \end{aligned}$$

Determine the predicted individual course and overall grades for this student, using the regression equations given in Table 5-2.

(h) Compare the two students described in f and g, explaining differences in their predicted course grades.

**Table 5-2.** Regression Equations for Predicting Course Grades and Overall Average from PACE Subscale Scores ($N = 53$)*

| Dependent Variable (Course or Overall Grade) | Independent Variable (PACE Subscale) | Regression Equation | Correlation Coefficient |
|---|---|---|---|
| Nursing principles and skills | Science and health | $y' = 74.54 + .35x$ | .598 |
| Dosages and solutions | Reading | $y' = 71.45 + .57x$ | .614 |
| First aid | Vocabulary | $y' = 78.50 + .30x$ | .420 |
| Body structure and function | Reading | $y' = 64.30 + .63x$ | .598 |
| Nutrition | Science and health | $y' = 75.20 + .38x$ | .588 |
| Personal and community health | General information | $y' = 86.34 + .22x$ | .498 |
| Personal and vocational relations | Vocabulary | $y' = 80.00 + .25x$ | .487 |
| Introduction to medical–surgical nursing | General information | $y' = 74.76 + .29x$ | .596 |
| Maternal–child health | Reading | $y' = 77.65 + .39x$ | .598 |
| Medical–surgical nursing laboratory | Science and health | $y' = 76.59 + .32x$ | .539 |
| Overall average | General information | $y' = 78.99 + .25x$ | .641 |

*$p < .01$ for all significance tests.

(i) Of what practical use is the information shown in this regression analysis?

6. Consider a regression of increase in birth weight on birth weight between 70 and 100 days after birth (expressed as a percentage of birth weights) for newborns.

# Regression Analysis

(a) Do you expect these two variables to be related, and if so, what do you expect to be the direction of the relationship?

(b) Data on these two variables are collected for 32 babies, and a regression equation calculated, with the following results:

$$n = 32, \quad b = -.86, \quad a = 167.87, \quad s^2_{y \cdot x} = 316.74, \quad s^2_x = 331$$

What is the prediction equation?

(c) What is the predicted increase in birth weight for a baby with a birth weight of 8 pounds?

(d) Calculate the $t$ value and test the null hypothesis $H: \beta = 0$, using the .05 level of significance.

(e) How could this relationship between birth weight and increase in weight be useful to a pediatrician, or is this sort of relationship interesting only to a statistician?

7. Refer to Table D in the Appendix to answer the following questions. Which of the following calculated $F$-test statistics would lead to rejection of the null hypothesis at the .05 level of significance?

(a) $F = 5.00$, with 1 and 8 degrees of freedom
(b) $F = 7.11$, with 1 and 8 degrees of freedom
(c) $F = 0.37$, with 1 and 25 degrees of freedom
(d) $F = 8.37$, with 1 and 25 degrees of freedom

8. Refer to Table D in the Appendix to answer the following questions. For a regression ANOVA, using the procedure described in this chapter, what $F$ value would be required for significance at the .01 level

(a) for a sample size of 20?
(b) for a sample size of 30?
(c) for a sample size of 102?
(d) for a sample size larger than 1000?

9. In a study of the effects of discussion of stress experience and traditional coronary heart disease risk factors on blood pressure, Smyth et al.[40] studied 33 inner-city black women. The researchers used Friedman and Rosenman's (15) standard interview technique to classify the women as either type A or type B (type A represents the coronary-prone individual). Included in the data presented by the investigators in their article were the age and resting systolic blood pressure for each subject. These figures are given in Table 5-3.

**Table 5-3.** Age and Resting Systolic Blood Pressure by Personality Type ($N = 33$)

| \multicolumn{2}{c}{Type A ($N = 16$)} | \multicolumn{2}{c}{Type B ($N = 17$)} |
|---|---|---|---|
| Age | Resting Systolic Blood Pressure | Age | Resting Systolic Blood Pressure |
| 40 | 128 | 60 | 140 |
| 53 | 127 | 52 | 153 |
| 35 | 141 | 59 | 159 |
| 50 | 151 | 47 | 192 |
| 40 | 149 | 58 | 148 |
| 47 | 162 | 34 | 106 |
| 54 | 156 | 27 | 113 |
| 49 | 142 | 25 | 110 |
| 36 | 126 | 33 | 120 |
| 36 | 121 | 43 | 97 |
| 35 | 115 | 34 | 113 |
| 62 | 113 | 41 | 135 |
| 42 | 116 | 26 | 125 |
| 27 | 100 | 38 | 132 |
| 37 | 108 | 23 | 124 |
| 33 | 110 | 20 | 95 |
|    |     | 24 | 104 |

(a) For the relationship generally hypothesized to exist between age and blood pressure, which variable is considered the independent variable and which is considered the dependent variable?

(b) For subjects classified as type A, construct a graph to illustrate the data (i.e., plot all the points).

(c) Using the method of least squares, calculate $b_{y \cdot x}$ and $a_{y \cdot x}$ for the type A subjects, and write the regression equation.

(d) What would be the predicted blood pressure for a subject of age 40, according to the regression equation?

(e) Calculate the mean-square deviation from regression, using the formula for $s^2_{y \cdot x}$ given in the text.

(f) Calculate the sample variance for the $x$ variable, $s^2_x$, using the ordinary formula for sample variance.

(g) What null hypothesis can be tested using the figures you have calculated? State the null hypothesis in substantive terms.

(h) Test the null hypothesis stated in item g, using a $t$ test at the .01 level of significance.

(i) State your conclusion in substantive terms.

# Regression Analysis

(j) Repeat questions b through i, using the data on age and blood pressure for the subjects classified as type B.

10. For Problem 9, the analysis can be done in the form of analysis of variance, by developing a regression ANOVA table like the one shown in the text. Carry out the following steps:
- (a) For the type A subjects, calculate the total sum of squares, the regression sum of squares, and the deviations sum of squares required for the regression ANOVA procedure.
- (b) Construct the regression ANOVA table and fill in the degrees of freedom, mean squares, and $F$-test statistic.
- (c) Test the null hypothesis, using the .01 level of significance.
- (d) Explain how the $F$-test statistic corresponds to the $t$-test statistic calculated for question h in Problem 9.
- (e) Repeat questions a through d, using the data on age and blood pressure for the subjects classified as type B.

# Chapter 6

## CORRELATION AND PARTIAL CORRELATION

**CORRELATION COEFFICIENT**

The term "correlation" refers to the statistical association or relationship between two variables. To say that two variables are correlated is to say that knowledge of the value of one gives some indication of what the value of the other is likely to be. For example, the statement that height and weight are positively correlated just means that tall people tend to be heavier than short people. Or a positive correlation between age and blood pressure indicates that older people tend to have higher blood pressure than younger people. By the nature of these examples, it should be obvious that correlation analysis is appropriate for the same kinds of research situations as regression analysis. In fact, correlation analysis is really just an alternative way of conceptualizing regression analysis.

Recall for a moment the mathematical model for regression analysis:

$$y = \alpha + \beta x$$

In this equation, $\beta$ represents the slope of the regression line. The unit of measurement of $\beta$ is "change in $y$ per unit change in $x$." If we are predicting weight in pounds from height in inches, for example, the unit of measurement of $\beta$ is "pounds per inch." If it happens that measures of height are obtained in units of feet rather than inches, the unit of measurement of $\beta$ is "pounds per feet." The actual numerical value of $b$, the estimate of the slope, depends on the units of measurement used for the two variables. If height is measured in feet instead of inches, the slope for the regression of weight on height will be much larger than if height is measured in inches. Because the value of $b$ depends so directly on the units of measurement used in collection of the data, it is difficult to get a feeling for how closely two variables are related just by inspection of the sample regression coef-

# Correlation and Partial Correlation

ficient. A large value of $b$ does not necessarily indicate a stronger relationship than a small value of $b$. Correlation analysis is a way of getting around this problem by an approach to the data that is slightly different from regression analysis.

The technique of correlation analysis requires calculation from the sample data of a quantity referred to as a *correlation coefficient* or *product moment correlation coefficient,* which can be used to evaluate the strength of a relationship between two variables. A correlation coefficient is actually just a standardized form of a regression coefficient ($\beta$ or its estimate $b$). The correlation coefficient can then be used as a unit free measure for quantifying the strength of the relationship between two variables $x$ and $y$. The actual population correlation between two variables is denoted by rho ($\rho$). The value of $\rho$ is estimated by the sample correlation coefficient, which is denoted as $r_{x \cdot y}$. The following formulas show how $r_{x \cdot y}$ is calculated from sample data and how it is related to the sample regression coefficient, $b_{y \cdot x}$.

For a sample of $x$ and $y$ values, $r_{x \cdot y}$ is calculated as

$$r_{x \cdot y} = \frac{\sum_{i=1}^{n} x_i y_i - \left\{ \sum_{i=1}^{n} x_i \sum_{i=1}^{n} y_i \right\}/n}{(n-1) s_x s_y}$$

Recall that $b_{y \cdot x}$, the sample regression coefficient, is

$$b_{y \cdot x} = \frac{\sum_{i=1}^{n} x_i y_i - \left\{ \sum_{i=1}^{n} x_i \sum_{i=1}^{n} y_i \right\}/n}{(n-1) s_x^2}$$

Combination of these two formulas shows the mathematical relationship between $r_{x \cdot y}$ and $b_{y \cdot x}$:

$$r_{x \cdot y} = \frac{\sum_{i=1}^{n} x_i y_i - \left\{ \sum_{i=1}^{n} x_i \sum_{i=1}^{n} y_i \right\}/n}{(n-1) s_x s_y} \cdot \left\{ \frac{s_y}{s_y} \right\} \left\{ \frac{s_x}{s_x} \right\}$$

$$= \frac{\sum_{i=1}^{n} x_i y_i - \left\{ \sum_{i=1}^{n} x_i \sum_{i=1}^{n} y_i \right\}/n}{(n-1) s_x^2} \cdot \left\{ \frac{s_x}{s_y} \right\}$$

$$= b_{y \cdot x} \left\{ \frac{s_x}{s_y} \right\}$$

or

$$b_{y \cdot x} = r_{x \cdot y} \left\{ \frac{s_y}{s_x} \right\}$$

The preceding equations show that $r_{x \cdot y}$ is a function of $b_{y \cdot x}$, the estimated slope, but that it is adjusted to account for the different units of measurement of the variables $x$ and $y$. Referring to the above example of height $(x)$ and weight $(y)$, $b_{y \cdot x}$ is measured in pounds per inch, or pounds/inch. Multiplication of $b_{y \cdot x}$ by $s_x/s_y$ is multiplication by inches/pounds, and the result is that $r_{x \cdot y}$ has no units. It is also apparent from the last previous equation that in situations where $b_{y \cdot x}$ is close to 0, which we would expect when there is no relationship between the variables, that $r_{x \cdot y}$ will also be close to 0, and that the larger $b_{y \cdot x}$ is, the larger $r_{x \cdot y}$ will tend to be.

The sample correlation coefficient, $r_{x \cdot y}$, turns out to be scaled in such a way that it always lies between $-1$ and $+1$. A correlation of $+1$ represents a perfect positive correlation between $x$ and $y$, whereas a correlation of $-1$ represents a perfect negative correlation between $x$ and $y$. Either of these cases corresponds to a regression analysis in which all the points lie on a straight line, so that there is no error in the prediction (no deviations from regression). This situation obviously happens infrequently, if ever, when real data are examined.

A value of $r_{x \cdot y}$ equal to 0 indicates no relationship between $x$ and $y$ and corresponds to $b_{y \cdot x}$ equal to 0, or zero slope for the estimated regression line. This situation thus represents the case where there is no predictability of $y$ given $x$. The case of $r_{x \cdot y}$ equal exactly to 0 happens infrequently in reality because there is normal random variation in the values of each variable, even when the variables are not associated with each other. The usual situation is that $r_{x \cdot y}$ is nonzero and lies somewhere between $-1$ and $+1$, and it is the task of correlation analysis to determine whether $r_{x \cdot y}$ is far enough from 0 to indicate an association between the variables $x$ and $y$.

The fact that $r_{x \cdot y}$ has no units is very useful when relationships between several variables are being considered simultaneously. The correlation between height and weight, for example, can be compared with the correlation between age and blood pressure, in terms of relative size. The two corresponding regression coefficients cannot be directly compared since their magnitudes are not adjusted to account for difference in units of measurement for these variables.

Research articles sometimes contain a large number of sample correlation coefficients presented in a form that is referred to as a *correlation matrix*. A correlation matrix is just an array of correlation coefficients computed on different pairs of variables measured on one sample. Consider the following example:

|  | Serum Cholesterol | Weight | Systolic BP | Age | Height |
|---|---|---|---|---|---|
| Serum cholesterol | 1.000 | .382 | .675 | .311 | .265 |
| Weight |  | 1.000 | .904 | .207 | .369 |
| Systolic blood pressure |  |  | 1.000 | .437 | .324 |
| Age |  |  |  | 1.000 | .105 |
| Height |  |  |  |  | 1.000 |

According to this matrix, the correlation between serum cholesterol and weight is .382, between age and height is .105, and so forth. The highest correlation among these variables is between weight and systolic blood pressure (.904), and the lowest is between age and height (.105). These comparisons give an idea of which of these variables are most closely related or correlated. A table of regression coefficients for these variables would not yield such comparisons, since the actual values of the regression coefficients would vary in each case depending on the units of measurement of the two variables involved.

The mathematical theory behind the development of the statistical test for the significance of a correlation coefficient includes the assumption that the two variables to be correlated are metric in nature and have a linear relationship. Other correlation coefficients, such as rank correlation coefficients, point biserial correlation coefficients, and so on, have been developed for cases where the variables are not metric; for instance, they might be ranks, or ordinal, or dichotomous. As long as the sample size is not too small, the tests for these alternative coefficients, which are really just product moment correlation coefficients calculated on nonmetric data, give essentially the same results in terms of hypothesis testing as if these coefficients were treated as product moment correlations. The nature of these variables may be such that the linear model cannot hold precisely, which means that the sample correlation coefficient cannot be as high as +1 or as low as −1. In testing for significance of such coefficients, however, one can treat them with the same procedure described in the next section for product moment correlations (for sample sizes ≥ 30). Cohen and Cohen[8] discuss these issues in some detail.

## TESTING A CORRELATION HYPOTHESIS

Suppose that a researcher wants to study the relationship between education and health-seeking behavior, to test the idea that people in higher socioeconomic levels tend to obtain more health care than others. He or she collects data on number of physician visits during a given year and number of years of education for a sample of 50 adults. The sample correlation coefficient $r_{x \cdot y}$ is computed to provide an estimate of the strength of the relationship between the two variables. A statistical test is then required to determine whether the correlation is significant, that is, whether education can be used to predict number of physician visits with success better than expected by chance.

The null hypothesis $H: \rho = 0$ is formed to test significance of the correlation coefficient. Here, $\rho$ represents the correlation coefficient in the population from which the sample was taken. If the variables are not related, $r_{x \cdot y}$ will generally differ slightly from 0 because of sampling error but will tend to be close to 0. The test is designed so that a large departure of $r_{x \cdot y}$ from 0 will result in rejection of $H: \rho = 0$. Suppose, for example, that a sample correlation coefficient of .40 is obtained. A correlation of .40 is greater than 0 but not equal to a perfect correlation of +1. The fact that .40 is positive indicates that the relationship between the two variables, if it is real, is a positive or direct one. In other words, the more education people have, the more physician visits they are likely to report. Use of the proper statistical test will determine whether the value of .40 most likely represents a deviation from 0 that is due to a nonzero value of $\rho$ or a deviation that is due to sampling error.

Recall that to test a hypothesis about a population value, we must know the nature of the sampling distribution of the sample estimate of the unknown population value. If we consider all possible random samples of size 50 on two variables from a population where the correlation between those two variables is equal to 0, it turns out that $r_{x \cdot y}$, the sample correlation coefficient, has a distribution such that

$$t = \frac{r_{x \cdot y} \sqrt{n - 2}}{\sqrt{1 - r_{x \cdot y}^2}}, \text{DF} = n - 2$$

where DF = degrees of freedom, is the appropriate test statistic. This $t$ is distributed according to the $t$ distribution, with $n - 2$ degrees of freedom, when the null hypothesis is true. In our sample, since $r_{x \cdot y} = .40$ and $n = 50$,

$$t = \frac{.40 \sqrt{50 - 2}}{\sqrt{1 - (.40)^2}}$$

$$= 3.02$$

Critical values for rejection of $H: \rho = 0$, obtained from Table B in the Appendix (using 40 degrees of freedom, since the values for 48 degrees of

Correlation and Partial Correlation

freedom are not given), are shown in Figure 6-1. The value of $t = 3.02$ computed for this sample is outside the value of 2.704 required for rejection of $H: \rho = 0$ at the .01 level of significance. Thus the null hypothesis is rejected, with $p < .01$. We can conclude that there is a significant relationship between number of years in school and number of physician visits.

The effects on the test statistic $t$ of changes in $r_{x \cdot y}$ and $n$ can be seen by inspection of the formula for calculation of the $t$ value. The larger $r_{x \cdot y}$ is, the larger $t$ is likely to be. The larger $n$ is, the larger $t$ is likely to be. It is apparent that a large sample size can offset a fairly small correlation coefficient enough to make the $t$ value significant. Thus a correlation coefficient must be interpreted in relation to the size of the sample from which it was computed. A very high correlation coefficient may be statistically meaningless if obtained from a very small sample. This issue of the effect of sample size on power of a statistical test is discussed further in Chapter 14.

Consider a sample correlation of size .40. This correlation may be significant or not, depending on the size of the sample from which it was obtained. The following figures show, for several different sample sizes, the degrees of freedom, required $t$ value at the .05 level, and the test statistic that would result from data with a sample correlation coefficient of .40:

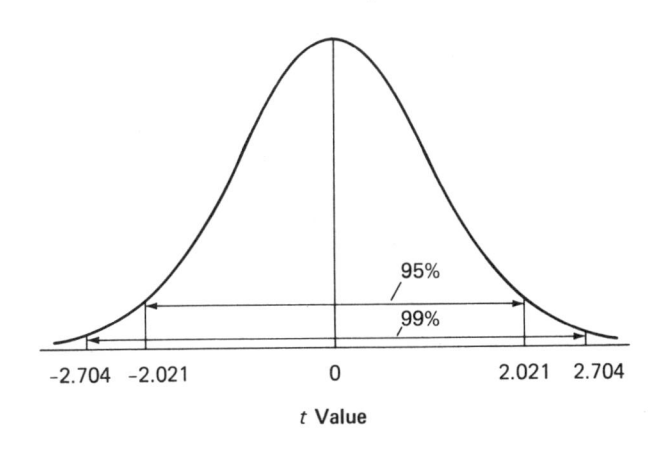

**Figure 6-1.** Cutoff points for 95% and 99% of the $t$ distribution with 40 degrees of freedom.

| Sample Size | Degrees of Freedom | Required $t$ (.05 Level) | Calcualted $t$ |
|---|---|---|---|
| 10 | 8 | 2.31 | 1.23 |
| 20 | 18 | 2.10 | 1.85 |
| 30 | 28 | 2.05 | 2.32* |
| 40 | 38 | 2.02 | 2.69* |
| 50 | 48 | 2.01 | 3.02* |

*$p < .05$.

In other words, for a correlation of .40 to be significant at the .05 level, the minimum sample size must be somewhere between 20 and 30.

The correlation coefficient is only the regression coefficient in standardized form. This means that a hypothesis test of $H: \rho = 0$ must be equivalent to the regression hypothesis test of $H: \beta = 0$. The $t$ test we have just described can, in fact, be shown to be algebraically the equivalent to the $t$ test used for $H: \beta = 0$ in Chapter 5. The problem to determine whether number of physician visits correlates with education could be redone as a regression problem, using education as the independent variable $x$ and number of physician visits as the dependent variable $y$. Exactly the same results as far as statistical significance would be obtained, since the resulting $t$ test statistic would be the same.

You may find that your own statistics book has a table of correlation coefficients that tells you the minimal value of the correlation required for different levels of significance and for different sample sizes. Each of the correlations given in the table is the correlation coefficient that, when substituted along with the corresponding sample size into the formula for the $t$ statistic, would produce the value of $t$ required for significance at the given level. If your sample correlation coefficient exceeds the tabled one, you know authomatically that if you calculated the $t$ statistic, it would be larger than the critical $t$ value from the table, and thus you can reject without calculating the test statistic. If your sample correlation coefficient is lower than the tabled one, you can retain $H: \rho = 0$ without going through the calculations. Either a table for the $t$ distribution or a direct table of correlation coefficients can be used to test $H: \rho = 0$, with equivalent results.

Occasionally, you may want to make a hypothesis test of the form $H: \rho = \rho_0$, where $\rho_0$ is some constant value other than zero. If you know that the correlation between two variables is generally .60, for example, you might want to test a sample correlation from a specific population to determine whether it differs from .60. In such a case, $r_{x \cdot y}$ is distributed in such a way that the test statistic given above is invalid; that is, it does not have a $t$ distribution. A test of the form $H: \rho = \rho_0$ ($\rho_0 \neq 0$) requires the

# Correlation and Partial Correlation

use of what is called *Fisher's z transformation*, in which a normally distributed test statistic is obtained. Refer to a statistics book such as Snedecor and Cochran[41] or Cohen and Cohen[8] for a discussion of this procedure.

Fisher's $z'$ transformation is also used to calculate confidence limits for a sample correlation coefficient. The $z'$ transformation is given by the formula

$$z' = \frac{1}{2}[\ln(1+r) - \ln(1-r)]$$

where ln is the natural logarithm and $r$ is the sample correlation coefficient. An $r$ to $z'$ table may be available that lists the corresponding value of $z'$ for each $r$, or you can use the above formula to calculate the value. The $z'$ score has a normal distribution with standard error

$$S_{z'} = \frac{1}{\sqrt{n-3}}$$

where $n$ is the sample size. For example, therefore,

$$z' \pm z_{.05}\left(\frac{1}{\sqrt{n-3}}\right)$$

are the 95% confidence limits for $z'$. Conversion of these confidence limits for $z'$ back to $r$ gives the 95% confidence limits for $r$.

## PROPORTION OF VARIANCE EXPLAINED

In a correlation or regression problem, $r^2_{x \cdot y}$ is sometimes interpreted as the "proportion of variance" of $y$ explained by $x$. This is commonly done for multiple regression (introduced in Chapter 7) but is discussed here because the idea can be most simply explained when only 2 variables are used. The mathematical relationship between $s^2_{y \cdot x}$, the mean-squared deviation from regression, and $r^2_{x \cdot y}$ is

$$s^2_{y \cdot x} = s^2_y(1 - r^2_{x \cdot y})$$

This formula can be algebraically transformed to

$$\frac{s^2_{y \cdot x}}{s^2_y} = 1 - r^2_{x \cdot y}$$

or

$$r_{x\cdot y}^2 = 1 - \frac{s_{y\cdot x}^2}{s_y^2}$$

Now $s_y^2$ is just the sample variance of the variable $y$, or the total amount of variation in $y$, and $s_{y\cdot x}^2$ represents variance of $y$ observations from values predicted by the regression equation. Therefore,

$$\frac{s_{y\cdot x}^2}{s_y^2}$$

is the proportion of the total variance of $y$ that is *not* explained by the regression. This means that

$$1 - \frac{s_{y\cdot x}^2}{s_y^2}$$

or $r_{x\cdot y}^2$ is the proportion of the variance of $y$ that *is* explained by the regression.

For example, consider a regression calculated to predict weight from height. Suppose that the correlation coefficient between height and weight turns out to be $r_{x\cdot y}^2 = .70$. This indicates that $(.70)^2 = 49\%$ of the variation in weight is explained by variation in height. Or 51% of the variation in weight is due to factors other than height. This concept will become clearer when we discuss multiple regression (in Chapter 7), in which several predictor variables are added to the regression equation to increase the proportion of variance explained. Before discussing the statistical procedure of partial correlation, we digress here briefly to make a distinction between association between variables and causal relationships between variables. This distinction will help to clarify the use of partial correlation in certain research situations.

## ASSOCIATION VERSUS CAUSATION

In our discussion of correlation, we have described a procedure for testing the statistical significance of the relationship between two variables. We have said that rejection of the null hypothesis $H: \rho = 0$ corresponds to rejection of the null hypothesis $H: \beta = 0$ in regression analysis and indicates predictability better than chance for one variable, given the value of the other variable. In the last section we described $r_{x\cdot y}^2$ as an indicator of the proportion of variance of the variable $y$ "explained by" the variable $x$. The words used to describe correlation and regression analyses suggest causal relationships between the variables studied. A note of caution should be interjected here, because a statistically significant relationship between two variables, demonstrated by using correlation or regression analysis, does not necessarily indicate a causal relationship.

If an event $x$ causes an event $y$ to happen, the variables $x$ and $y$ will be related statistically. For example, an excess of caloric intake causes obesity (an unfortunate, but truly causal relationship). If we measured average excess intake of calories and weight gain over a year for a sample of adults, the two variables would be significantly related, according to the statistical analysis. A regression equation could be calculated, and the slope would be significantly different from zero. Equivalently, the correlation would be significant. It is not true, however, that a statistically significant relationship between two variables proves causation. Demonstration of a causal relationship between two variables requires other evidence in addition to a statistical relationship between the variables. Refer to a text on research design, such as that by Smith[39], for a discussion of how causal relationships are established.

Most pertinent to our discussion is the requirement that one must be able to rule out alternative (noncausal) explanations for the relationship between the variables to establish a causal relationship. In other words, one must be able to show that the relationship is nonspurious, that is, not due to some other uncontrolled factor or variable. A common procedure for eliminating spurious factors in a research study is the randomization of subjects into groups. In a well-controlled, randomized study, it may be reasonable to conclude that a difference between a control group and an experimental group at the end of the study is due to, or caused by, the experimental treatment.

In most nonrandomized studies, causation is very difficult to establish because it is difficult to rule out alternative explanations of why variables are related and because there are often multiple causes for the dependent variables. In such studies, however, claims for causal relationships are often made without considering alternative explanations for relationships between variables. This is a common occurrence in studies where data on several variables have been collected for a large number of individuals and analyzed by use of regression or correlation techniques. When you are evaluating such studies or using such techniques for your own research, you should keep in mind that statistical association between variables does not in itself demonstrate causation.

In situations where the possible influences of many variables on the relationship under consideration have not been controlled by the study design, it is sometimes possible to use analytic procedures to statistically remove the effect of some variables. If a statistically significant relationship between two variables has been demonstrated and you suspect that the relationship is a causal one, you can strengthen the evidence of causality if you can show that the relationship is not due to the influence of other, extraneous variables. If data are available on such variables, they can be incorporated into the analysis in such a way that their effect on the causal relationship can be controlled or accounted for. If the statistical relationship between the study variables persists after extraneous factors are controlled, the evidence for causality is increased. Partial correlation, the subject of the final section of this chapter, is one statistical procedure that can be used to control for the effects of such extraneous variables.

## PARTIAL CORRELATION

In much research, data are collected on a large number of variables on subjects who are not under the manipulative control of the investigator. For example, in a study of previous hospitalization experiences and anxiety among surgical patients, a researcher might find a negative relationship between the number of previous hospitalizations and anxiety on admission. The researcher would like to conclude that previous experience with hospitals makes patients more familiar with what to expect and thus less anxious than patients without such previous experience, that is, a causal relationship. However, if patients with a large number of previous hospitalizations tend to be older than those with few previous hospitalizations and also tend to be less anxious because of their age, the apparent relationship between number of previous hospitalizations and anxiety would be a spurious one, a function of age rather than a causal relationship. In a situation where it is not possible to control extraneous variables by the research design, it is sometimes possible to exert some kind of statistical control over such variables. One way of doing this is through the use of a procedure called *partial correlation*.

"Partial correlation" refers to the correlation between two variables with a third variable controlled. Consider the study described previously, where data have been obtained for a sample of surgical patients on the following variables:

$x_1$ = age
$x_2$ = number of previous hospitalizations
$x_3$ = admission anxiety score

Suppose that a researcher is interested in the relationship between number of previous hospitalizations and admission anxiety and has found

# Correlation and Partial Correlation

a negative correlation between these two variables. The researcher then theorizes that admission anxiety can be decreased by previous hospitalization experience, that is, that there is a causal relationship. But the patients in the study are of different ages. It may be that older people have more previous hospitalizations and are also generally less anxious than younger people, so that the number of previous hospitalizations and anxiety appear to be correlated because both are affected by age.

In order to eliminate or "control for" the effect of age, it would be possible to compute the correlation between number of previous hospitalizations and admission anxiety for patients at each specific age. If age were not the cause of an apparent relationship between these two variables, these correlations would be negative and significant, like the original correlation between the two variables with age ignored. An alternative way of combining all the data to obtain a measure of the relationship between number of previous hospitalizations and admission anxiety with the effect of age controlled is to use what is known as *partial correlation*. Partial correlation is actually obtained by a series of regression analyses, as you will see by the following example.

The study described above would result in three measures for each patient, as described by the following notation:

| Age ($x_1$) | Number of Previous Hospitalizations ($x_2$) | Admission Anxiety Score ($x_3$) |
|---|---|---|
| $x_{11}$ | $x_{21}$ | $x_{31}$ |
| $x_{12}$ | $x_{22}$ | $x_{32}$ |
| $x_{13}$ | $x_{23}$ | . |
| . | . | . |
| . | . | . |
| . | . | . |
| $x_{1n}$ | $x_{2n}$ | $x_{3n}$ |

For each symbol, the first subscript represents the variable and the second subscript stands for the individual. For example, $x_{11}$ is the age of the first patient, $x_{1n}$ is the age of the $n$th patient, $x_{23}$ is the number of previous hospitalizations of the third patient, $x_{33}$ is the admission anxiety score of the third patient, and so on.

An ordinary correlation coefficient between number of previous hospitalizations and admission anxiety would measure the relationship between these two variables without taking the effect of age into account. The calculation and testing of $r_{x \cdot y}$ would be as described in this chapter, with the age values, $x_{11}, x_{12}, \ldots, x_{1n}$, ignored. To control for the effect of age, we would like measures of numbers of previous hospitalizations and admission anxiety from which the effects of age have been removed. This is accomplished by two regression analyses, using age as the independent or predictor variable in each case.

First, the least-squares criterion is used to compute a regression line for predicting number of previous hospitalizations from age. The resulting prediction equation can be written

$$x'_2 = a_2 + b_2 x_1$$

For any specific patient, say, patient $i$, $x'_{2i}$ is the number of previous hospitalizations of the patient, as predicted by that patient's age, $x_{1i}$. Since the actual number of previous hospitalizations of the patient is $x_{2i}$, the quantity

$$(x_{2i} - x'_{2i})$$

represents the deviation of the patient's observed number of previous hospitalizations from the number predicted on the basis of age. This deviation is the residual, or the part that is *not* related to age. Similarly, a second regression of admission anxiety on age yields the prediction equation

$$x'_3 = a_3 + b_3 x_1$$

Again, for patient $i$, $x'_{3i}$ is the admission anxiety predicted by that patient's age, $x_{1i}$. The deviation of the actual admission anxiety, $x_{3i}$, from the value predicted by age, $x'_{3i}$, is written as

$$(x_{3i} - x'_{3i})$$

This deviation represents the residual, or the part that is not related to age, that is, with the effect of age removed.

The partial correlation of number of previous hospitalizations with admission anxiety is the correlation coefficient between the two residuals just described: $(x_{2i} - x'_{2i})$ and $(x_{3i} - x'_{3i})$. This correlation measures the association between the number of previous hospitalizations and admission anxiety with the effect of age removed and is represented symbolically as:

$$r_{x_2 x_3 \cdot x_1}$$

It is not necessary to go through the two regression analyses shown earlier, in order to calculate a partial correlation coefficient, because a

# Correlation and Partial Correlation

formula is available by which $r_{x_2x_3 \cdot x_1}$ can be calculated directly from correlations between each pair of the three variables involved. This formula is

$$r_{x_2x_3 \cdot x_1} = \frac{r_{x_2x_3} - r_{x_2x_1}r_{x_3x_1}}{\sqrt{(1 - r^2_{x_2x_1})(1 - r^2_{x_3x_1})}}$$

Here, $r_{x_2x_3}$ is just the correlation between the number of previous hospitalizations and admission anxiety, $r_{x_2x_1}$ is the correlation between age and number of previous hospitalizations, and so forth. These correlations between two variables, with no third variable considered, are sometimes referred to as *zero-order* correlations. A partial correlation between two variables with a third controlled may be referred to as a *first-order* correlation.

The significance of a partial correlation coefficient is tested by the formula

$$t = \frac{r_{x_2x_3 \cdot x_1}\sqrt{n - 3}}{\sqrt{1 - r^2_{x_2x_3 \cdot x_1}}}, \qquad DF = n - 3$$

Notice that this formula is the same as that used to test a zero-order correlation, except that it has $n - 3$ degrees of freedom instead of $n - 2$ degrees of freedom. The null hypothesis tested by this $t$ test is $H: \rho_{x_2x_3 \cdot x_1} = 0$, that is, there is no correlation between the variables $x_2$ and $x_3$ with the effects of $x_1$ controlled.

The effect of controlling for the third variable can be understood by comparing the test results for the first-order partial correlation with the test results for the zero-order correlation. For the example given, suppose that the zero-order correlation between number of previous hospitalizations and admission anxiety is negative and significant, indicating that one decreases as the other increases, ignoring the effect of age on this relationship. Suppose that the partial correlation with age controlled or "partialled out" is not significantly different from zero. Such a result indicates that the apparent relationship indicated by the zero-order correlation is only a reflection of the fact that both of these variables are correlated with age. Suppose, on the other hand, that the partial correlation is negative and significant. This indicates that the relationship is either a causal one or is due to some variables other than age; the relationship between the two variables has not been explained by age. Often the partial correlation is lower than the zero-order correlation but still significant. This indicates that part of the relationship is due to the third variable, but that there is still a relationship that has not been completely explained away by the third variable.

The idea of partial correlation can be extended to allow for control of more than one variable. A second-order partial correlation between two variables is one in which two other variables are controlled. This can be written

$$r_{x_3x_4 \cdot x_1x_2}$$

that is, the partial correlation between variables $x_3$ and $x_4$ with the effects of variables $x_1$ and $x_2$ removed. The same $t$ test is used as for zero-order and first-order correlations, substituting the second-order partial correlation in the formula and using $n - 4$ degrees of freedom. The formula is

$$t = \frac{r_{x_3x_4 \cdot x_1x_2} \sqrt{n-4}}{\sqrt{1 - r^2_{x_3x_4 \cdot x_1x_2}}}, \quad DF = n - 4$$

The null hypothesis is

$$H: \rho_{x_3x_4 \cdot x_1x_2} = 0$$

and rejection of the null hypothesis indicates that the relationship between $x_3$ and $x_4$ is not explained by $x_1$ or $x_2$. The method can be extended indefinitely. However, a degree of freedom is lost each time a new control variable is added. If the data come from a relatively small sample, one can quickly reduce the degrees of freedom to such an extent that the critical $t$ value becomes excessively large.

Partial correlation is a powerful analytic technique that is very useful in nonexperimental studies where there are many extraneous variables present that might be responsible for the relationship of real interest to the researcher. In such studies, although it may not be possible to actually demonstrate a causal relationship, it may be possible through partial correlation to greatly reduce the number of competing explanations for relationships between variables. Partial correlation also forms the basis for the common procedure of stepwise multiple regression, to be described in Chapter 7.

## PROBLEMS

1. In Problem 5 in Chapter 5, results of several regression analyses are given. Table 5-2, which shows the regression equations, includes correlation coefficients for each of the pairs of variables for which regression analysis was done.

(a) Write the dependent variables in order from the one with the strongest correlation with its PACE subscale (overall average, $r_{x \cdot y} = .641$) to the one with the weakest correlation with its PACE subscale (first aid, $r_{x \cdot y} = .420$).

(b) Write the dependent variables in order from the one with the highest regression coefficient (body structure and function, $b_{y \cdot x} = .63$) to the one with the lowest regression coefficient (personal and community health, $b_{y \cdot x} = .22$).

(c) Compare the lists from a and b, explaining why they differ and which is more indicative of relative strength of the various relationships. Pay particular attention to the difference in position on the two lists of the overall average.

2. In Problem 9 in Chapter 5, age and resting systolic blood pressure data were listed for 16 type A subjects and 17 type B subjects.

(a) Calculate the sample variance of age, $s_x^2$, for the type A subjects (or refer to your calculations for Problem 9, Chapter 5, question f).

(b) Calculate the sample variance of resting systolic blood pressure, $s_y^2$, for the type A subjects.

(c) Use your calculations from a and b to determine the correlation coefficient between age and resting systolic blood pressure for type A subjects, according to the formula

$$r_{x \cdot y} = \frac{\sum_{i=1}^{n} x_i y_i - \left\{ \sum_{i=1}^{n} x_i \sum_{i=1}^{n} y_i \right\}/n}{(n-1) s_x s_y}$$

(d) Use the value for $b_{y \cdot x}$ calculated in Problem 9, Chapter 5, question c, along with your values for $s_x$ and $s_y$ to calculate $r_{x \cdot y}$ by the alternative formula

$$r_{x \cdot y} = b_{y \cdot x} \left\{ \frac{s_x}{s_y} \right\}$$

(e) State the null hypothesis that can be tested using this correlation coefficient.

(f) Test the null hypothesis stated in e, using a $t$ test at the .01 level of significance.

(g) Compare the results of this hypothesis test with the results obtained in Problem 9, Chapter 5, question h. Explain the correspondence.

(h) Repeat a through g for the data for the type B subjects.

3. Hegedus[18] conducted an investigation designed to examine the empirical basis for the belief that a written nursing care plan is necessary for the delivery of good nursing care. Using a sample of 80 patients with diagnosed myocardial infarction, she gathered data on characteristics of patients and their nurses, measures of how adequately each patient's nursing care plan was done, and several patient outcome measures. Patient characteristics included age, level of education, sex (1 = male, 2 = female), and coronary prognostic index (a lower score indicates better prognosis than higher score). Nurse characteristics included age, length of experience in nursing, and length of experience in primary care nursing. Each nursing care plan was scored on assessment, statement of nursing diagnoses, and evidence of documentation of nursing activities. The patient outcome variables were length of stay, psychological state, health knowledge, and incidence of complications and temperature elevation. The nursing care plan variables were scored so that a high score represents a more complete care plan than a low score. For patient outcome variables, high scores indicated greater length of stay, better psychological state, more health knowledge, greater incidence of complications, and more days of elevated temperature than low scores. Table 6-1 indicates the correlations between the patient outcome measures and all the other study variables.

(a) What null hypothesis can be tested by using the correlation coefficient −.21 between patient's age and psychological state?
(b) Calculate the $t$-test statistic for testing the null hypothesis stated in a.
(c) Should the null hypothesis stated in a be accepted or rejected? Why? Consider both the .05 and .10 levels of significance.
(d) State your conclusion about how the patient's age and psychological state are related, based on your answers to a, b, and c.
(e) For practice, answer questions a through d for the other correlation coefficients shown in Table 6-1.
(f) Which patient outcome variables are associated with nursing care plan assessment, and how, according to the data?
(g) Which patient outcome variables are associated with nursing care plan diagnosis, and how, according to the data?
(h) Which patient outcome variables are associated with nursing care plan documentation, and how, according to the data?
(i) Explain why partial correlation would be useful for further investigation of the relationships between nursing care plan variables and patient outcomes.

4. In a study of the association between selected patient characteristics and psychosocial stress experiences during hospitalization, Volicer

**Table 6-1.** Correlations Between Patient Characteristics, Nurse Characteristics, Nursing Care Plan Variables, and Patient Outcome Variables ($N = 80$)

| Independent and Extraneous Variables | Temperature | Length of Stay | Complications | Psychological State | Health Knowledge |
|---|---|---|---|---|---|
| **Patient Characteristics** | | | | | |
| Age | .27 | .20 | .04 | −.21 | −.12 |
| Education | −.16 | −.08 | −.05 | .19 | .23 |
| Coronary prognostic index (CPI) | .37 | .22 | −.04 | −.20 | −.10 |
| Sex (1 = male, 2 = female) | .22 | .02 | .25 | −.13 | .09 |
| **Nurse Characteristics** | | | | | |
| Age | .24 | .04 | .16 | −.24 | −.11 |
| Years as a nurse | .15 | .02 | .07 | −.13 | −.04 |
| Years in primary nursing | .16 | .18 | .15 | .01 | .01 |
| **Nursing Care Plan Variables** | | | | | |
| Assessment | .27 | −.09 | .01 | .22 | .26 |
| Diagnosis | .04 | −.21 | .03 | .05 | .07 |
| Documentation | −.16 | −.00 | −.21 | −.10 | .13 |

and Burns[44] interviewed 252 patients on two medical wards of a community hospital. Patients were interviewed to obtain data on four types of variables that might affect hospital stress, as follows:

1. Demographic (age, sex, marital status, education)
2. Prior hospitalization experience (number of years since last hospitalization, number of previous hospitalizations)
3. Life stress prior to hospitalization (during the year prior to hospitalization)
4. Present illness (seriousness of illness, reported pain)

Each patient also received a score on a hospital stress rating scale, as an indicator of stress during hospitalization. A correlation matrix for the study variables is given in Table 6-2.

(a) What null hypothesis can be tested using the correlation coefficient $-.27$ between age and life stress during the year prior to hospitalization (state in your own words)?

(b) Calculate the $t$-test statistic for testing the null hypothesis stated in a.

(c) Should the null hypothesis stated in a be accepted or rejected? Why?

(d) What conclusion can you make on the basis of your answer to c?

(e) For practice, answer questions a through d with reference to other correlation coefficients shown in Table 6-2.

(f) According to the data, what independent variables used in this study are significantly correlated with scores on the hospital stress rating scale? Describe the nature of each significant correlation in your own words.

(g) What proportion of variance in the hospital stress rating scores is explained by life stress during the year prior to hospitalization? For practice, answer this question for other independent variables as they relate to hospital stress scores.

(h) Calculate the partial correlation coefficient between number of previous hospitalizations and hospital stress, controlling for years since last hospitalization.

(i) Test the partial correlation coefficient calculated in h for significance.

(j) Discuss the partial correlation results, comparing the partial correlation calculated in h with the zero-order correlation between number of previous hospitalizations and hospital stress.

5. Denton and Wisenbaker[10] conducted a study to investigate the common assumption in educational programs that the more experience nursing students have with death and dying, the less anxiety about death they are likely to have. Death anxiety was measured by a scale ranging from 0 to 15, with 0 indicating the least anxiety and 15 indicating the greatest anxiety. Three measures of death experience were obtained for 76 nurses and nursing students, as follows:

1. DE1—death of a close friend or relative (1 = yes, within past year, 0 = other responses)
2. DE2—having seen a violent death (1 = yes, 0 = no)

**Table 6-2.** Correlation Matrix for Patient Demographic Characteristics, Prior Hospitalization Variables, Life Stress Variables, Present Illness Variables, and Hospital Stress Scores ($N = 252$)

| | AGE | SEX | MAR | ED | LAST | NO | YR1 | YR2 | SIS | PAIN | HSRS |
|---|---|---|---|---|---|---|---|---|---|---|---|
| Demographic Characteristics | | | | | | | | | | | |
| Age (AGE) | 1.00 | −.14 | .12 | −.24 | −.06 | .11 | −.27 | −.08 | .28 | −.21 | −.17 |
| Sex (SEX) | | 1.00 | −.26 | .12 | .03 | −.17 | −.01 | −.03 | .02 | −.08 | .06 |
| Marital status (MAR) | | | 1.00 | −.12 | .03 | −.07 | .00 | .02 | .01 | −.01 | .00 |
| Education (ED) | | | | 1.00 | .04 | −.01 | .11 | −.09 | .06 | −.07 | .02 |
| Prior Hospitalization Variables | | | | | | | | | | | |
| Years since last hospitalization (LAST) | | | | | 1.00 | −.38 | −.14 | −.10 | −.06 | −.14 | −.17 |
| Number of prior hospitalizations (NO) | | | | | | 1.00 | .14 | .03 | .00 | .16 | .13 |

Table 6-2. Continued

|  | AGE | SEX | MAR | ED | LAST | NO | YR1 | YR2 | SIS | PAIN | HSRS |
|---|---|---|---|---|---|---|---|---|---|---|---|
| Life Stress |  |  |  |  |  |  |  |  |  |  |  |
| Past year (YR1) |  |  |  |  |  |  | 1.00 | .07 | −.10 | .19 | .20 |
| 1–2 years ago (YR2) |  |  |  |  |  |  |  | 1.00 | −.18 | .11 | .20 |
| Present Illness Variables |  |  |  |  |  |  |  |  |  |  |  |
| Seriousness (SIS) |  |  |  |  |  |  |  |  | 1.00 | −.14 | −.04 |
| Pain (PAIN) |  |  |  |  |  |  |  |  |  | 1.00 | .22 |
| Hospital Stress Score (HSRS) |  |  |  |  |  |  |  |  |  |  | 1.00 |

# Correlation and Partial Correlation

3. DE3—being in a situation where one thinks death is imminent (0 = never, 1 = once, 2 = twice, 3 = three or more times)

Age and work experience (0 = nursing student, 1 = nurse) were also measured, since the researchers felt that these might be potentially confounding variables. The data were analyzed by calculation of a measure called *Yule's Q*. For purposes of this problem, treat the figures as ordinary correlation coefficients. Since the measures are not metric scales, you must refer back to the coding descriptions to interpret the meaning of the direction of each correlation in substantive terms (e.g., the zero-order correlation of $-.39$ between death anxiety and DE2 shown below indicates that those who did see a violent death had lower death anxiety scores than those who did not). Correlation coefficients reported by the investigators are given in Table 6-3.

Assume that, because of some missing data, the number of observations in each case is 56.

(a) Test each of the above correlations for significance, using the .05 level. Remember that the formula for the $t$ test and corresponding degrees of freedom change according to the number of control variables used.

(b) Which of the death experience variables used in this study were found to be correlated with death anxiety, according to the zero-order correlations? State your conclusions about each of these relationships in substantive terms, that is, explain the nature of the relationships.

(c) What is the effect of age on the relationship between death anxiety and each of the death experience variables?

(d) What is the effect of work experience on the relationship between death anxiety and each of the death experience variables?

**Table 6-3.** Zero-, First-, and Second-Order Correlations of Death Experience Variables with Death Anxiety

| Death Experience Variable | Zero-Order Correlations (No Control Variables) | First-Order Correlations, Age Controlled | First-Order Correlations, Work Experience Controlled | Second-Order Correlations (Age and Work Experience Controlled) |
|---|---|---|---|---|
| DE1 | −.14 | −.08 | −.13 | −.02 |
| DE2 | −.39 | −.32 | −.54 | −.57 |
| DE3 | −.42 | −.38 | −.41 | −.27 |

(e) Among the three death experience variables, which is the best predictor of death anxiety, ignoring other variables?
(f) Among the three death experience variables, which is the best predictor of death anxiety, taking the effects of age and work experience into account?
(g) Does the analysis support the assumption that was being tested by the researchers, that is, that the more experience nursing students have with death and dying, the less anxiety about death they are likely to have?

6. Suppose that you have calculated a correlation coefficient of $r_{x \cdot y}$ = .30 for a set of sample observations.

(a) Calculate a $t$ value and test for significance at the .05 level, assuming a sample size of $n = 5$.
(b) Repeat a, assuming a sample size of $n = 10$.
(c) Repeat a, assuming a sample size of $n = 20$.
(d) Repeat a, assuming a sample size of $n = 50$.
(e) Explain differences in results for a through d.

7. Correlation coefficients are often computed to evaluate reliability of measurement tools in a research study. A highly reliable tool or instrument is one in which the same or very nearly the same observations are obtained by different observers using the same methods, or by the same observer at different points in time.

(a) Suggest a situation where correlation might be used to judge reliability.
(b) Explain what variables would be correlated.
(c) Why do you think that researchers expect that such correlations should be very high (e.g., $\geq .80$), that is, generally much higher than correlations required to reach statistical significance? For example, explain why a researcher might be very unhappy with a correlation coefficient of .30 in this situation but might also be perfectly happy with a correlation coefficient of .30 between two study variables.

# Chapter 7

# MULTIPLE REGRESSION

## MULTIVARIATE ANALYSIS

We have already discussed the use of regression analysis to predict the value of one variable from that of another and correlation to describe the strength of a relationship between two variables. Both $t$ Tests and chi-square tests have been described as methods for assessing the relationship between two variables. There are many research situations in which more than two variables are to be analyzed simultaneously; partial correlation, one such procedure, has already been described in the previous chapter. Those statistical techniques that involve the analysis of more than one independent variable or more than one dependent variable or both are referred to as *multivariate analysis* procedures. Occasionally, this term is restricted to cases where there is more than one dependent variable. The broader definition just given will be used in this text. This chapter provides an introduction to multiple regression analysis, the most general and commonly used multivariate analysis procedure.

Multiple regression is an extension of bivariate regression analysis to the case where more than one independent variable is to be considered as a predictor. Instead of one independent variable $x$ predicting the dependent variable $y$, we will now consider two independent predictors simultaneously, $x_1$ and $x_2$ (or $x_1$, $x_2$, $x_3$, and so on if there are more than two predictors). The multiple regression procedure, like the procedure with one predictor already discussed, provides for the estimation of parameters of a regression equation from the sample data, calculation of a prediction equation, and hypothesis tests about relationships among variables.

As an example of the type of problem appropriate for analysis by a multiple regression procedure, consider a study of factors affecting the number of physician visits per year made by individuals in a particular city. There are several independent variables that might affect the dependent variable, the number of times people see their physicians during a year's time. These might include age, number of previous hospitalizations, education, income, and so forth. In an analysis of variables influencing number of physician visits, using the simple regression and correlation procedures presented in earlier chapters, one could determine relationships between age and number of physician visits, between education and number of physician visits, and so forth. Multiple regression analysis allows the researcher to use all the independent variables together as predictors of the dependent variable, rather than considering them one at a time.

In any research study with several independent variables, the investigator usually wants to study relationships among the independent variables themselves, as well as determining how each of them is related to the dependent variable. In examples like the one in the previous paragraph, the independent variables, such as age, education, and income are likely to be intercorrelated. This means that their combined predictive value is usually less than the sum of the predictive value of each, since they don't add independent pieces of information to the prediction of number of physician visits. Multiple regression analysis accounts for these intercorrelations, so that the resulting regression equation does not contain redundant information.

Multiple regression analysis in this example would allow the researcher to determine, through evaluation of how closely the regression equation fits the data points, how well the number of physician visits can be predicted using information about age, number of previous hospitalizations, education, and the other independent variables combined. The general procedure for this sort of analysis is described in the first several sections of this chapter. The analytic technique will be introduced by discussion of situations where two independent variables are to be used as predictors. Extensions to the case of more than two independent variables will subsequently be made.

More common in nursing research than multiple regression analysis, where two or more independent variables are used simultaneously as predictors, is a variation called *multiple stepwise regression analysis*. In nursing and other behavioral research, data are often collected on a large number of variables thought to be related to the dependent variable, and the researcher's intent is to make as good a prediction as possible, using a relatively small number of independent variables. Often many of the variables are intercorrelated, and one can select a small subset from all of the variables which will have predictive power nearly as large as that obtained by the entire set of variables. A stepwise procedure would, for example, allow the investigator to determine how well number of physician visits can be predicted by age, how education increases prediction of

# Multiple Regression

number of physician visits with the effect of age already controlled, how income increases prediction with age and education already controlled, and so on. This is further described in later sections of this chapter.

## DETERMINING A REGRESSION EQUATION

The additive model for multiple regression with two independent variables is written as follows:

$$y = \alpha + \beta_1 x_1 + \beta_2 x_2 + e$$

This equation, which is geometrically the equation for a plane, expresses $y$ as a function of the two variables $x_1$ and $x_2$. The quantity $\beta_1$ is the average increase in $y$ for an increase of 1 unit in $x_1$, with $x_2$ remaining constant, and is called the *partial regression coefficient* of $y$ on $x_1$. And $\beta_2$, similarly, is the partial regression coefficient of $y$ on $x_2$.

The actual values of $\alpha$, $\beta_1$, and $\beta_2$ are, of course, unknown for the population under consideration. Using sample data, however, it is possible to calculate estimates for these parameters. The actual procedure is quite complicated and is not presented here. If a packaged computer program for multiple regression analysis is not readily available, try very hard to locate one. If necessary, refer to Overall and Klett[35] or Kerlinger and Pedhazur[26] for procedures for hand calculations.

The procedure for estimation of the regression equation parameters is based on the method of least squares described in Chapter 5. This means that the sample estimates are calculated in such a way that the sum of the squared differences between each observed and predicted $y$ is minimized. The effect of the least-squares criterion can be stated in another way. The method determines the linear combination of predictors, that is, the regression equation, that will maximize the correlation between the observed and predicted values of the dependent variable.

The sample estimates for $\alpha$, $\beta_1$, and $\beta_2$ are denoted as $a$, $b_1$, and $b_2$. The sample regression equation, therefore, can be written as follows:

$$y' = a + b_1 x_1 + b_2 x_2$$

Substituting values for $x_1$ and $x_2$ for any individual into this equation, one can calculate $y'$, the predicted score on the dependent variable. Correspondence between the predicted and observed scores can then be used to evaluate the relationship between the independent and dependent variables.

The strength of the relationship between the independent and dependent variables in multiple regression is estimated by a sample quantity called the *multiple correlation coefficient,* denoted by a capital $R$. The multiple correlation coefficient is just an ordinary correlation coefficient calculated to show the relationship between two variables. In this case the two "variables" are the observed values of the dependent variable $y_i$ and the values of $y_i'$ predicted by the regression equation. The value of $R$ goes from 0 to 1, since there can be either no prediction or some prediction (a negative $R$ cannot occur). The quantity $R^2$, by extension of the interpretation of $r^2_{x \cdot y}$ given in the previous chapter, is the proportion of variance of $y$ that is explained by all the independent variables included in the regression equation.

A significant departure of $R$ from 0 indicates that the regression equation does have predictive power, and the statistical test for such a departure is described in the next section of this chapter. Note that bivariate regression analysis, as presented in Chapter 5, is really just a special case of multiple regression, in which there is only one predictor variable. The formulas and procedures to be described for testing for significance of prediction in multiple regression are generalizations of those given in Chapter 5, and the basic idea of partitioning total variation into a part due to regression and a part due to deviations from regression is the same as described in that earlier chapter.

## TESTING A MULTIPLE REGRESSION HYPOTHESIS

Consider a study where we wish to determine whether use of marijuana can be predicted from information on alcohol and cigarette use. Since use of marijuana is to be predicted, a variable representing frequency of use of marijuana will be the dependent variable. There will be two independent variables, those representing frequency of alcohol use and frequency of cigarette use. Suppose that we have data on number of times per week marijuana, alcohol, and cigarettes are used for a sample of size $n = 40$. (These data are from an unpublished study done by students in Boston University School of Nursing, Research Methods, Fall 1972.)

The following notation will be used for the variables observed:

$y$ = number of times marijuana is used per week
$x_1$ = number of times alcohol is used per week
$x_2$ = number of times cigarettes are used per week

# Multiple Regression

Computer output provides the following estimates of values needed to write the regression equation:

$$\begin{aligned} a &= -.04894 \sim -.05 \\ b_1 &= .38779 \sim .39 \\ b_2 &= .13276 \sim .13 \\ R &= .46834 \sim .47 \end{aligned}$$

Since the regression equation is of the form

$$y' = a + b_1 x_1 + b_2 x_2$$

we can write

$$y = -.05 + .39 x_1 + .13 x_2$$

According to the equation, use of marijuana increases as use of alcohol increases, since $b_1 = .39$ is positive. Also, use of marijuana increases as use of cigarettes increases, since $b_2 = .13$ is also positive. Predicted values can be calculated as in the following example. Suppose that an individual uses alcohol 3 times per week and cigarettes 8 times per week. Since

$$\begin{aligned} y' &= -.05 + .39(3) + .13(8) \\ &= -.05 + 1.07 + 1.04 \\ &= 2.06 \end{aligned}$$

we would predict that this individual uses marijuana about 2 times per week. By the same procedure, predicted values could be calculated for all the individuals in the sample. The multiple correlation coefficient $R = .47$ given above is the correlation between the predicted number of times marijuana is used per week and the actual number of times reported by the subjects, calculated across all the subjects in the sample.

The test for significance of the multiple correlation coefficient utilizes the null hypothesis

$$H: \rho = 0$$

where $\rho$ (rho) stands for the multiple correlation coefficient in the population. This null hypothesis is equivalent to the hypothesis

$$H: \beta_1 = \beta_2 = 0$$

If the regression equation does not have any predictive value, there will be no correlation between the observed and predicted values. Then $R$, the estimate of $\rho$, will tend to be close to 0, deviating from 0 only because of sampling error. This will indicate that no meaningful values of $\beta_1$ and $\beta_2$ can be found to express the relationship between the independent and dependent variables, or that use of marijuana does not vary as a function of use of alcohol and use of cigarettes. The sample estimates of $b_1 = .39$ and $b_2 = .13$ in the equation given earlier do deviate from 0, suggesting that the equation may indeed have predictive power. A significance test is necessary to determine whether these values are far enough from zero that $H: \beta_1 = \beta_2 = 0$ can be rejected.

The test for significance of $R$ in multiple regression is a generalization of the $F$ test described in Chapter 5. In that chapter, the total sum of squared deviations of $y$ from the mean,

$$\sum_{i=1}^{n} (y_i - \bar{y})^2$$

was partitioned into two parts. These are

$$\sum_{i=1}^{n} (y_i' - \bar{y})^2$$

the regression sum of squares, and

$$\sum_{i=1}^{n} (y_i - y_i')^2$$

the deviations sum of squares. Since multiple regression yields a regression equation and thus predicted values of $y$, the same quantities can be calculated as before; therefore, the same partition of total variation is made.

The difference between multiple regression and regression in the bivariate case is that in multiple regression, the predicted values of $y$ are based on information from two or more independent variables, rather than one. The effect of this is a change in the degrees of freedom associated with each of the two sources of variation used for the analysis. The degrees of freedom for the regression sum of squares (1 in the bivariate case) become equal to the total number of independent variables, which will be denoted by the letter $k$. Since the total degrees of freedom remains $n - 1$, the degrees of freedom for the deviations sum of squares ($n - 2$ in the bivariate case) becomes $n - k - 1$. Obviously, when there is only one

# Multiple Regression

predictor, $k = 1$, and the degrees of freedom revert to 1 and $n - 1 - 1 = n - 2$.

The generalized form of the regression ANOVA table is therefore similar to the bivariate table, but with changes in the degrees of freedom column and thus in the mean-square column, as shown in this example:

### Regression ANOVA

| Source of Variation | Sum of Squares | Degrees of Freedom | Mean Square |
|---|---|---|---|
| Regression | $\sum_{i=1}^{n}(y_i' - \bar{y})^2$ | $k$ | $\sum_{i=1}^{n}(y_i' - \bar{y})^2/k$ |
| Deviation | $\sum_{i=1}^{n}(y_i - y_i')^2$ | $n - k - 1$ | $\sum_{i=1}^{n}(y_i - y_i')^2/(n - k - 1)$ |
| Total | $\sum_{i=1}^{n}(y_i - \bar{y})^2$ | $n - 1$ | $\sum_{i=1}^{n}(y_i - \bar{y})^2/(n - 1)$ |

The quantity

$$\frac{\sum_{i=1}^{n}(y_i' - \bar{y})^2}{k}$$

is called the *mean-square regression*, or $MS_R$, and the quantity

$$\frac{\sum_{i=1}^{n}(y_i - y_i')^2}{(n - k - 1)}$$

is called the *mean-square deviation from regression*, or $MS_D$. The *total mean square*

$$\frac{\sum_{i=1}^{n}(y_i - \bar{y})^2}{(n - 1)}$$

is the ordinary sample variance of the dependent variable $y$ and is the same, of course, as in the bivariate case.

The test statistic, as for the bivariate case, is

$$F = \frac{\text{Mean-square regression}}{\text{Mean-square deviation from regression}}$$

or, in multiple regression,

$$F = \frac{\sum_{i=1}^{n} (y_i' - \bar{y})^2 / k}{\sum_{i=1}^{n} (y_i - y_i')^2 / (n - k - 1)}$$

For this particular $F$ distribution, the numerator degrees of freedom are $k$, and the denominator degrees of freedom are $n - k - 1$. In determining whether the calculated $F$ is large enough to reject the null hypothesis, therefore, one would look in the row and column of the $F$ table that correspond to $k$ and $n - k - 1$ degrees of freedom. It is the number of independent variables in the regression equation *(k)* that determines both the numerator and denominator degrees of freedom. The various $k$ and $n - k - 1$ combinations determine the different $F$ distributions that constitute the "family" of $F$ distributions referred to in Chapter 5.

For the data on use of alcohol, cigarettes, and marijuana, substitution of the actual data yields the following table:

| Source of Variation | Sum of Squares | Degrees of Freedom | Mean Square | F |
|---|---|---|---|---|
| Regression | 7.84690 | 2 | 3.92345 | 5.198 |
| Deviation | 27.92810 | 37 | 0.75481 | |
| Total | | 39 | | |

In this table, the $F$ value has been included in a separate column and has been calculated as

$$F = \frac{\text{Mean-square regression}}{\text{Mean-square deviation from regression}}$$

$$= \frac{\sum_{i=1}^{n} (y_i' - \bar{y})^2 / k}{\sum_{i=1}^{n} (y_i - y_i')^2 / (n - k - 1)}$$

$$= \frac{3.92345}{0.75481}$$

$$= 5.198$$

# Multiple Regression

The $F$ statistic has $k = 2$ and $n - k - 1 = 40 - 2 - 1 = 37$ degrees of freedom, and the $F$ required for significance at the .05 level, with 2 and 37 degrees of freedom, is

$$F_{.05}(2,37) = 3.26$$

Thus the null hypothesis is rejected at the .05 level of significance.

We can conclude from the analysis that significant prediction of use of marijuana is obtained by using the two independent variables of alcohol and cigarette use. Significant prediction in multiple regression, as in bivariate regression, is identified when the calculated $F$-test statistic exceeds the tabled value at the chosen level of significance. The calculation formula for $F$ illustrates the logic behind this procedure for decision making. The numerator of the $F$, the mean-square regression, will tend to be small when there is no predictive power, since in this case the predicted values will lie on a horizontal line at the mean of $y$, and this will tend to make $F$ small. If there is predictive power, the numerator will tend to be larger and thus tend to increase $F$. The denominator of the $F$, the mean-square deviation from regression, will be relatively larger when the observed values are far from the predicted, resulting in a small $F$-test statistic. When the prediction is good, the denominator will be relatively small, reflecting the tendency of observed values to be close to predicted values, and resulting in a large $F$ value.

The proportion of variance explained ($R^2$) can be determined from the regression ANOVA table by the following formula:

$$R^2 = \frac{\text{Regression sum of squares}}{\text{Total sum of squares}}$$
$$= \frac{SS_R}{SS_T}$$

This means that the $F$-test statistic can be calculated directly from $R^2$, without calculating sums of squares. This formula is

$$F = \frac{R^2/k}{(1 - R^2)/(n - k - 1)}$$

In this formula, $R$ is the multiple correlation coefficient, $n$ is the sample size, and $k$ is the number of independent variables. This $F$, of course, has an $F$ distribution with $k$ and $n - k - 1$ degrees of freedom.

The calculation of $F$ by the above formula results in the same $F$-test statistic as that obtained by using the ratio of the mean-square regression to the mean square deviation from regression. Application of the formula to the data on use of marijuana, alcohol, and cigarettes, with the unrounded value of $R = .46834$ used instead of .47 to avoid roundoff error, yields a test statistic of

$$F = \frac{R^2/k}{(1 - R^2)/(n - k - 1)}$$
$$= \frac{(.46834)^2/2}{[1 - (.46834)^2]/37}$$
$$= 5.19$$

This is the same $F$ as the that resulting from the first method of calculation.

The logic of rejecting the null hypothesis $H: \rho = 0$ when the $F$-test statistic is large is even clearer for this formula than for the earlier one from the regression ANOVA table. When there is no predictive power, there will be no correlation between the observed and predicted values, and $R$ will tend to be close to 0, making $F$ small. Deviation of $R$ from 0 results from predictive power and will tend to make $F$ large, by increasing the numerator while simultaneously decreasing the denominator. The effect of sample size is also clear. For either formula for $F$, a large $n$ tends to increase $F$ and thus make it easier to reject the null hypothesis. In Chapter 14 we will return to a discussion of the effect of sample size on test statistics.

The overall $F$ test in multiple regression simply allows the researcher to make an overall statement about prediction. From the example shown earlier, one can conclude that use of marijuana can be predicted significantly by use of alcohol and cigarettes together. No conclusion can be made about the effect of either independent variable alone or how they interrelate in their effect on use of marijuana. Such relationships are often of greater interest to the researcher than the overall effect, and they can be investigated by use of partial correlation or by a stepwise multiple regression procedure such as that described in the following section.

## STEPWISE SELECTION OF VARIABLES

The multiple regression procedure just described can be used to determine whether the regression equation has any predictive power, regardless of the number of independent variables used. Often the investigator does not wish simply to answer this question, but rather to select the best predictors from a large number of independent variables on which data have been obtained. In nursing research, sociological research, research in education, and other related fields, data are often collected in many

# Multiple Regression

variables in an attempt to find important correlates of the particular dependent variable under consideration. Stepwise multiple regression is a procedure by which the predictive value of all of the potential predictor variables can be considered sequentially, and the combination of those providing the best predictive power can be selected. Commonly, three or four of a large number of variables will explain almost as much of the variation in the dependent variables as can be explained by a much larger number of variables.

Several different stepwise multiple regression procedures are possible, and the variety of procedures reported in published studies has increased with the availability of canned statistical programs, which make it possible to enter and delete independent variables in regression equations in virtually any order or manner desired. The most common procedure is called the *forward inclusion solution,* a technique in which the independent variables are entered into the analysis one after the other. Another alternative is referred to as the *backward solution,* in which an equation that includes all the independent variables is first calculated, and then these variables are deleted one at a time. A combination of these procedures, which allows for the later removal of variables that were previously entered, is also possible. Another type of analysis determines a subset of independent variables, among all possible sets, which will result in the greatest degree of explained variance. The forward inclusion procedure is the most commonly used, and therefore is described in this text in detail. See Kerlinger and Pedhazur[26] for discussion and examples of the other procedures.

As an example, consider the study described in Chapter 6, problem 4. The researchers have used responses to a list of questions to score each of several hundred hospital patients on a scale measuring level of hospital stress experienced. They want to determine which of the many characteristics of patients known at the time of admission might be useful in the prediction of level of hospital stress. Variables known for patients in the study include age, education, sex, marital status, number of previous hospitalizations, number of years since last hospitalization, pain, and seriousness of illness. Using stepwise multiple regression, the investigator in such a study can evaluate the contribution of each of these potential predictors to the explanation of variation in hospital stress and determine which ones form a set of independent variables with good predictive power.

Stepwise multiple regression is just one particular form of the multiple regression procedure described in Chapter 6. In discussing multiple regression, we described a procedure for calculating a regression equation using several independent variables simultaneously. We then used an $F$ test to evaluate whether the equation was able to provide significant prediction of the dependent variable, based on the value of the sample multiple correlation coefficient, $R$. The stepwise multiple regression procedure also yields a final regression equation, but the independent variables are entered into the equation one at a time, in a specific order, according to their ability to predict the dependent variable, instead of being entered altogether. The procedure thus consists of a sequence of multiple regressions, and the criteria for which independent variable will be entered at each step will be described in detail by application to the example used earlier for multiple regression.

Respondents in the study on drug use described earlier were asked to estimate the number of times they used alcohol, cigarettes, and marijuana each week. They were also asked about use of aspirin, although this variable was not used in the earlier analysis. As an example of multiple regression, you may recall that we calculated a regression equation with alcohol and cigarette use as predictors of use of marijuana. The $F$ test allowed us to conclude that information on the use of alcohol and use of cigarettes did indeed provide significant prediction of use of marijuana. To consider how the same data could be approached using a stepwise multiple regression procedure, assume that we are interested in obtaining an equation that can provide us with significant prediction of use of marijuana. We are willing to use any of the independent variables but want to eliminate those that do not contribute significantly to the prediction of marijuana use.

The first step of a stepwise multiple regression is to pick from all the independent variables the best single predictor of the dependent variable. This is, by definition, the independent variable that has the highest zero-order correlation with the dependent variable and can be determined by examining the correlation matrix for all the variables. The correlation matrix for the drug study is as follows:

|            | Aspirin | Alcohol | Cigarettes | Marijuana |
|------------|---------|---------|------------|-----------|
| Aspirin    | 1.00    | 0.27    | −0.23      | 0.17      |
| Alcohol    |         | 1.00    | 0.24       | 0.40      |
| Cigarettes |         |         | 1.00       | 0.34      |
| Marijuana  |         |         |            | 1.00      |

Since we are considering use of marijuana as the dependent variable and use of the other drugs as the independent variables, we are interested in how each of the variables (use of aspirin, use of alcohol, and use of cigarettes) correlates with use of marijuana. These correlations appear in the last column of the correlation matrix. The highest correlation is between use of alcohol and use of marijuana, indicating that, among the three independent variables, use of alcohol is the best predictor. A simple regres-

# Multiple Regression

sion for use of marijuana on use of alcohol is calculated, and the results are:

$$n = 40 \qquad R = .39661 \sim .40$$
$$a = .16527 \sim .17 \qquad R^2 = .15730 \sim .16$$
$$b = .45845 \sim .46 \qquad y' = .17 + .46x_1$$

In the prediction equation, $x_1$ now represents the independent or predictor variable, use of alcohol; and $y$ represents the dependent variable, use of marijuana. Since use of alcohol was chosen as the independent variable correlating best with the dependent variable, the value of $R$, the multiple correlation coefficient, is as high as possible. Neither of the other independent variables would give as high a value for $R$; that is, neither would provide as good prediction of use of marijuana. Of course, with only one predictor, $R$ is the same as the correlation between use of alcohol and use of marijuana that appears in the correlation matrix (.40).

The criterion for the second step in stepwise multiple regression is to select, from among the remaining independent variables, the one that will improve the prediction the most, when used simultaneously with the independent variable that has been selected on the first step. Since $R$ is used as the measure of how good the prediction is, this criterion requires that we select as the second predictor the independent variable that will result in the largest increase in $R$ for the prediction equation using both the first and second independent variables, compared to the $R$ obtained with just one predictor. Another way of stating this is to say that we want the increase in $R$, using the two predictors compared with one predictor to be larger than the increase in $R$ that would be obtained by adding any other independent variable as the second predictor.

On first glance, it would seem that one could merely select as the second independent variable that one among the remaining variables that correlates best with the dependent variable. But recall that the zero-order correlations, that is, the correlations between pairs of variables, do not account for relationships with any other variables. In this example, we want to choose a second variable that will increase the explained variance in use of marijuana, given that the variable use of alcohol has already been used. If we choose as a second variable one that happens to correlate highly with use of alcohol as well as use of marijuana, the explained variation will not increase as much as one might suspect by inspection of the zero-order correlation between that second variable and use of marijuana. In a sense, some of the explanatory power of this second variable will have already been accounted for by the inclusion of use of alcohol in the regression equation.

The second variable that will improve prediction the most (increase $R$ or $R^2$ the most) is the one that has the highest correlation with use of marijuana with use of alcohol removed, or controlled. This variable can be identified by considering the partial correlation of each of the remaining independent variables with use of marijuana, controlling for use of alcohol. We look for the variable that will increase predictability most, given the one that has already been used. For these data, the partial correlations of the remaining independent variables with use of marijuana, controlling for use of alcohol, are

$$\begin{array}{ll} \text{Aspirin} & .07 \\ \text{Cigarettes} & .27 \end{array}$$

Examination of these partial correlations indicates that use of cigarettes has the highest partial correlation with use of marijuana, with use of alcohol controlled. The two variables, use of cigarettes and use of alcohol, will thus together provide a better prediction equation for use of marijuana than an equation including the two variables use of aspirin and use of alcohol, as predictor variables. Calculation of a multiple regression for use of marijuana on use of alcohol ($x_1$) and use of cigarettes ($x_2$) gives the following equation:

$$\begin{aligned} y' &= -.05 + .39x_1 + .13x_2 \\ R &= .47 \\ R^2 &= .22 \end{aligned}$$

These values are, of course, exactly the same as those obtained in the section on multiple regression, with use of alcohol and use of cigarettes as predictors, since the second step of the stepwise procedure is just an ordinary multiple regression with two independent variables.

Consider the $R$ value of .47 (or $R^2$ value of .22) shown above. These can be compared with the corresponding values obtained with use of alcohol alone as a predictor, to show the effect of including use of cigarettes as a second predictor. The $R$ for use of alcohol alone was .40 ($R^2 = .16$). The increase in $R$ from .40 to .47 (or the increase in proportion of variance explained from 16% to 22%) represents the effect of including use of cigarettes as a second predictor.

Comparison of the zero-order correlation between use of cigarettes and use of marijuana that appears in the correlation matrix (.34) with the partial correlation controlling for use of alcohol (.27) is also instructive. The decrease in the correlation from .34 to .27 represents the part of the zero-order correlation between use of cigarettes and use of marijuana that

# Multiple Regression

is due to the relationship of both of these variables to the use of alcohol. The difference between the zero-order correlation between use of aspirin and use of marijuana (.17) and the first-order partial correlation, controlling for use of alcohol (.07) also indicates a relationship between use of aspirin and use of alcohol.

The stepwise procedure can be continued indefinitely until all the potential variables have been included. At each step, one calculates the partial correlation between each independent variable not yet included in the equation and the dependent variable, controlling for all independent variables included on previous steps. The third step requires the calculation of second-order partial correlations, the fourth step requires the calculation of third-order partial correlations, and so forth. In the example used here, use of aspirin is the only remaining variable and would thus be the only one that could be added at the third and last step. There are often many more than three independent variables to be considered, however, and inclusion of all the independent variables will usually require many more than three steps.

In the next section we will consider statistical tests that can be used to evaluate the results of such a stepwise procedure. Recall that in the multiple regression procedure described earlier, all the independent variables were used simultaneously, and the $F$ test provided a method of determining whether significant prediction resulted. In stepwise multiple regression, the researcher can test the results obtained at each step of the procedure and specifically, can determine whether there has been a significant improvement in prediction at each step, as measured by the amount of increase in $R$ (or $R^2$). Often, after a sequence of three or four steps, the researcher will find that inclusion of the next independent variable does not cause a significant increase in $R^2$, the proportion of variance explained. At this point the procedure is usually terminated and the remaining independent variables are not entered into the regression equation. These tests are now described in detail, by application to the drug study data.

## STEPWISE SIGNIFICANCE TESTS

On the first step of the stepwise multiple regression just described, use of alcohol alone was selected as a predictor of use of marijuana. The regression equation produced by this analysis is not of major interest, and the equation will not be given here. What is important for us to know at this point is what the regression ANOVA looks like, because information from the ANOVA table will be useful in evaluation of change on the second step of the stepwise procedure. Canned computer programs for stepwise multiple regression usually include the ANOVA table for each step as well as the regression equation. The ANOVA table resulting from considering the use of alcohol as the only predictor of use of marijuana was as follows:

Regression ANOVA

| Source of Variation | Sum of Squares | Degrees of Freedom | Mean Square | F |
|---|---|---|---|---|
| Regression | 5.62747 | 1 | 5.62747 | 7.09 |
| Deviations | 30.14753 | 38 | 0.79336 | |
| Total | 35.77500 | 39 | | |

Since there was only one predictor in this analysis, the value of $k$, the number of predictors, is 1, corresponding to 1 degree of freedom for the regression sum of squares, as indicated in the table. Also, the value of $n - k - 1$ is 38, which corresponds to 38 degrees of freedom for the deviations sum of squares. For 1 and 30 degrees of freedom (using 30 because 38 is not listed in many $F$ tables), an $F$ value of 4.17 is required for significance at the .05 level. The $F$ of 7.09, since it is larger than the required 4.17, is thus significant at the .05 level, indicating that use of alcohol is a significant predictor of use of marijuana. This test, of course, gives the same result that would be obtained by either a $t$ test for the significance of the correlation coefficient or for the significance of the regression coefficient.

The second step in the stepwise procedure resulted in selection of use of cigarettes as the second predictor. The resulting regression ANOVA, with the two independent variables, use of alcohol and use of cigarettes, appeared on the computer printout as

Regression ANOVA

| Source of Variation | Sum of Squares | Degrees of Freedom | Mean Square | F |
|---|---|---|---|---|
| Regression | 7.84690 | 2 | 3.92345 | 5.198 |
| Deviations | 27.92810 | 37 | 0.75481 | |
| Total | 35.77500 | 39 | | |

If you refer back to the earlier section on multiple regression hypothesis testing in this chapter, which describes the regression ANOVA for ordinary multiple regression with two predictors, you will see that the same regression ANOVA table resulted from this analysis as from that earlier one.

# Multiple Regression

The interpretation of the significant $F$ value of 5.198 is the same as before. That is, use of alcohol and use of cigarettes together result in predicted values for use of marijuana that correlate significantly with the observed values. The hypothesis $H: \rho = 0$ is rejected. In stepwise multiple regression, however, our intent is not to determine whether $R^2$ differs from zero, but to determine whether $R^2$ has increased with the addition of the second variable. In order to make this determination, we compare the two regression ANOVA tables and consider the change in the regression sum of squares from one to the other.

In the first regression ANOVA table, where use of alcohol alone was entered as a predictor of use of marijuana, the regression sum of squares was

$$\sum_{i=1}^{n} (y'_i - \bar{y})^2 = 5.62747$$

This quantity represents that part of the total variation in $y$ that can be attributed to the effect of use of alcohol on use of marijuana. The regression sum of squares from the second table,

$$\sum_{i=1}^{n} (y'_i - \bar{y})^2 = 7.84690$$

represents that part of the total variation in $y$ that can be attributed to the effects of both use of alcohol and use of cigarettes on use of marijuana. The difference between these two values,

$$7.84690 - 5.62747 = 2.21943$$

represents that part of the regression sum of squares using the two predictors that is due to the addition of the second variable, use of cigarettes. In other words, given use of alcohol as a predictor, we can increase the regression sum of squares by 2.21943 by the addition of use of cigarettes as a second predictor.

Note that the increase in the regression sum of squares of 2.21943 does not represent the effect of use of cigarettes on use of marijuana by itself. A regression ANOVA with use of cigarettes as a single predictor would not give 2.21943 as a regression sum of squares, but would give a larger regression sum of squares. This is because of the correlation between the two independent variables, use of alcohol and use of cigarettes. The value of 2.21943 represents an addition to the regression sum of squares gained by adding use of cigarettes as a predictor, over and above the amount due to use of alcohol alone. Use of cigarettes apparently has some predictive value that is due to more than just its correlation with use of alcohol. Note also that since the total sum of squares remains the same, an increase in the regression sum of squares means a corresponding decrease in the deviations sum of squares (the unexplained part of the variation in y). The test to be described now is used to determine whether this increase in the regression sum of squares (the part of the total variation explained by the predictors) is statistically significant.

Symbolically, the null hypothesis tested in this case is

$$H: \beta_2 = 0$$

The $F$ statistic used to determine whether adding the second variable has made a significant increase in prediction is

$$F = \frac{\text{Regression sum of squares (2 var)} - \text{Regression sum of squares (1 var)}}{\text{Mean square deviations (2 var)}}$$

which has an $F$ distribution with 1 and $n - 3$ degrees of freedom, when the null hypothesis is true. Acceptance of the null hypothesis is equivalent to concluding that the second variable does not contribute significantly to the prediction, given the first. Rejection of the null hypothesis means that the researcher concludes that the regression sum of squares and consequently $R^2$ is increased significantly by the addition of the second variable.

For our data, the calculation is

$$F = \frac{7.84690 - 5.62747}{0.75481} = 2.94$$

Comparison of the calculated $F$ statistic with the tabulated value for the .05 level of $F = 4.11$, with 1 and 37 degrees of freedom, shows that the calculated $F$ is not large enough for rejection of the null hypothesis $H: \beta_2 = 0$. We conclude that use of cigarettes and use of alcohol together do not explain significantly more of the variation in use of marijuana than that explained by use of alcohol alone.

If you look back to the correlation matrix, you can see that the correlation between use of cigarettes and use of marijuana is .34. For a sample of size 40, .34 is a significant correlation; thus, use of cigarettes does correlate significantly with use of marijuana. The inclusion of cigarettes as a second predictor in the regression equation does not significantly improve the prediction because use of cigarettes is correlated with the first

# Multiple Regression

predictor, use of alcohol. By entering the variable use of alcohol as a predictor, we are using up some of the predictive power in the variable use of cigarettes, because of this correlation. Analysis of the same data using the test for partial correlation would yield comparable results. The $t$ test for significance of the partial correlation between use of cigarettes and use of marijuana with use of alcohol controlled (.27) would lead to acceptance of the null hypothesis. As you might suspect, this $t$ test for partial correlation is equivalent to the $F$-test just described for testing the addition of a variable in stepwise multiple regression ($t = \sqrt{F}$).

In our particular example, only two predictor variables were used. However, as we said earlier, a stepwise multiple regression can be carried on indefinitely with a test for significant increase in $R^2$ at each step. The $F$ test for the addition of a third variable

$$F = \frac{\text{Regression sum of squares (3 var)} - \text{Regression sum of squares (2 var)}}{\text{Mean-square deviations (3 var)}}$$

with 1 and $n - 4$ degrees of freedom when the null hypothesis is true, can be used to test

$$H: \beta_3 = 0$$

An analogous $F$ value can be computed at each step. The degrees of freedom are always 1 for the numerator and $n - k - 1$ for the denominator.

The stepwise $F$ tests can also be calculated directly from the values of $R$ at the different steps. Let $R_k$ stand for the multiple correlation coefficient with $k$ predictors, and let $R_{k-1}$ stand for that with $k - 1$ predictors. Then the formula

$$F = \frac{R_k^2 - R_{k-1}^2}{(1 - R_k^2)/(n - k - 1)}$$

can be used to calculate the $F$-test statistic. Applying this formula to the example described earlier in this chapter, $R_k$ ($k = 2$) is the multiple correlation between observed use of marijuana and that predicted by use of alcohol and use of cigarettes together, and $R_{k-1}$ is the multiple correlation coefficient with use of alcohol alone as a predictor. Thus

$$R_k \cong .47 \ (R_k^2 \cong .22)$$

and

$$R_k - 1 \cong .40 \ (R_{k-1}^2 \cong .16)$$

Substitution of these values into the formula for $F$ just given leads to

$$F = \frac{R_k^2 - R_{k-1}^2}{(1 - R_k^2)/(n - k - 1)}$$

$$= \frac{.22 - .16}{(1 - .22)/37}$$

$$= 2.85$$

which deviates from the $F$ calculated from the ANOVA tables ($F = 2.94$) only because of rounding error.

In stepwise regression, then, we continue to add predictor variables, testing the $F$ at each step to determine whether the increase in sum of squares due to regression is significant. The new independent variable considered at each step is that one which has the highest partial correlation with the dependent variable, with the effects of independent variables already included controlled ("partialled out"). A significant $F$ value means a significant increase in $R$ (and thus $R^2$) and indicates that the newly added variable has contributed to the prediction. At some point the increase in $R^2$ will no longer be significant. This often happens on about the third or fourth step. When the increase in $R^2$ is no longer significant, it is common to terminate the stepwise procedure and omit the remaining variables from the regression equation.

When stepwise multiple regression is done by using a packaged program, such as that available under the *Statistical Package for the Social Sciences*,[34] it is sometimes possible to set a criteria (e.g., minimal level of significance of the stepwise $F$) for stopping the procedure. If this is not done, the computer continues to enter the variables one by one until all the independent variables have been used. In such a case, you can look at each step to determine the one on which the increase in $R^2$ is no longer significant and eliminate that step and subsequent steps from your presentation of findings. The computer output usually includes the overall $F$ value (to test significance of prediction by using all the variables entered at that point) as well as the stepwise $F$ (to test the increase in prediction at that particular step). The overall $F$ is not particularly useful for interpretation and should not be confused with the stepwise $F$. In fact, the overall $F$ tends to decrease as variables are added because of loss of degrees of freedom in the denominator (deviations from regression). This is related to the problem of shrinkage, to be discussed shortly.

Sometimes a research report will contain a statement about the relative importance of the independent variables in the final regression equation. If the equation is of the form

$$y' = .3 + 1x_1 + 2x_2 + 3x_3$$

# Multiple Regression

for example, a statement is sometimes made that, according to the regression coefficients, $x_3$ is the best predictor, $x_2$ the second, and $x_1$ the third. This is not valid, since the values of the regression coefficients depend on the scales of the variables used. One way of correcting for this is to convert the regression coefficients into what are called *standard regression coefficients*. For each independent variable $x_i$,

$$b_i \sqrt{\frac{\sum_{i=1}^{n}(x_i - \bar{x})^2}{\sum_{i=1}^{n}(y_i - \bar{y})^2}}$$

is called the *standard partial regression coefficient*. These standardized coefficients are then used to measure the relative importance of variables. The standardized coefficients, however, measure relative importance of the variables only if they are independent from each other. This is seldom the case, and this makes the interpretation of the regression coefficients very difficult.

It should be noted that the final equation in a stepwise multiple regression is not necessarily the best, in terms of prediction, that could be obtained with the same number of independent variables. As already mentioned, there are other procedures for selecting variables to include in a regression equation. One alternative method is to work backward, beginning with a regression on all the independent variables and eliminating them one by one to get down to a smaller set. By eliminating at each step that variable whose elimination causes the least decrease in $R^2$, one can continue as long as variables can be eliminated with no significant decrease in $R^2$. The final set of variables obtained by this or by other alternate procedures would be similar, but not necessarily identical, to those obtained by the forward inclusion procedure we have described in this chapter.

The most commonly used procedure is the one we have presented, in which variables are added one at a time, with a test for significant increase in $R^2$ at each step. Nie et al.[34] provide clear and detailed discussion of many different forms of multiple regression analysis. In addition to the possibilities of either adding or eliminating one variable at a time, one can add or eliminate more than one variable at a time. The authors just mentioned describe many of these variations in detail and include the appropriate tests for significance for many different situations. They also explain how the various $F$ tests can be written as functions of $R$ rather than as functions of the sums of squares.

A final note is that the researcher can control the order of entering variables into a stepwise multiple regression as much or as little as desired.

We have described situations where the partial correlations determine the order of entry of variables at every step. However, more control may be exercised if it is appropriate to the situation. For example, suppose one subgroup of independent variables occurs prior in time to a second subset. In this situation, it would be logical to first consider the effect on $R^2$ of all the variables in the first subset and then the effect of all those in the second subset, given those in the first subset. The researcher could enter all the variables from the first subset in a stepwise fashion according to the partial correlations and a subsequently enter those from the second subset, again in a stepwise fashion. Numerous variations are available to fit various forms of data and research questions of interest to the investigator.

## SHRINKAGE IN MULTIPLE REGRESSION

The predictive power of the equation produced by multiple regression is judged by the value of $R$, the multiple correlation coefficient. Recall that $R$ is the correlation between the observed values and those predicted by the equation, and $R^2$ is the proportion of variance of $y$ that is explained by the independent variables. Because of the way in which the $R$ is calculated, there tends to be an upward bias in the values of $R$ and $R^2$. This problem is referred to as *shrinkage* in multiple regression.

One factor that influences the amount of overestimation of the value of $R$ is the ratio of the number of predictor variables used to the sample size. The larger this ratio is, the more overestimation there tends to be in the value of $R$. In other words, use of a large number of predictor variables with data from a small sample results in an inflated value of $R$ and consequently of $R^2$, the proportion of variance explained. The following formula can be used to obtain an estimate of $R^2$ that takes account of the shrinkage in multiple correlation:

$$\hat{R}^2 = 1 - (1 - R^2) \left\{ \frac{n-1}{n-k-1} \right\}$$

In this formula, $R$ is the sample multiple correlation coefficient, $n$ is the sample size, and $k$ is the number of independent variables. The value of $\hat{R}^2$ is an estimate of the squared multiple correlation coefficient in the population which is more accurate than the original $R^2$.

Application of this formula to the $R$ value calculated in the previous section of this chapter is shown below. The calculated $R$ value was

$$R = .46834 \sim .47$$

or

$$R^2 \sim .22$$

# Multiple Regression

for a sample of size $n = 40$, using $k = 2$ predictor variables. The estimated population squared multiple correlation is, therefore,

$$\hat{R}^2 = 1 - (1 - R^2) \left\{ \frac{n - 1}{n - k - 1} \right\}$$

$$= 1 - [1 - (.47)^2] \left\{ \frac{40 - 1}{40 - 2 - 1} \right\}$$

$$= 1 - (1 - .22) \left\{ \frac{39}{37} \right\} = .18$$

The shrinkage in $R^2$ in this instance is the difference between .22 and .18, or about 4% of the variance.

Multiple regression is commonly used in research situations where the sample size is small relative to the number of predictor variables, and shrinkage should be taken into account in estimating what proportion of the variance in the dependent variable can be realistically associated with the independent variable. A very common procedure in regression analysis of a large set of variables is to continue adding predictor variables indefinitely for the purpose of increasing the value of $R$, the multiple correlation coefficient (and consequently $R^2$). The value of $R$ always increases when a new variable is added to the regression, so that one can increase $R^2$ as much as desired by adding enough independent variables. But when the shrinkage in $R^2$ is taken into account, a large $R^2$ may not be as impressive as it seems. Instances where this is a problem, of course, are those in which the sample size is small relative to the number of independent variables.

## PROBLEMS

1. Suppose that data on age, weight, and blood pressure are obtained for a sample of 20 adults. A regression procedure is used to obtain an equation for predicting blood pressure from age and weight, and results in the regression ANOVA shown in Table 7-1.
   (a) Complete the ANOVA table.
   (b) Explain in your own words what null hypothesis can be tested.
   (c) Suppose that the multiple correlation coefficient in this analysis is $R = .71$. Show how this $R$ can be used to calculate the $F$-test statistic.
   (d) Explain the conclusion in substantive terms.
   (e) Estimate the population $\hat{R}^2$ by using the formula given in this chapter to account for shrinkage.

**Table 7-1.** Regression ANOVA for Prediction of Blood Pressure from Age and Weight ($N = 20$)

| Source of Variation | Sum of Squares | DF | Mean Square | F |
|---|---|---|---|---|
| Regression | 83.4 | | | |
| Deviations | 81.6 | | | |
| Total | 165.0 | | | |

(f) What questions about the effects of age and weight are not answered by this analysis but could be answered by a stepwise multiple regression analysis?

2. In the section on stepwise significance tests earlier in this chapter, an $F$-test statistic was given for determining whether addition of a second variable in the stepwise multiple regression procedure results in a significant increase in $R^2$, the proportion of variance explained. For the prediction of use of marijuana by use of other drugs, use of alcohol was entered on the first step and use of cigarettes on the second, and the $F$ statistic for the second step was $F = 2.94$. It was stated that a $t$ test for significance of the partial correlation between use of cigarettes and use of marijuana, controlling for use of alcohol, would lead to equivalent results, and that $t = \sqrt{F}$. Using the partial correlation of .27 between use of cigarettes and use of marijuana and the $t$-test formula for partial correlation given in Chapter 6, demonstrate the correspondence between these tests by calculating $t$. Since $F = 2.94$, the value should be $t = \sqrt{F} \cong 1.7146$, with slight allowance for roundoff error.

3. In a study of relationships between husband–wife compatibility and couple's health, Hong[20] hypothesized that in cases where compatibility of husband and wife is high, health status of the husband and wife should be higher than in cases where compatibility is low. Compatibility was scored according to a standardized scale (FIRO-B) on which high scores represent lower compatibility than low scores. Health status was scored by the Cornell Medical Index, which yields high scores for poor health status and low scores for good health status. This researcher found a significant positive correlation between marital compatibility and wife's health status, but no correlation between marital compatibility and husband's health status, and she wished to conduct further investigation into the relationship between these two variables for wives. Specifically, she wished to determine what effect the wife's age, socioeconomic status, education, number of children, religion, duration of marriage, and location of residence might have on the apparent relationship between marital compatibility and wife's health status. These extraneous variables were

# Multiple Regression

chosen on the basis of earlier research suggesting that they might influence either marital compatibility or health. Table 7-2 shows which of these extraneous variables were significantly correlated with either marital compatibility or wife's health. The researcher used stepwise multiple regression to combine all the variables into one analysis. The independent variables included all the extraneous variables and marital compatibility, and the dependent variable was the wife's health status. The variables were allowed to enter without any constraints on their order imposed by the researcher. At each step an $F$ test was calculated to determine whether the explained variance ($R^2$) had increased significantly. The analysis selected the variable "residence" on the first step and "marital compatibility" on the second step. The variable selected on the third step did not result in a significant increase in $R^2$, and thus the procedure was terminated after two steps. The regression ANOVA for residence and marital compatibility as predictors of wife's health is shown in Table 7-3.

(a) Explain in substantive terms what is indicated by the positive correlation between marital compatibility and wife's health, taking into account how the variables were scored.

(b) What effect do age and duration of marriage have on marital compatibility, according to the correlation coefficients?

(c) What effect do socioeconomic status, religion, years of education, and residence have on wife's health status, according to the correlation coefficients?

(d) How can you tell by examination of the correlation coefficients that, among the extraneous variables, residence will be selected as the best predictor of health status?

**Table 7-2.** Significant Correlates of Extraneous Variables with Wife's Health and Marital Compatibility

| Extraneous Variables | Wife's Health | Marital Compatibility |
|---|---|---|
| Age | — | .20* |
| Number of children | — | — |
| Socioeconomic status | −.28* | — |
| Religion (1 = Catholic, 2 = Protestant) | −.39* | — |
| Years of education | −.30* | — |
| Duration of marriage | — | .18* |
| Residence (1 = low-income housing, 2 = suburbia) | −.42* | — |

*$p < .05$.

**Table 7-3.** Regression ANOVA for Prediction of Wife's Health by Residence and Marital Compatibility

| Source of Variation | Sum of Squares | DF | Mean Square | F |
|---|---|---|---|---|
| Regression | 2910.54 | 2 | | |
| Residual | 11056.14 | 75 | | |

(e) Why do you suppose that socioeconomic status, religion, and years of education did not enter into the regression equation for prediction of health status, even though the correlation analysis shows that these three variables are all significant correlates of health status?

(f) Calculate the mean squares and $F$ value and complete the regression ANOVA table.

(g) What null hypothesis can be tested by the $F$ value.

(h) Test the $F$, using the .01 level of significance.

(i) Explain your findings in substantive terms.

4. In Chapter 6, Problem 4, a study of the relevance of patient characteristics for psychosocial stress experienced during hospitalization was described. Data from this study were subjected to a multiple stepwise regression procedure to further investigate the effects of hospital stress on patient characteristics, as indicated by the correlations given in Chapter 6. Refer to that chapter for further description of the study variables. The regression procedure was carried out using a sequence of four stages, corresponding to the four types of independent variables listed in Chapter 6. That is, the demographic variables were entered into the equation first, in stepwise fashion, followed by the prior hospitalization variables, in stepwise fashion, and so forth. Results of the regression analysis are given in Table 7-4.

If necessary, refer back to the correlation matrix in Chapter 6 to answer the following questions:

(a) Which of the demographic variables is the best predictor of hospital stress, and how do you know?

(b) How could the answer to a have been determined by examination of the correlation matrix?

(c) What is the multiple correlation coefficient between observed hospital stress scores and those predicted by the equation using the demographic variables together?

(d) What proportion of variance in the hospital stress scores is explained by the demographic variables?

(e) Why does the number of previous hospitalizations not contribute significantly to the prediction of hospital stress in this analysis,

# Multiple Regression

**Table 7-4.** Multiple Stepwise Regression for Prediction of Hospital Stress by Demographic Characteristics, Prior Hospitalization Experience, Life Stress, and Present Illness Variables ($N = 252$)

| Stages | Variables (in Order Entered) | R | $R^2$ | $R^2$ Increase |
|---|---|---|---|---|
| I. Demographic characteristics | Age | .17 | .03 | .03* |
| | Sex | .17 | .03 | .00 |
| | Marital status | .17 | .03 | .00 |
| | Education | .18 | .03 | .00 |
| II. Prior hospitalization experience | Years since last hospitalization | .25 | .06 | .03* |
| | Number of prior hospitalizations | .27 | .07 | .01 |
| III. Life stress | 1–2 years prior to hospitalization | .32 | .10 | .03* |
| | Year prior to hospitalization | .35 | .12 | .02* |
| | (Year prior to hospitalization)²‡ | .38 | .14 | .02* |
| IV. Present illness | Pain | .40 | .16 | .02† |
| | Seriousness of illness | .40 | .16 | .00 |

*$p < .05$
†Nonsignificant, that is, rounded value.
‡Ignore this entry. It will be discussed in Chapter 8.

even though the correlation matrix indicates a significant association between these two variables?

(f) The correlation between life stress 1–2 years prior to hospitalization and hospital stress is .20, according to the correlation matrix. In other words, 4% of the variance in hospital stress is explained by life stress 1–2 years prior to hospitalization. Why, then, is the increase in $R^2$ on the step where this life stress predictor is entered only equal to 3%?

(g) The correlation matrix for the study variables indicates that life stress the year prior to hospitalization decreases as age increases ($r_{x \cdot y} = -.27$) and also that hospital stress decreases as age increases ($r_{x \cdot y} = -.17$). Does this mean that the significant contribution of this life stress variable to the explained variance of hospital stress, as indicated in the regression analysis, could be due to age, that is, could be explained by the effect of age on both life stress and hospital stress?

(h) The pain variable is significantly correlated with hospital stress according to the correlation matrix. Why, then, does entry of the pain variable in the multiple regression analysis not lead to a significant increase in $R^2$?

(i) State in your own words the substantive meaning of the final $R$ of .40 and $R^2$ of .16 resulting from the regression analysis.

(j) Determine an estimate of the population proportion of variance explained in this analysis, taking account of shrinkage. How could the researchers reduce the amount of shrinkage?

5. Problem 3 in Chapter 6 was based on a study of the use of nursing care plans and variations in patient outcomes. Data given in that problem consisted of correlation coefficients between patient outcome variables and the other study variables. The nursing care plan variables were the independent variables of interest to the researcher, since she wanted to study how patient outcomes might be affected by use of nursing care plans. The other study variables, which included selected patient and nurse characteristics, were included because of their possible effects on the nursing care plan and patient outcome variables. To examine the effects of the nursing care plan variables on patient outcomes with patient and nurse characteristics taken into account, the researcher investigated each significant association between a nursing care plan variable and a patient outcome variable using stepwise multiple regression. For each regression procedure, the patient characteristics significantly correlated with the patient outcome were entered first, in stepwise fashion, followed by the nurse characteristics significantly correlated with the patient outcome, also in stepwise fashion. At the third stage, the nursing care plan variable was entered, so that at that point the effects of the relevant patient and nurse characteristics had been accounted for. In selecting patient and nurse characteristics to be included, the researcher chose any of either patient or nurse characteristics that correlated significantly with the patient outcome at the .10 level or better. The stepwise multiple regression for prediction of patient's psychological status by the assessment score for the nursing care plan resulted in the analysis shown in Table 7-5.

Refer back to the correlation matrix for this study to answer the following questions as necessary.

(a) What proportion of the variation in patient's psychological status can be explained by the patient characteristics used in the regression analysis?

# Multiple Regression

**Table 7-5.** Stepwise Multiple Regression Analysis for Prediction of Patient's Psychological Status by Assessment Score ($N = 80$)

| Stage | Variables in Order Entered | R | $R^2$ | $R^2$ Increase |
|---|---|---|---|---|
| Patient characteristics | Age | .21 | .04 | .04 |
|  | Education | .25 | .06 | .02 |
|  | Coronary prognostic index | .27 | .07 | .01 |
| Nurse characteristics | Age | .34 | .11 | .04 |
| Nursing care plan variable | Assessment | .41 | .17 | .06 |

(b) Is the proportion of variance explained by the variables mentioned in a significant? Carry out the appropriate hypothesis test and discuss the conclusion in substantive terms.

(c) Among the three patient characteristics used in the analysis, why was age entered into the regression first?

(d) The correlations between these three patient characteristics and patient's psychological status are $-.21$, $.19$, and $-.20$, respectively. Why is it that the multiple correlation between patient's observed psychological status and that predicted by these three variables together is $R = .27$, that is, substantially lower than the sum of the three zero-order correlations?

(e) Determine whether the prediction of patient's psychological status is significantly improved by the use of the nurse's age on the fourth step. Explain any difference between the effect of the nurse's age according to the regression analysis and the effect according to the zero-order correlation between nurse's age and patient's psychological status.

(f) Determine whether the prediction of patient's psychological status is significantly improved by the use of the nursing assessment score on the fifth step of the regression analysis.

(g) Summarize the results of the analysis. Explain what has been demonstrated about the relationship between the completeness with which an assessment is done and the patient's psychological status.

6. For the study just described in Problem 5, the stepwise regression procedure for prediction of incidence of complications by the documentation score for the nursing care plan led to the analysis given in Table 7-6.

**Table 7-6.** Stepwise Multiple Regression Analysis for Prediction of Incidence of Complications by Documentation Score ($N = 80$)

| Stage | Variables in Order Entered | R | $R^2$ | $R^2$ Increase |
|---|---|---|---|---|
| Patient characteristics | Sex | .25 | .06 | .06 |
| Nurse characteristics | Age | .31 | .09 | .03 |
|  | Years in primary nursing | .32 | .10 | .00 |
| Nursing care plan variable | Documentation | .37 | .14 | .04 |

Refer back to the correlation matrix for this study in Problem 3, Chapter 6, as necessary, to answer the following questions:

(a) Why is sex the only patient characteristic included in this analysis?

(b) Why is the $R$ on the first step the same as the zero-order correlation between sex and incidence of complications shown in the correlation matrix?

(c) Do the nurse characteristics significantly improve the prediction of incidence of complications, controlling for sex?

(d) Do the patient and nurse characteristics used in this analysis together provide any significant prediction of incidence of complications?

(e) Determine whether the prediction of incidence of complications is significantly improved by use of the nursing documentation score on the fourth step of the regression analysis.

(f) Summarize the results of the analysis. What can you say about the effect of the completeness with which documentation is made on the incidence of complications?

# Chapter 8

## MULTIPLE REGRESSION, CONTINUED

In the last several chapters we have introduced the analytic techniques of regression and correlation and have discussed the use of multiple regression analysis to simultaneously examine the effects of several independent variables on the dependent variable of interest. We have presented examples in which linear relationships were used as models, in which the absence of interaction effects between independent variables was assumed, and in which independent variables were described as quantitative in form. The intent of this chapter is to demonstrate the applicability of multiple regression in situations where nonlinearity is suspected, where interaction may be present, or where independent variables are qualitative in nature.

A nonlinear relationship between two variables is one that can be best approximated by a curve rather than a straight line. As you will recall, an ordinary linear regression analysis yields a line to approximate the relationship between two variables and a statistical test of the null hypothesis of no linear relationship between the variables. Failure to reject the null hypothesis in regression or correlation analysis is commonly and erroneously thought to demonstrate that there is no relationship between the variables studied. If there is a relationship that is in fact nonlinear, it is quite reasonable that the line determined by linear regression analysis will fit the data poorly and thus that the null hypothesis will be retained. Either a theoretical rationale or inspection of the data by graphing the values may lead the researcher to suspect that there is a relationship between the variables that is not being detected by linear regression analysis.

For example, consider a nursing study of the effect of periodic turning of bedfast patients on the rate of wound healing. Suppose that patients are randomized into eight treatment groups and the treatment consists of turning once, twice, three times, and so on, per hour, respectively. One might predict that the time for wound healing (measured as number of days to healing) would decrease rapidly with increased turning up to a point, after which additional turning would have no effect. A graph of the

171

data might look something like the one in Figure 8-1. Clearly, the relationship is nonlinear. A simple linear regression analysis might result either in nonsignificance or in poor predictive power. In this chapter we will describe how to improve predictability in such a situation by taking nonlinear effects into account.

Another situation that may occur in nursing research is one in which interaction between the independent variables is suspected on either experiential or logical grounds. Consider a study of the effects of age and education on patients' desire for information about treatment procedures. Let us assume that the nurse researcher has a scale to measure "need for information," scored so that a high score represents need for detailed information and low score represents no desire for any information at all. A stepwise regression procedure like the one we have used up to this point would select the best predictor of need for information, let us say age, and then indicate the increase in predictability due to addition of the second variable, education, given the presence of age in the regression equation. However, let us assume a situation like the following. Suppose that need for information decreases with age among subjects with less than a high school education, but does not decrease with age for subjects with high school education or more. In other words, the effect of age is dependent on or varies with educational level. This suggests that there is interaction between the independent variables, and predictability of the regression equation may be increased if this interaction can be taken into account. A procedure for incorporating a measure of such an interaction effect will be presented shortly.

In this chapter we will also explore the use of regression analysis when the independent variable of interest is qualitative in form. We have used examples in earlier chapters in which the independent variables were quantitative, but there are many variables relevant to nursing research

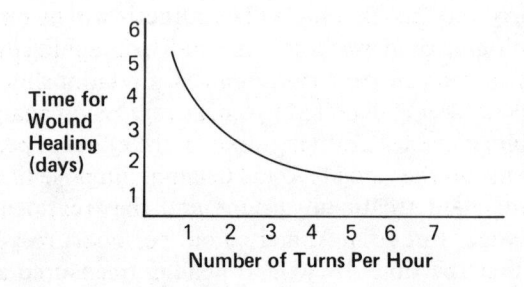

**Figure 8-1.** Hypothetical relationship between number of turns per hour and time for wound healing in days.

# Multiple Regression, Continued

that are simple categorical ones without even ordinal scaling. Examples of such variables include:

1. Type of patient (medical vs surgical)
2. Nursing intervention (given vs not given)
3. Patient awareness of diagnosis (yes vs no)
4. Sex (Male vs Female)
5. Type of nurse education (associate degree vs diploma vs baccalaureate)
6. Type of medical care (clinic, vs private M.D. vs emergency room)

As you will see shortly, such variables can be incorporated into regression analysis by the use of coding systems to represent the various categories of each variable. The analysis of variance procedures to be discussed in later chapters of this book are really just special cases of multiple regression analyses using independent variables that are categorical. A procedure for combining qualitative and quantitative independent variables into a single multiple regression analysis is also discussed.

## NONLINEAR RELATIONSHIPS

Correlation and regression analysis, as we have already pointed out, are useful for the study of linear relationships among variables. In regression of a variable $y$ on a variable $x$, the model is written as an equation for a straight line,

$$y = \alpha + \beta x + e$$

The least-squares criterion is used to calculate estimates of $\alpha$ and $\beta$ so that the relationship between $x$ and $y$ can be expressed as a straight line. If the variables $x$ and $y$ are not linearly related, the regression coefficient or the correlation coefficient will (with high probability) not differ significantly from zero.

However, suppose that $x$ and $y$ are related, but that the relationship is not linear. In this case, the relationship cannot be very well expressed by a straight line, so that deviations of observed values from the least-squares line will be substantial. Therefore, the statistical test will indicate either a nonsignificant regression coefficient or correlation coefficient or one with significant but low predictive power. The nonlinear nature of the relationship will be missed unless some additional sort of analysis can be done.

There are many examples relevant for nursing research that might illustrate nonlinear relationships. The example given in the introduction to this chapter, the relationship between time for wound healing and number of turns per hour, is one. Two other examples are shown in Figures 8-2 and 8-3.

Figure 8-2 represents findings of Janis[22] that are often cited by nurse researchers. Janis studied patients both before and after surgery and found that patients with a moderate level of preoperative fear had lower postoperative anxiety than patients with either low or high preoperative fear. The relationship that Janis observed between preoperative fear and postoperative anxiety was nonlinear, and a regression analysis of the relationship between these two variables would almost certainly result in nonsignificant findings. The relationship between the two variables apparent in Figure 8-2 is a second degree or quadratic one, as represented by the curve, and we will momentarily see how analysis of this relationship can be incorporated into a multiple regression analysis.

The second example shown in Figure 8-3 is a hypothetical one that you might call a "backfire experiment." The researcher in this study wanted to speak with patients prior to surgery to give them information about procedures to be carried out during the operation, and she hypothesized that the more often she described the details of the operation, the lower the patients' postoperative anxiety would be. She varied the number of times that patients were seen preoperatively from one to six. However, she became so involved in vivid descriptions of the gory details of the surgery that her intervention had the effect of increasing postoperative anxiety. In fact, three descriptions were enough to make the postoperative

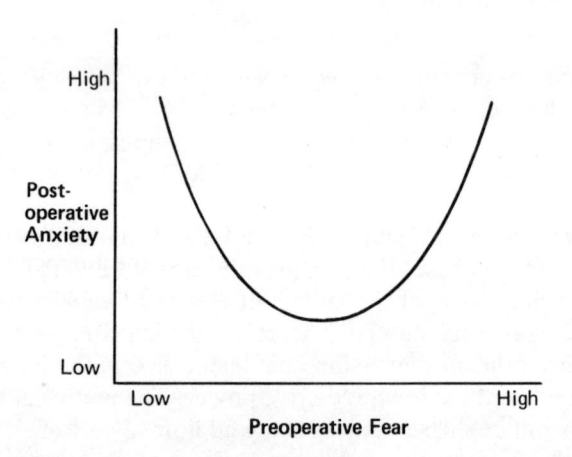

**Figure 8-2.** Hypothetical relationship between preoperative fear and postoperative anxiety.

# Multiple Regression, Continued

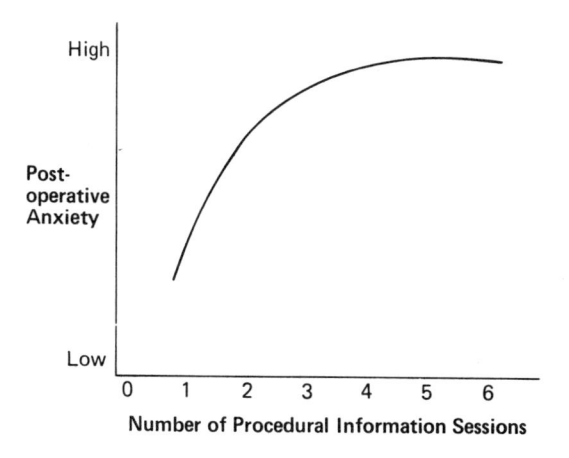

**Figure 8-3.** Hypothetical relationship between number of procedural information sessions and postoperative anxiety.

anxiety scores go as high as possible on the anxiety scale so that patients receiving four, five, and six descriptions scored about the same as those receiving three because the score just couldn't go any higher than it already was with three descriptions. A regression analysis of these data might yield a significant regression coefficient, but probably one with low predictive power, which could be improved by taking the nonlinear nature of the relationship into account.

Both of the above examples illustrate a quadratic relationship between two variables, which can be represented by the following mathematical model:

$$y = \alpha + \beta_1 x + \beta_2 x^2$$

The above equation is the equation for a curve or parabola. According to the model, the dependent variable, $y$, is related to the independent variable, $x$, in such a way that it changes as a function of both $x$ and $x^2$. In terms of our examples, $y$ represents postoperative anxiety, and $x$ represents either preoperative fear. (Fig. 8-2) or number of procedural descriptions (Fig. 8-3). Note that the above equation looks very much like a multiple regression analysis with two independent variables, $x$ and $x^2$. This is, in fact, precisely the method by which such a situation can be handled. The researcher simply treats the variable $x$ as one independent variable and the variable $x^2$ as a second independent variable.

A stepwise regression with $x$ entered at step 1 followed by $x^2$ at step 2 is carried out by the usual procedures. For computer analysis, of course, one would first instruct the computer to compute the $x^2$ variable by squaring the value of $x$ for each subject. The usual $F$ test for significance of $R^2$ on step 1 is calculated, indicating whether the linear model provides any significant prediction. This is followed by step 2, where $x^2$ is added as a second term and the significance test for addition of the second variable is done. Recall from our discussion of stepwise multiple regression that a test can be made at each step to determine whether there has been a significant increase in $R^2$. In this case, a significant increase at step two means that prediction is increased by addition of the quadratic term, that is, that the quadratic model fits the data better than the linear model. Nonsignificance on step 2 indicates that addition of the quadratic term has not improved the prediction and suggests that the researcher might as well stick with the original linear model.

The possibility of nonlinear relationships was investigated by Volicer and Burns[44] in a study of patient characteristics that might affect hospital stress. This study was described in problem 4 of Chapter 6 and was also discussed in problem 4 of Chapter 7. One of the relationships investigated for possible nonlinearity was that between life stress and hospital stress. For medical patients, a zero-order correlation of $r_{x \cdot y} = .20$ was found between the life stress score the year prior to hospitalization and the hospital stress score, indicating that this life stress score was a significant predictor of hospital stress, using a linear model. The positive and significant correlation suggested that hospital stress tended to increase as life stress the year prior to hospitalization increased. The researchers decided to extend the analysis to determine whether a nonlinear model might fit the data better than a linear model.

A nonlinear model of the relationship between life stress and hospital stress could be based on relationships such as those shown in either Figure 8-4 or 8-5.

Figure 8-4 depicts a situation where hospital stress not only increases as life stress increases, but increases at a faster rate as life stress increases. Figure 8-5 suggests that, although hospital stress tends to increase with increasing life stress, the rate of increase decreases as life stress increases. As you might suspect, the model in Figure 8-4 would result in a positive regression coefficient for the squared term and that in Figure 8-5 in a negative regression coefficient for the squared term.

The researchers determined the existence of a nonlinear relationship in this study by use of partial correlation rather than by regression analysis. As you recall from Chapter 7, these procedures are equivalent. First, a new variable was created by squaring the life stress score for each individual. Call the life stress variable $x$, the life stress variable squared $x^2$,

# Multiple Regression, Continued

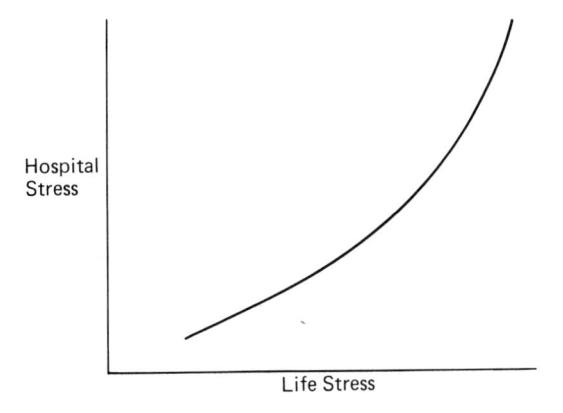

**Figure 8-4.** Hypothetical relationship between life stress and hospital stress indicating increasing rate of increase.

and the hospital stress variable $y$. Next, the investigators determined the partial correlation between $x^2$ and $y$, controlling for $x$. This partial correlation

$$r_{x^2 y \cdot x} = .19$$

was statistically significant at the .05 level. In other words, there was a significant positive correlation between life stress squared and hospital

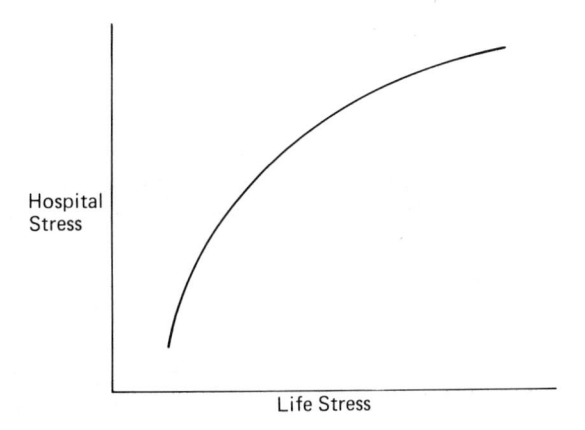

**Figure 8-5.** Hypothetical relationship between life stress and hospital stress indicating decreasing rate of increase.

stress, with life stress controlled. The fact that the partial correlation was positive indicated a relationship like that shown in Figure 8-4. Of course, these results indicate what would have happened had the data been subjected to stepwise multiple regression analysis. The increase in $R^2$ from the addition of life stress squared on the second step would have been significant according to the $F$ test, since that test is equivalent to the $t$ test for partial correlation. Thus in this example, better prediction of hospital stress could be attained by accounting for the nonlinear relationship rather than using the customary linear model.

Mathematically, it is possible to extend the analysis of nonlinearity beyond the squared or quadratic term used in the example just given. This is accomplished in stepwise multiple regression by the addition of more terms. The value of $x^3$ can be added on step 3, $x^4$ on step 4, and so on, and the $F$ test can be done at each step to see whether prediction is significantly increased. Each additional term allows for another curve in the line, making the modeling of extremely complicated relationships possible. In research dealing with behavioral variables such as those common to nursing research, however, significant increases in prediction after the squared term are unusual and very difficult to interpret. Readers are referred to Kerlinger and Pedhazur[26] for discussion of extension of nonlinear regression analyses beyond the quadratic term.

You may recall a discussion at the end of Chapter 5 regarding the effect of the range of values of a variable studied on the results of the statistical analysis. In that discussion it was pointed out that many variables of interest to nurse researchers do not have simple linear relationships over a wide range of values. In this section you have seen examples of how curvilinear relationships can be studied by incorporating quadratic terms into the model. Note that for any variable, the range of values that you choose to investigate can result in very different outcomes in terms of the model that best fits the data. Examples given in this section illustrate this problem clearly.

The hypothetical data shown in Figure 8-2 indicate a U-shaped relationship between preoperative fear and postoperative anxiety. If your study sample happened to consist of patients with preoperative fear scores on the lower half of the possible range for this variable, your data would not show a curvilinear relationship, but rather an inverse relationship between preoperative fear and postoperative anxiety. However, if your study sample consisted of patients with preoperative fear scores in the upper half of the range, your data would show a positive relationship between preoperative fear and postoperative anxiety. Care should be taken in interpretation of such results, since the clinical implications would likely be the opposite. The computer, in number-crunching your data, has no notion of what part of the range of a variable is being studied, and even less idea about clinical implications. The choice of an analytical model and interpretation of results is the researcher's responsibility, and it is important to think carefully about how the study was designed, as it relates to interpretation of the findings.

The example shown in Figure 8-3 also illustrates this problem. Suppose that in designing this study, you decide to use experimental groups receiving 0, 1, 2, or 3 procedural information sessions only. Your data are likely to fit a linear regression model quite well, since it appears that postoperative anxiety increases directly with the number of information sessions, going from 0 to 3. However, suppose that your experimental groups receive 4, 5, or 6 sessions only. In this case, your analysis would suggest that there is no relationship between number of procedural information sessions and postoperative anxiety, since the line is quite horizontal over this range of values. In designing any study like this, you will want to keep in mind that you should use, as levels of the experimental variable, values in a range where you expect maximal effect, on the basis of previous research, your clinical expertise, or both. In interpretation of results, avoid generalizing to levels of the experimental variable that were not actually used in the study.

An alternative procedure for handling nonlinear relationships is to transform the original variables. Sometimes when the relationship between $y$ and $x$ is nonlinear, for example, that between $y$ and $\log x$, between $y$ and $1/x$, or between $y$ and some other mathematical function of $x$ may be linear in form. In such cases, one may carry out linear regression analysis by using the transformed $x$ variable instead of the original $x$ value for each individual. Such procedures are not described in detail here, but the reader is referred to Nie et al.[34] for more detailed discussion of such data transformations. Snedecor and Cochran[41] describe several typical nonlinear relationships and explain what transformations are needed to produce linear relationships.

## INTERACTION

The multiple regression procedures described in earlier chapters are based on the assumption that the effects of the independent variables are additive. Effects are additive when any specific independent variable has the same relationship with the dependent variable for each value of the other independent variables. For the example given on the introduction to this chapter on the effects of age and education on patients' desire for information about treatment procedures, the additive model assumes that age has the same relationship with need for information at every educational level. If this were true, one could do a separate analysis with the dependent variable need for information regressed on the independent variable age for each level of the independent variable education (e.g., less than high school, high school or more). The result would be two regression lines, and, if there were no interaction effects, the lines would be parallel; that is, they would have the same slope (regression coefficient). In other words, the relationship between age and need for information would be the same, regardless of level of education.

When interaction is present, the additive model presented in Chapter 7 is not adequate to describe the data, and the separate regression lines would not be parallel. For example, if need for information increased with age for those with high school education or more but decreased with age for those with less than high school education, the two lines could cross, since one would have a positive slope and one would have a negative slope. Or, if both relationships were positive but with different slopes, that is, different strengths of relationship, the lines might move toward each other or away from each other, with or without actually crossing. Allowing for sampling error, of course, we would not expect two sample regression lines to be exactly parallel, even in the absence of interaction. Statistically, we are interested in determining whether there is *significant* interaction, that is, evidence that the two population lines, which are estimated from the sample data, are not parallel.

For a second example, consider a study of the effects of life stress prior to delivery and length of labor on Apgar scores of newborns. Assume that life stress has been measured on a continuous scale by an index such as the Social Readjustment Rating Scale devised by Holmes and Rahe[19]. Suppose, for example, that high life stress scores are associated with low Apgar scores, but that this is true only when length of labor is relatively long. In other words, when labor is short, Apgar scores are high, regardless of whether life stress prior to delivery was high or low. One could calculate separate analyses for the dependent variable Apgar score regressed on the independent variable life stress, for those with long labors and those with short labors. In the first case, the relationship is negative, and the analysis would yield a regression line with a negative slope. In the second case, there is no relationship, and the slope of the line would be zero, so the two lines would not be parallel.

In cases where there is interaction between the independent variables, the additive model does not adequately describe the relationship among the variables. Better prediction of the dependent variable can be attained by incorporating the interactive effect into the model. The contribution of interaction to prediction is most commonly handled by the inclusion of *multiplicative terms* into the regression equation. For a situation with two independent variables, the model takes the following form:

$$y = \alpha + \beta_1 x_1 + \beta_2 x_2 + \beta_3 x_1 x_2$$

The last term, which is the multiplicative term, is the product of the two variables and represents the effect of the two variables jointly, that is, in addition to their independent effects. Applying this equation to the above example, $y$ represents Apgar scores, $x_1$ represents life stress scores, $x_2$ represents length of labor, and $x_1 x_2$ represents the product of life stress and length of labor for each individual. The equation is in the form of a multiple regression with three predictor variables and is handled analytically as just that.

To accomplish such an analysis, one first creates the variable $x_1 x_2$ for each subject by multiplying the life stress score by length of labor. This value does not have to be entered into the computer as raw data, of course. Any standard packaged program should have a data manipulation procedure that can be used to compute the variable $x_1 x_2$ by multiplication of the values for $x_1$ and $x_2$ for each subject. Then the usual multiple regression procedure is performed, treating the values of $x_1$, $x_2$, and $x_1 x_2$ as three independent variables. The logical procedure is to first run a multiple regression analysis using $x_1$ and $x_2$ as independent variables, that is, the additive model. Next, run multiple regression with three independent variables, $x_1$, $x_2$, and $x_1 x_2$. This can be easily accomplished by using a packaged program for stepwise multiple regression with $x_1 x_2$ constrained to enter on step 3.

A nonsignificant change in the regression sum of squares between the two regressions would indicate that the additive model with only the two predictors $x_1$ and $x_2$ is adequate to describe the data. When there is significant interaction, graphical presentation of the data is useful in interpreting the nature of the interaction. See Winer[46] for a more detailed discussion of procedures to follow a finding of significant interaction effects.

If there are more than two independent variables and if all possible interactions are to be considered, the model immediately becomes more complicated. For three independent variables, for example, there are 3 main effects ($x_1$, $x_2$, $x_3$), 3 two-way interactions ($x_1 x_2$, $x_1 x_3$, $x_2 x_3$) and 1 three-way interaction ($x_1 x_2 x_3$), and 7 steps in the multiple regression would be necessary to account for all of these possible kinds of interaction. Unless the researcher has an extremely large sample, it may not be possible to use so many independent variables without considerable shrinkage in $R^2$ due to loss of degrees of freedom. Furthermore, just as for higher terms in nonlinear regression, significant results at higher levels than two-way interaction are uncommonly observed in behavioral research and difficult to interpret substantively.

## DUMMY CODING

To this point, multiple regression procedures have been described for cases in which all the independent variables were continuous. Many variables commonly encountered in nursing research are not continuous, but rather qualitative or categorical in form. They include variables such as sex, type of nursing education, and others like those listed in the first section of this chapter, and may have either two or more categories. Also, in any experimental study in which subjects are assigned to either a control or an experimental group, the group assignment is a categorical variable. Categorical variables can be accommodated in multiple regression analysis by the use of a coding system to represent group membership.

A code is a set of symbols (such as letters or numbers) to which meanings have been assigned. You probably created "secret" codes when you were a child, by arbitrarily assigning numbers to letters of the alphabet, which allowed you to write secret messages to your friends. Most of you have heard of the Morse Code, in which a sequence of dots and dashes is used to represent each letter. Coding systems are useful in statistical analysis of categorical data because they allow for numerical representation of any kind of information. Once all the data of interest have been put into numerical form, it is possible to calculate and carry out significance tests. The simplest of these systems, and the one to be described here, is referred to as *dummy coding*.

For example, consider dummy coding for a dichotomous variable such as sex. In this case, all the members of one category are assigned the number 1 arbitrarily, and the others are assigned the number 0. The variable sex, for example, can be represented by the dummy variable $x$, coded as

$$1 = \text{Female}$$
$$0 = \text{Male}$$

The variable $x$ can be used in multiple regression in the same way as other variables. For example, one can compute a regression using $x$ (1 = female, 0 = male) as a predictor of $y$ (e.g., length of hospital stay). A significant result has the same interpretation as for any regression analysis; in this case, that sex is a correlate of length of hospital stay. Since the variable

# Multiple Regression, Continued

is dichotomous, one could also describe significant results by stating that women tend to stay longer in the hospital than men, or the opposite, whichever the case may be.

When the categorical variable can take on three values, two dummy variables are used to represent the variable. For example, consider type of nurse education as a variable with the categories of associate degree, diploma, and baccalaureate. The first dummy variable will be $x_1$, coded as

$$1 = \text{Associate degree}$$
$$0 = \text{Not associate degree}$$

and the second will be $x_2$, coded as

$$1 = \text{Diploma}$$
$$0 = \text{Not diploma}$$

The type of education for each subject is specified by the two dummy variables, according to the following codes:

Associate degree: $x_1 = 1, x_2 = 0$
Diploma: $x_1 = 0, x_2 = 1$
Baccalaureate: $x_1 = 0, x_2 = 0$

The number of dummy variables necessary to define membership on a categorical variable is always 1 less than the number of categories.

After dummy variables are created, they can be used to carry out a multiple regression analysis in the same manner as any other variables. For example, a regression equation can be computed by using $x_1$ and $x_2$ as independent variables in the prediction of salary. A significant $R^2$ using both of these predictors would indicate that salary is significantly related to type of education. To be able to interpret such results in substantive terms, one would have to examine mean salary levels to determine the nature of the relationship between salary and type of education (i.e., who makes the most money).

It is possible to determine group means on the dependent variable in regression analysis with categorical variables by examination of the regression equation. For each individual, the predicted score is equal to the mean of the group to which that individual belongs. For example, the best estimate of length of stay for a female patient would be the mean length of stay for all females. This is reflected in the regression equation, as indicated by the following fictitious illustration.

Suppose that men stay on the average 4 days and women 6 days, and that the dummy variable $x$ (1 = female, 0 = male) is used for sex in the regression analysis. The resulting prediction equation would be

$$y = 4 + 2x$$

For males, $x = 0$, resulting in 4, the mean length of stay for men, as the predicted value. Generally, then, with one dummy variable, the $y$ intercept is the mean for the variable coded 0. For females, $x = 1$, resulting in 6, the mean length of stay for women, as the predicted value. The value of the slope $b$ (which in this case is 2) is the amount by which the mean for the group coded 1 deviates from the mean for the group coded 2. Similar interpretations from the regression equation can be made when more than one dummy variable is used.

Readers who recall the use of $t$ tests for the difference between means may be puzzled at this point at the use of regression analysis to examine the same thing (e.g., sex differences in length of stay for two groups). Others familiar with ANOVA for examination of differences in more than two means may also be perplexed by the use of regression analysis to test differences in salary for three different types of nurse as presented above. In fact, regression analysis incorporates both of these procedures as special cases and yields identical statistical inferences to that obtained by a $t$ test for the difference between two means or ANOVA for the difference in two or more group means. The relationship between regression analysis results and ANOVA results is discussed further in Chapter 9.

Various additional coding systems have been devised to allow for the inclusion of categorical variables representing group membership in regression analysis. A procedure called *effect coding* is similar to dummy coding but uses codes of 1s, 0s, and −1s to represent the groups. An advantage of effect coding is that each of the regression coefficients in the resulting regression equation reflects a treatment effect, so that a predicted score is composed of the grand mean plus the treatment effect of the group to which a particular subject belongs. A third type of coding, called *orthogonal coding,* allows for testing for significant differences between specific groups, rather than simply one overall test of significance. Both Kerlinger and Pedhazur[26] and Cohen and Cohen[8] discuss these alternative coding systems in detail. Although effect and orthogonal coding generally require simpler calculations than dummy coding when group sample sizes are equal, this factor should not be a major consideration, since it is assumed that you are very likely to be using a computer for calculating the regression equation. The sample sizes are only likely to be equal if the groups are treatment groups to which subjects have been assigned by randomization.

# Multiple Regression, Continued

The results of the statistical analysis are the same, regardless of the coding system used, as are predictions made from the regression equations.

Coding systems are also useful for the analysis of data collected over a long period, when one wants to determine whether there has been a change over time. There are many situations in which it is important to analyze the change over time in indicators such as number of patients coming to a clinic or hospital or incidence of various diseases, both for purposes of future planning and for investigation of the determinants of change. Such problems fit under the general heading of *time series*. A simple example of a time series is the number of patients seen in an outpatient clinic for treatment of hypertension over a 5-year period. To determine whether there has been a change during the 5-year period, the researcher can treat the data by a regression analysis, using time as the independent variable and number of cases as the dependent variable. The values for time (the independent variable) are coded as $-2, -1, 0, +1$, and $+2$, where $-2$ represents the first year and $+2$ represents the last year, and an ordinary regression equation is calculated. Note that for the situation just described, the data obtained at different time points represent different individuals. This type of problem should not be confused with cases where before–after measures or other repeated measures are obtained for the same people.

Both qualitative and quantitative variables can be included in a single multiple regression analysis. For example, suppose that a researcher wants to study the effects of both sex and duration of operation on length of hospital stay for a group of patients undergoing cholecystectomy. The first step would be to create a dummy variable for sex (e.g., call it $d$). With duration of operation denoted by $x$ and length of hospital stay by $y$, one could then write the model as

$$y = \alpha + \beta_1 d + \beta_2 x + \beta_3 dx$$

The three terms on the right-hand side represent sex ($\beta_1 d$), duration of operation ($\beta_2 x$) and interaction between sex and duration of operation ($\beta_3 dx$). The procedures for analysis and for determining whether the interaction term can be dispensed with are fairly complicated, and the reader is referred to Nie et al.[34] for further discussion. If interaction is not a factor, the additive model

$$y = \alpha + \beta_1 d + \beta_2 x$$

can be used. In this case, an ordinary stepwise multiple regression will determine the effect of sex and duration of operation on length of hospital stay.

## SUMMARY

In the last few chapters, several techniques for examining multivariate relationships have been described. These include ordinary multiple regression, partial correlation, and stepwise multiple regression. By now you should be appreciative of the interrelationships among these various procedures, which are often erroneously regarded as distinct and unrelated techniques. We have also discussed how to test for nonlinear relationships and interaction and how to incorporate qualitative variables into regression analysis by use of coded variables. As you probably have begun to surmise, most multivariate situations can be handled by some form of regression analysis.

In the next several chapters, we turn to analysis of data with the use of what is traditionally called *analysis of variance* (ANOVA). Models for ANOVA originated for use in well-controlled, experimental studies, where true causal hypotheses can be tested. Compared with multiple regression analysis, the ANOVA techniques are often viewed as more precise or more scientific. As you know from the last several chapters, regression analysis itself is ANOVA, and you will see in the next few chapters that the traditional ANOVA designs are just special cases of multiple regression analysis. We present the ANOVA designs in this text as separate topics, only because that is how they are generally conceptualized. Keep in mind as you read further that the degree to which one can infer causal relationships is not dependent on how the data are analyzed, that is, what particular analytic technique is used. The judgments made about causality have to be made in terms of the study methodology, including how subjects were chosen, how much the investigator controlled the experimental treatment to exclude extraneous effects, how all the variables were measured, and so forth. As Cohen and Cohen[8] point out (in a very good discussion of multiple regression analysis in relation to analysis of variance) "the logical status of causal inference is a function of how the data were produced, not how they are analyzed."

Evidence for causality should particularly be kept in mind when stepwise multiple regression is used for data analysis. This procedure is sometimes used to control for extraneous variables that might influence both the dependent variable and the independent variable of interest in such a way as to make them appear to be related (by zero-order correlation). Once the extraneous variables are controlled (by entering them into a prediction equation) the subsequent entry of the independent variable may not result in a significant increase in $R^2$, suggesting that the relationship is spurious, that is, it is due to the fact that both the independent and dependent variable are affected by the extraneous variables. In making judgments like this, the researcher should always refer back to the study methodology and to the theoretical rationale that might account for relationships among variables. Multiple regression analysis has a way of making the structure of interrelationships appear deceptively simpler than they may be in actuality. If results of an analysis lead the researcher to conclude that the relationship between two variables is explained by a third variable, there should be logical as well as analytic evidence that the explanatory (third) variable really does affect the other two variables.

Stepwise multiple regression also is often used to determine how well a dependent variable may be predicted by a set of independent variables. In behavioral sciences such as nursing, it is often reasonable to hypothesize a multiplicity of causes; that several variables may have some influence on a given outcome. The significance of the relationship of each independent variable with the dependent variable can be determined by correlation analysis. If all the independent variables are used together in a stepwise multiple regression procedure, some may not lead to a significant increase in $R^2$ when they are entered. This often happens, of course, because of the interrelationships among the independent variables themselves. The researcher cannot conclude that those variables that fail to contribute significantly to the prediction of the dependent variable in stepwise multiple regression have been shown to have no causal effect. To reiterate, statistical evidence for or against causality should be interpreted by reference back to the theoretical and methodological framework on which the study is based.

## PROBLEMS

1. Price and Collins[36] collected data from nursing students at the University of Wyoming to study factors that might affect smoking behavior. A traditionally accepted view that the most significant factor influencing young people to smoke is the model of smoking parents in the home, along with more recent research suggesting that peer influences might represent a stronger influence than parent modeling, led these researchers to question their subjects about smoking behavior of both their parents and friends. The respondents were asked to answer yes or no to the following questions:
   1. Does your father smoke?
   2. Does your mother smoke?
   3. Does your best friend smoke?
   4. Do most of your friends smoke?

as well as to provide information about their own smoking behavior. In their article, the researchers presented a tabulation of responses to the above questions by smoking behavior of the respondent, as shown in Table 8-1.

(a) If necessary for review, calculate and test the null hypothesis of no association between father's smoking behavior and respondent's smoking behavior. The same analysis can also be carried out for the mother, best friend, and most friends variables.

(b) According to the chi-square values given above (as indicated by the $p$ value), which parent or peer smoking behaviors are associated with smoking among the respondents?

(c) How can you explain the relationship between best friend's smoking behavior and respondent's smoking behavior substantively; that is, what is the direction of the relationship?

(d) Answer question c for most friends' smoking behavior.

(e) Suppose that the researchers want to use a multiple regression analysis to predict smoking behavior, using the smoking behavior of father, mother, best friend, and most friends as independent variables. Use a dummy coding system to create four variables that could be used as predictors for such an analysis. (Ignore the dependent variable, which is itself categorical. This situation is discussed in Chapter 13 under the section on discriminant analysis).

(f) According to the chi-square data above, which of the dummy variables would you expect to be entered first, if a stepwise multiple regression procedure were used?

Table 8-1. Smoking Behavior of Respondent by Parent or Peer Smoking Behavior

| Parent or Peer Smoking Behavior | | Never | Quit | Smoke Now | N | Chi-Square |
|---|---|---|---|---|---|---|
| Father smokes | Yes | 18 (25%) | 26 (36%) | 28 (39%) | 72 | 2.87 |
| | No | 35 (36%) | 35 (36%) | 28 (28%) | 98 | |
| Mother smokes | Yes | 14 (23%) | 21 (35%) | 25 (42%) | 60 | 4.22 |
| | No | 40 (36%) | 39 (35%) | 31 (29%) | 110 | |
| Best friend smokes | Yes | 8 (14%) | 19 (32%) | 32 (54%) | 59 | 22.48* |
| | No | 45 (41%) | 41 (38%) | 23 (21%) | 109 | |
| Most friends smoke | Yes | 10 (15%) | 24 (35%) | 34 (50%) | 68 | 23.00* |
| | No | 42 (43%) | 37 (38%) | 18 (19%) | 97 | |

*$p < .001$.

# Multiple Regression, Continued

(g) Why would it be reasonable to predict that father's smoking behavior and mother's smoking behavior would not contribute significantly to $R^2$, the proportion of variance in respondent smoking behavior explained by the four predictor variables?

2. Refer back to the study of the influence of husband–wife compatibility on couples' health by Hong[20], described in Problem 3 in Chapter 7.

(a) Suggest how two of the extraneous variables used in this study might have an interactive effect on wife's health (e.g., socioeconomic status and year of education).
(b) Explain how you would create a new variable to represent the interaction term.
(c) Write the model that would be used and explain how the analysis would be carried out.

3. In this chapter, a study by Volicer and Burns[44] was used to illustrate the investigation of a nonlinear relationship between life stress and hospital stress. These researchers looked for possible nonlinear relationships between hospital stress and each of their study variables. This analysis was carried out separately for medical patients and surgical patients since the correlates of hospital stress were different for these two patient groups. The technique of partial correlation was used to test for a significant correlation between the square of each study variable and hospital stress, controlling for the original study variable itself. Refer back to the example from the study given in this chapter for more detail about how this procedure was carried out. Results of the analysis are given in Tables 8-2 and 8-3.

(a) For medical patients, what substantive relationship is indicated by the correlation of $r_{x \cdot y} = -.17$ between age and hospital stress?
(b) What can be concluded from the nonsignificant partial correlation of $r_{x^2 y \cdot x} = -.07$ between age squared and hospital stress, controlling for age, for medical patients?
(c) For a stepwise regression analysis, predicting hospital stress among medical patients, using age as the first predictor and age squared as the second predictor, what would be the results of the $F$ test on the first step? How do you know this?
(d) For the regression analysis described in c, what would be the results of the $F$ test for significant increase in $R^2$ on the second step, and how do you know?
(e) Answer questions a through d for the other analyses indicated in the tables.

**Table 8-2.** Partial Correlation of Squared Study Variables with Original Study Variables, Controlling for Original Study Variables, for Medical Patients ($N = 252$)

| Variable $x$ | Correlation of $x$ with Hospital Stress | Partial Correlation of $x^2$ with Hospital Stress, Controlling for $x$ |
|---|---|---|
| Age | −.17* | .07 |
| Number of previous hospitalizations | .13* | .10 |
| Years since last hospitalization | −.17* | .11 |
| Life Stress 1 year prior to hospitalization | .20* | .19* |
| Life stress 1–2 years prior to hospitalization | .20* | .07 |
| Pain | .22* | .06 |

*$p < .05$.

4. In a study of psychologic and sociologic phenomena that might interact with physical factors during pregnancy in such a way as to adversely affect neonatal outcome, Kirgis et al.[28] gathered data on 51 pregnant women during either the second or third trimester of pregnancy. The variables measured that might affect pregnancy outcome included:

1. Life stress during the preceding 6 months.
2. Illness-proneness (major illnesses in the last 10 years)
3. Number of frequently occurring pregnancy symptoms in each trimester
4. Number of past pregnancy complications
5. Months since last delivery
6. Number of medications
7. Hemoglobin at discharge
8. Length of labor—stage I

The measure used as an indicator of outcome was the 5-minute Apgar score which, according to the authors, is an indicator of the health of the mother and fetus during pregnancy and a predictor of neurologic outcome for the infant. Since the authors were interested in certain interactive effects of stress with other variables, they used some of the original variables to calculate several interactive terms that were included in a

## Multiple Regression, Continued

**Table 8-3.** Partial Correlation of Squared Study Variables with Original Study Variables, Controlling for Original Study Variables, for Surgical Patients ($N = 216$)

| Variable $x$ | Correlation of $x$ with Hospital Stress | Partial Correlation of $x^2$ with Hospital Stress, Controlling for $x$ |
|---|---|---|
| Age | −.27* | −.09 |
| Life stress 1 year prior to hospitalization | .22* | .10 |
| Life stress 1–2 years prior to hospitalization | .28* | .15* |
| Pain | .26* | .00 |

*$p < .05$.

multiple regression analysis. As you will see below, neither all of the original variables, nor all possible interaction terms were included, but only those of interest to the researchers. Data included in Table 8-4 are from the published analysis.

(a) Which of the independent variables in this analysis is the single best predictor of Apgar scores?

**Table 8-4.** Stepwise Multiple Regression Analysis for Prediction of Infant Apgar Scores at 5 minutes ($N = 51$)

| Predictor Variables | $R$ | $R^2$ | $r_{x \cdot y}$ (Zero-Order Correlation with Apgar Score) |
|---|---|---|---|
| 1. Stress × illness-proneness | .3291 | .1083 | −.3291 |
| 2. Stress × pregnancy symptoms in first trimester | .4361 | .1901 | −.4338 |
| 3. Stress × pregnancy symptoms in third trimester | .4754 | .2260 | −.4325 |
| 4. Stress × number of past pregnancy complications | .7413 | .5496 | −.6748 |
| 5. Months since last delivery | .8685 | .7542 | .4591 |
| 6. Number of medications | .8828 | .7794 | −.2313 |
| 7. Hemoglobin at discharge | .8902 | .7925 | .2574 |
| 8. Length of labor—stage I | .8960 | .8028 | −.2736 |

(b) What is the significance of the fact that some of the zero-order correlations are negative and some are positive?
(c) How much of the variation in Apgar scores can be explained by the interaction between stress and illness-proneness?
(d) How can you tell that the researchers exerted some control over the order in which variables were entered in this analysis, that is, that it is not an ordinary stepwise regression with order of entry determined by relationships in the data?
(e) Determine for each step of this analysis whether the increase in $R^2$ is significant.
(f) Explain in your own words the substantive meaning of the increase in $R^2$ from the first to the second step of the regression analysis.
(g) Repeat f for the other steps in the analysis.
(h) Taking shrinkage into account, what proportion of the population variance can be explained by the eight variables used in the above analysis?
(i) What sort of analysis would you have to carry out to determine whether the interaction between stress and illness-proneness contributes significantly to the prediction of Apgar scores over and above the effects of these two variables considered individually?

# Chapter 9
# ANALYSIS OF VARIANCE AND MULTIPLE COMPARISONS

**USES OF ANALYSIS OF VARIANCE**

In an earlier chapter we discussed the use of $t$ tests to study differences between two means. When the data are such that more than two means are to be tested, the $t$ test is no longer applicable. Analysis of variance, usually called *ANOVA,* is designed to allow for the simultaneous comparison of several means. The general ANOVA procedure allows for a test of the null hypothesis that all the group means are equal. It is also usually of interest to the researcher to study differences between various groups in detail, since some may be alike and some different. There are many different techniques for making these comparisons among the various group means, referred to by the general name of *multiple comparisons.* This chapter includes a detailed discussion of the general ANOVA technique, as well as an introduction to several different multiple comparison procedures.

One common situation in which ANOVA may be used is controlled experimental studies. For example, consider a study of the effects of a new antihypertensive drug on blood pressure. Suppose that the investigator wants to determine whether the new drug is better at reducing blood pressure than a commonly used standard drug and also whether the dosage of the new drug makes any difference. The investigator randomizes patients into four groups:

Group 1:  Control, standard drug
Group 2:  Low level of new drug
Group 3:  Medium level of new drug
Group 4:  High level of new drug

The patients are kept on the drugs for a month, and then blood pressures are obtained. The analytic procedure usually done in such a situation is

ANOVA, to test the null hypothesis of no difference in mean blood pressure among the four groups. If the effect of the new drug is the same as that of the standard drug, this null hypothesis would be retained. Additionally, the researcher would want to determine whether the three different doses of the new drug considered have different effects on blood pressure, and this could be tested by use of a multiple comparison procedure.

Analysis of variance can also be used in nonexperimental situations where more than two means are to be compared. Suppose that data on samples of patients from three general hospitals are used to calculate average length of stay for each hospital. In such a case, ANOVA could be used to determine whether there is a significant difference in mean length of stay for the three hospitals. Or suppose that a researcher collects data on salary level and type of education for a large sample of nurses. Then ANOVA would be used to determine whether there is any difference in salary among the various nurse groups (e.g., associate degree, diploma, baccalaureate). In any similar situation, where means of one variable are to be compared for groups classified according to another variable, ANOVA is appropriate.

The $t$ test for the difference between two means is really just a special case of ANOVA. You will see that when only two means are compared, the test used for the ANOVA procedure is equivalent to the $t$ test for the difference between two means. The general ANOVA procedure covers any situation where group means are to be compared. It should be noted here that for the ANOVA procedure to be discussed in this chapter, the groups to be compared are assumed to be independent. If observations are correlated (e.g., before–after measures on the same individuals), the methods to be presented here are not valid. Such data would be handled by *repeated measures ANOVA,* to be described in Chapter 11. The model we discuss here is called *one-way ANOVA,* as distinguished from more complicated ANOVA designs to be presented in subsequent chapters.

## THE ONE-WAY ANOVA MODEL

For the ANOVA situation, we can think of observations on $x_{ij}$, the continuous variable, for individuals in each of several independent groups, where each group is assumed to be a random sample from the corresponding population. The notations of these observations are shown in Table 9-1.

For example, $x_{24}$ represents the observation on the fourth individual listed in group 2, $n_3$ is the symbol for the number of individuals in group 3, and $\bar{x}_7$ refers to the mean value of all the observations in group 7.

# Analysis of Variance and Multiple Comparisons

**Table 9-1** Conventional Notation System for One-Way ANOVA With $k$ Groups

| Group 1 | Group 2 | | Group $k$ |
|---|---|---|---|
| $x_{11}$ | $x_{21}$ | . . . . . . . . . . . . . . . . . . . . . . . . | $x_{k1}$ |
| $x_{12}$ | $x_{22}$ | . . . . . . . . . . . . . . . . . . . . . . . . | $x_{k2}$ |
| . | . | . . . . . . . . . . . . . . . . . . . . . . . . | . |
| . | . | . . . . . . . . . . . . . . . . . . . . . . . . | . |
| . | . | . . . . . . . . . . . . . . . . . . . . . . . . | . |
| $x_{1n_1}$ | $x_{2n_2}$ | . . . . . . . . . . . . . . . . . . . . . . . . | $x_{kn_k}$ |
| $\bar{x}_1$ | $\bar{x}_2$ | | $\bar{x}_k$ |

$k$ = number of groups ($k \geq 2$)   $i$ = group number ($i = 1, 2, \ldots, k$)   $j$ = observation number   $x_{ij}$ = observation $j$ in group $i$   $n_i$ = number of observations in group $i$   $\bar{x}_i$ = mean of observations in group $i$   $\bar{x}$ = mean of all observations   $N$ = total number of observations ($N = n_1 + n_2 \cdots + n_k$)

The most commonly used type of ANOVA is referred to as *model I*, or the *fixed-effects model*, and this is the model to be used in this chapter (other models will be discussed in subsequent chapters). In the fixed effects model, the observations ($x_{ij}$) within each group ($i$) are assumed to be normally distributed around a population mean ($\mu_i$) with population variance $\sigma^2$, variance in all groups assumed equal. Each observation in group $i$ can, therefore, be expressed as

$$x_{ij} = \mu_i + e_{ij}$$

where $e_{ij}$ represents the random element in each observation due to variation around the mean.

The mean of all the population values is referred to as $\mu$, and $\mu$ is, of course, the average of all of the group population means ($\mu_i$). The amount by which each group mean ($\mu_i$) deviates from the mean of all values ($\mu$) is assumed to be fixed, although unknown, and denoted by $\alpha_i$. In other words, for any $\mu_i$,

$$\mu_i = \mu + \alpha_i$$

Substituting this value for $\mu_i$ in the above equation for $x_{ij}$, we have

$$x_{ij} = \mu + \alpha_i + e_{ij}$$

the mathematical model for ANOVA.

The value of $\alpha_i$, the amount by which the mean in group $i$ deviates from the grand mean, is called the *treatment effect*, that is, the average effect on observation $x_{ij}$ due to the fact that it belongs to group $i$. Because of the treatment effects, each group may have a different mean, but the variance is assumed to be the same in each group. Real data seldom meet these assumptions precisely. The effect of departures from the assumptions of normality and homogeneity of variance depend on the extent of the deviation. Snedecor and Cochran[41] discuss this issue and situations in which nonnormality and heterogeneity of variance are likely to be problematical.

## PARTITIONING THE SUM OF SQUARES IN ONE-WAY ANOVA

As indicated in the ANOVA model, any observation $x_{ij}$ can deviate from the mean of all the observations because of a treatment effect ($\alpha_i$) and/or because of random variation within its group ($e_{ij}$). The ANOVA procedure allows us to separate and measure these two effects. Recall that for any sample of observations, the estimate of variance is the average of squared deviations of those observations from their mean, or

$$s^2 = \frac{\sum_{i=1}^{n} (x_i - \bar{x})^2}{n - 1}$$

Using the notation introduced above, we will now write the estimate of variance of observations in an ANOVA problem. Because of the classification of observations into groups, each value is noted as $x_{ij}$ instead of as $x_i$, and so the formula looks a little more complicated:

$$s^2 = \frac{\sum_{i=1}^{k} \sum_{j=1}^{n_i} (x_{ij} - \bar{x})^2}{N - 1}$$

The term "analysis of variance" means literally the analysis of this variation among all the observations in the study. In order to analyze this variation, we work with the numerator

$$\sum_{i=1}^{k} \sum_{j=1}^{n_i} (x_{ij} - \bar{x})^2$$

which is called the *total sum of squares*, denoted by $SS_T$.

Analysis of Variance and Multiple Comparisons    197

The total sum of squares can be partitioned, by simple algebraic manipulation, into three parts, so that

$$\sum_{i=1}^{k}\sum_{j=1}^{n_i} (x_{ij} - \bar{x})^2 = \sum_{i=1}^{k}\sum_{j=1}^{n_i} (x_{ij} - \bar{x}_i)^2$$
$$+ 2 \sum_{i=1}^{k}\sum_{j=1}^{n_i} (x_{ij} - \bar{x}_i)(\bar{x}_i - \bar{x})$$
$$+ \sum_{i=1}^{k} n_i (\bar{x}_i - \bar{x})^2$$

The middle term on the right, called the *cross-product*, can be shown to equal 0, and so

$$\sum_{i=1}^{k}\sum_{j=1}^{n_i} (x_{ij} - \bar{x})^2 = \sum_{i=1}^{k}\sum_{j=1}^{n_i} (x_{ij} - \bar{x})^2$$
$$+ \sum_{i=1}^{k} n_i (\bar{x}_i - \bar{x})^2$$

The total sum of squares, therefore, can be partitioned, or divided into two parts. These will be shown below to represent two different kinds of variation among the sample observations.

The first quantity,

$$\sum_{i=1}^{k}\sum_{j=1}^{n_i} (x_{ij} - \bar{x}_i)^2$$

is calculated by taking the deviation of each observation from the mean for its group, squaring each of these deviations, and adding them, first within each group and then across all the groups. For each group, the sum of squared deviations is the numerator of the variance estimate for that group, so that the above formula actually represents a variance estimate pooled across all the groups. It is a measure of variation among observations within groups, that is, around each group mean, and is called the *within-groups sum of squares* or the *error sum of squares*, and denoted by $SS_W$.

Remember that earlier we expressed each observation as

$$x_{ij} = \mu_i + e_{ij}$$

where $e_{ij}$ represents variation around the mean in group $i$. If the sample mean $\bar{x}_i$ is substituted for the unknown population mean $\mu_i$, this formula becomes

$$x_{ij} = \bar{x}_i + e_{ij}$$

or

$$x_{ij} - \bar{x}_i = e_{ij}$$

Therefore, we could write the within-groups sum of squares,

$$\sum_{i=1}^{k} \sum_{j=1}^{n_i} (x_{ij} - \bar{x}_i)^2$$

as

$$\sum_{i=1}^{k} \sum_{j=1}^{n_i} e_{ij}^2$$

which also indicates that this part of the total sum of squares represents variation of observations around their means within groups.

The second quantity in the partition of the total sum of squares

$$\sum_{i=1}^{k} n_i(\bar{x}_i - \bar{x})^2$$

is calculated by taking the deviation of each group mean from the grand mean, squaring, multiplying by the number of observations in each group, and adding across all the groups. Since $\bar{x}$ (the estimate of $\mu$) is the mean of all the group means, this quantity is also measure of variance (if the group means are considered as individual observations) since $\bar{x}$ can thus be interpreted as a sum of squared deviations of observations from their mean. The quantity is a measure of variation due to differences among the groups and is called the *between-groups sum of squares* or the *treatment sum of squares* and is denoted by $SS_B$.

Reference back to the notation used for the ANOVA model is again instructive. Recall that each group mean was expressed as $\mu_i = \mu + \alpha_i$, where $\alpha_i$ represents the treatment effect of group $i$. Substitution of the sample values for group means and for the grand mean changes this expression to

$$\bar{x}_i = \bar{x} + \hat{\alpha}_i$$

or

$$\bar{x}_i - \bar{x} = \hat{\alpha}_i$$

Therefore, we could write the between-groups sum of squares,

$$\sum_{i=1}^{k} n_i (\bar{x}_i - \bar{x})^2$$

Analysis of Variance and Multiple Comparisons

as

$$\sum_{i=1}^{k} n_i \alpha_i^2$$

which shows that the between-groups sum of squares represents the estimated treatment effects, weighted according to the number of observations in each group.

The total sum of squares has $N - 1$ degrees of freedom. The partition just described is associated with a partition of the total degrees of freedom into two parts. The within groups sum of squares is a pooled estimate of variance across all the groups, and one degree of freedom is lost for the variance estimate within each group. The degrees of freedom associated with the variance estimate in group $i$ is, therefore, $n_i - 1$. The within-groups degrees of freedom then becomes

$$(n_1 - 1) + (n_2 - 1) + \cdots + (n_k - 1) = (n_1 + n_2 + \cdots + n_k)$$
$$- (1 + 1 + \cdots + 1)$$
$$= N - k$$

The between-groups sum of squares is an estimate of variance of the group means from the grand mean, and the degrees of freedom for a variance estimate is the number of observations minus 1. In this case the number of observations is $k$, the number of groups, and thus the degrees of freedom for the between-groups sum of squares is $k - 1$. Note tht the degrees of freedom associated with the two pieces of the partition sum to the total degrees of freedom, that is,

$$(N - k) + (k - 1) = N - 1$$

The partition of the total sum of squares just described forms the basis for testing the ANOVA null hypothesis of no difference in group means. As in the regression analysis presented in earlier chapters, a ratio of mean squares forms a test statistic with an $F$ distribution. In the next section we describe how to use the ANOVA partition to test a hypothesis, with an application to an actual research situation. The fact that this ANOVA is a special case of regression analysis will also be shown.

## TESTING THE ONE-WAY ANOVA HYPOTHESIS

The $F$ ratio that provides the test statistic in ANOVA is a ratio of two mean squares, in this case the *mean square between groups* and the *mean square within groups.* The mean squares are formed as described in the regression chapters, by dividing each sum of squares by its corresponding degrees of freedom. Thus the mean square between groups, which is also called the *treatment mean square,* is calculated as

$$MS_B = \frac{\text{Between-groups sum of squares}}{\text{Between-groups degrees of freedom}}$$

$$= \frac{SS_B}{k-1}$$

$$= \frac{\sum_{i=1}^{k} n_i (\bar{x}_i - \bar{x})^2}{k-1}$$

And, the mean square within groups, sometimes referred to as the *error mean square,* is calculated as

$$MS_W = \frac{\text{Within-groups sum of squares}}{\text{Within-groups degrees of freedom}}$$

$$= \frac{SS_W}{N-k}$$

$$= \frac{\sum_{i=1}^{k} \sum_{j=1}^{n_i} (x_{ij} - \bar{x}_i)^2}{N-k}$$

The mean square within groups is actually a pooled estimate of variance. It is the weighted average of the sample variance within each group. If we refer to the within-group sample variances as $s_1^2, s_1^2, \ldots, s_k^2$, the pooled estimate of variance is

$$s_p^2 = \frac{(n_1 - 1) s_1^2 + (n_2 - 1) s_2^2 + \cdots + (n_k - 1) s_k^2}{n_1 + n_2 + \cdots + n_k - k}$$

which is another way of writing the mean square within groups. By looking back to Chapter 3, you can verify that when $k = 2$, that is, when there are two groups, the mean square within groups is the pooled estimate of variance used in the ordinary $t$ test for the difference between two groups.

The mean square between groups and the mean square within groups are used to form a test statistic for the null hypothesis of no difference

Analysis of Variance and Multiple Comparisons

among the group means. It can be shown mathematically that, when the null hypothesis is true,

$$F = \frac{MS_B}{MS_W}$$

$$= \frac{SS_B/(k-1)}{SS_W/(N-k)}$$

$$= \frac{\sum_{i=1}^{k} n_i (\bar{x}_i - \bar{x})^2/(k-1)}{\sum_{i=1}^{k}\sum_{j=1}^{n_i} (x_{ij} - \bar{x}_i)^2/(N-k)}$$

has an $F$ distribution with $k - 1$ and $N - k$ degrees of freedom. The following example illustrates the use of this $F$ ratio in an ANOVA situation with four group means.

In a study designed to investigate the effect of different instructional methods on student achievement[16], one hundred students enrolled in an introductory microbiology class were randomly assigned to one of four treatment groups. Three of the groups were given a minicourse designed to inform hospital personnel about problems involved in contamination and decontamination of respiratory therapy equipment, and the fourth group, which served as a control, received a commercial programmed instruction booklet to read. The three experimental groups received programmed instruction (PI), and audiovisual instruction (AV), and a combination of both kinds of instruction (AV-PI), respectively. Scores on the subject matter achievement test were obtained for each subject at the end of the instruction period. The investigator used ANOVA for an overall test for differences in mean achievement scores in the four groups.

The null hypothesis for ANOVA, just like the null hypothesis for a $t$ test, is that there is no difference among the group means. For ANOVA, this is written

$$H: \mu_1 = \mu_2 = \cdots = \mu_k$$

According to this hypothesis, the population means are all equivalued. In other words, for the example described, the null hypothesis is that there is no difference in mean achievement test scores for the hypothetical populations represented by the four treatment groups.

The mean achievement test scores for the four groups were calculated as indicated in Table 9-2.

**Table 9-2** Post-test Scores on Achievement Test ($N = 100$)

| Group | N | Mean score | SD* |
|---|---|---|---|
| Programmed instruction | 28 | 71.00 | 8.35 |
| Audiovisual instruction | 30 | 68.13 | 10.79 |
| Programmed and audiovisual instruction | 16 | 71.38 | 9.65 |
| Control | 26 | 52.85 | 8.30 |

*Standard deviation.

According to the sample data, all three experimental forms of instruction resulted in higher mean scores on the achievement test than the control group. Inspection of Table 9-1 leads one to suspect that there may be no differences in achievement means for the three experimental groups. A hypothesis test for a significant difference in means, taking standard errors into account, is now needed.

The results of ANOVA are customarily presented in a table such as Table 9-3. The figures for our example are given in Table 9-4. You can verify the mean-square figures and the $F$ value by your own calculations.

Using the $F$ ratio from the above table, and the fact that this ratio is known to have an $F$ distribution with $k - 1$ and $N - k$ degrees of freedom, you can easily test the null hypothesis $H: \mu_1 = \mu_2 = \mu_3 = \mu_4$. With

$$k - 1 = 4 - 1 = 3$$

**Table 9-3.** Analysis of Variance for Differences among Group Means

| Source of Variation | Sum of Squares | DF | Mean Square | F |
|---|---|---|---|---|
| Between groups (treatment) | $\sum_{i=1}^{k} n_i (\bar{x}_i - \bar{x}^2)$ | $k - 1$ | $MS_B$ | $MS_B/MSW$ |
| Within groups (error) | $\sum_{i=1}^{k} \sum_{j=1}^{n_i} (x_{ij} - \bar{x}_i)^2$ | $N - k$ | $MS_W$ | |
| Total | $\sum_{i=1}^{k} \sum_{j=1}^{n_i} (x_{ij} - \bar{x})^2$ | $N - 1$ | | |

Analysis of Variance and Multiple Comparisons

**Table 9-4** Analysis of Variance for Group Differences in Posttest scores on achievement test ($N = 100$)

| Source of Variation | Sum of squares | D.F. | Mean square | F |
|---|---|---|---|---|
| Between groups | 6939.02 | 3 | 2312.010 | 29.920* |
| Within groups | 7418.34 | 96 | 77.274 | |
| Total | 14354.36 | 99 | | |

*$p < .01$.

degrees of freedom for the numerator and

$$N - k = 100 - 4 = 96$$

degrees of freedom for the denominator, the $F$ value required for significance at the .05 level is

$$F_{.05}(3, 80) = 2.72$$

The value of 96 degrees of freedom is usually not given in tables of the $F$ distribution, and so 80 was used here. The $F$-test statistic in this case is $F = 29.920$, which is clearly larger than 2.72, indicating that the null hypothesis should be rejected. There is a significant difference in post-test scores among the four instructional groups, according to the statistical test.

The $F$ test is always a one-tailed test, and the calculated $F$ value is always greater than zero, since it is a ratio of sums of squares. Recollection of what is represented by the between- and within-group sums of squares will clarify the nature of the $F$ value. Remember that

$$MS_B = \frac{\sum_{i=1}^{k} n_i (\bar{x}_i - \bar{x})^2}{k - 1}$$

The value of $MS_B$, which is the numerator of the $F$ value, tends to be small if the sample group means, which estimate $\mu_1$, $\mu_2$, $\mu_3$, and $\mu_4$, are close together. This is likely to happen if there is no difference between the population means. In this case, the differences between the sample means result from sampling error or chance, and the differences should be relatively small. If there really are differences between the population means, there should be larger discrepancies among the sample group means, reflecting the fact that different populations are being sampled. The result of this should be a relatively larger $MS_B$. The denominator of $F$, which is $MS_W$, estimates the normal variation in groups, regardless of their means, and does not change when means are unequal. In cases where the null hypothesis is false, therefore, the $F$ value will tend to be large. This is exactly what we want, because it is precisely in those cases where the null hypothesis is false that we want evidence to reject it.

Before we continue, let us note that the ANOVA we have just described is actually a special case of regression analysis. In the example just presented, type of group instruction can be considered a predictor of posttest achievement score. To analyze these data in regression form, we would need to create dummy variables, since the type of group instruction is a categorical variable. Because there are four categories for this variable, the number of dummy variables would be 3. A multiple regression analysis using the three dummy variables as predictors of posttest achievement scores would determine whether type of instruction significantly predicts achievement, and the regression table would be as indicated in Table 9-5.

Now, in Table 9-5, let us substitute $x_{ij}$ values for $y_{ij}$ values, $N$ for $n$, and 3 for $k$, since there are three predictors. In addition, recall that when predictors in regression are categorical, the predicted value for each individual is the mean of the group to which that individual belongs. This means that we can substitute $\bar{x}_i$ for $\bar{y}'_i$. With appropriate changes in the summation signs to account for the fact that we are labeling our observations $x_{ij}$ instead of $y_i$, the first three columns of the table become those shown in Table 9-6.

As you may have guessed by now, this is the ANOVA table we developed in this chapter! The mean square and the resulting $F$ value for regression analysis will yield the same results as the ANOVA. Analysis of variance is really just regression analysis with categorical independent

**Table 9-5** Regression Analysis of Variance with $k$ Predictors Using $y_i$ Notation

| Source of Variation | Sum of Squares | DF | Mean Square | F |
|---|---|---|---|---|
| Regression | $\sum_{i=1}^{n}(y'_i - \bar{y})^2$ | $k$ | $MS_R$ | $MS_R/MS_D$ |
| Deviation | $\sum_{i=1}^{n}(y_i - y'_i)^2$ | $n - k - 1$ | $MS_D$ | |
| Total | $\sum_{i=1}^{n}(y_i - \bar{y})^2$ | $n - 1$ | | |

Analysis of Variance and Multiple Comparisons

**Table 9-6** Regression Analysis of Variance with three Predictors Using $x_{ij}$ Notation

| Source of Variation | Sum of Squares | DF |
|---|---|---|
| Regression | $\sum_{i=1}^{k} n_i (\bar{x}_i - \bar{x})^2$ | 3 |
| Deviation | $\sum_{i=1}^{k} \sum_{j=1}^{n_i} (x_{ij} - \bar{x}_i)^2$ | 96 |
| Total | $\sum_{i=1}^{k} \sum_{j=1}^{n_i} (x_{ij} - \bar{x})^2$ | 99 |

variables, even though it is often presented as a method of analysis completely different from regression.

Although the null hypothesis in ANOVA is usually stated as "no difference in the group means," the correspondence of this analysis with regression analysis means that the null hypothesis can also be stated as "group membership does not account for a significant proportion of the variation in the dependent variable." In Chapter 7, the formula

$$R^2 = \frac{SS_R}{SS_T}$$

was given for calculating $R^2$ from the sums of squares in the regression ANOVA. For the traditional ANOVA presented in this chapter, the "regression" sum of squares is commonly called the "between-groups" or "treatment" sum of squares. Therefore, the proportion of variance in the dependent variable accounted for by group membership in ANOVA is

$$R^2 = \frac{\text{Between-groups sum of squares}}{\text{Total sum of squares}}$$
$$= \frac{SS_B}{SS_T}$$

It is not common to calculate $R^2$ for traditional ANOVA analyses, but it is often instructive. You may find cases where there is a highly significant difference among the means, according to the $F$ test, but where $R^2$ is fairly low. This is important because of the tendency to view significant ANOVA results as more impressive or more scientific than significant regression results, which typically have fairly low $R^2$ values. Often the corresponding $R^2$ for ANOVA is no larger than a typical $R^2$ for regression analysis (e.g.,

.25 or .30). The tendency for such low values to occur is due to the difficulty of precisely measuring variables characteristic of behavioral sciences, as well as to the multiplicity of causes likely to be responsible for the variation in the dependent variable. It should be clear now that the choice between ANOVA and regression analysis can be based on the form taken by the independent variables or even just on what particular computer programs are available.

We now come to the subject of multiple comparisons. The $F$ test in our example has indicated a significant difference in means. This does not mean that all of the population means are different from each other, but just that they are not all the same. Multiple comparisons are statistical procedures to identify which groups differ and which do not. Several different types of multiple comparison procedures will be introduced in the following section, and references for further study will be provided.

## MULTIPLE COMPARISONS

There are many research situations in which an investigator is unlikely to be satisfied with the overall $F$ test provided by the ANOVA procedure. For example, in the ANOVA problem described in the previous section, the study involved the four following groups, classified by type of instruction:

Group 1: Programmed instruction
Group 2: Audio-visual instruction
Group 3: Programmed and audiovisual instruction
Group 4: Control

Rejection of the null hypothesis $H: \mu_1 = \mu_2 = \mu_3 = \mu_4$ allows the researcher to conclude only that the four groups are not the same on posttest achievement scores. It is very likely that this researcher would want to know whether there are any differences in achievement between programmed and audiovisual instruction and whether both types of instruction together lead to higher achievement scores than either type alone. Such information can be determined from the data by use of what are called *multiple comparison procedures,* or procedures for making several comparisons among group means.

As another example, consider a design fairly common in nursing research. Several nursing studies have been done to test the effects of preoperative teaching procedures on various outcomes for surgical patients Often the investigator, in addition to a control group receiving no pre erative teaching and an experimental group receiving the teaching i. ⌣r-vention, will include a third group who receive attention and psychological support, but no teaching per se. The purpose for inclusion of the third group, of course, is to determine whether gains in the experimental group are due to the teaching itself or just to the extra attention. Ordinary ANOVA of such data yields a test of $H$: $\mu_1 = \mu_2 = \mu_3$ and rejection of this null hypothesis indicates that the three group means are not all the same. Questions about whether the teaching makes any difference in outcome, over and above that obtained by psychological support alone, require further analysis using some sort of multiple comparison procedure.

At first glance, it might not seem necessary to describe any new kinds of test for these multiple comparisons of group means. It would be possible to calculate a $t$ test for the difference in means for any two means of interest. If there were four groups in a study, for example, there would be six possible comparisons of two means. The problem with such a procedure is that as the number of $t$ tests increases, the likelihood of obtaining significant results by chance alone also increases. Thus in repeated application of $t$ tests to the same data base, the probability of finding statistically significant results, given no actual difference in population means, tends to increase (i.e., the Type I error tends to increase). It is for this reason that many different procedures for multiple comparisons have been devised, with the intent of allowing for several comparisons among group means while keeping the probability of Type I error low, so that the researcher is protected against falsely claiming too many significant differences in means.

A *contrast* or a *comparison* of group means is a linear combination of group means such as

$$\bar{x}_1 - \bar{x}_2$$

or

$$\bar{x}_1 - \bar{x}_3$$

or

$$\bar{x}_1 + \bar{x}_2 - 2\bar{x}_3$$

constructed in such a way that the sum of the coefficients of the $\bar{x}_i$ is equal to zero. Thus the general definition of a contrast can be written as

$$L = \lambda_1 \bar{x}_1 + \lambda_2 \bar{x}_2 + \cdots + \lambda_k \bar{x}_k, \qquad \sum_{i=1}^{k} \lambda_i = 0$$

In the example used earlier in the chapter, where several types of instruction were compared, suppose that one wanted to compare programmed instruction (Group 1) with audiovisual instruction (Group 2).

The contrast that would allow for such a comparison is

$$L_1 = \bar{x}_1 - \bar{x}_2$$

and in this case, $\lambda_1 = 1$, $\lambda_2 = -1$, $\lambda_3 = 0$, and $\lambda_4 = 0$. That is, groups 3 and 4 have been eliminated from the comparison by making $\lambda_3 = 0$ and $\lambda_4 = 0$. To compare the combination of programmed instruction plus audiovisual instruction (group 3) with the average of each method alone (groups 1 and 2), one would write the contrast

$$L_2 = \bar{x}_1 + \bar{x}_2 - 2\bar{x}_3$$

Note that $\lambda_4 = 0$, since the control group (group 4) is not included in the comparison, and also that

$$\sum_{i=1}^{k} \lambda_i = 1 + 1 - 2 + 0$$
$$= 0$$

Multiple comparison procedures allow one to define, for any situation, several comparisons such as those above, and then to carry out hypothesis tests related to population values of the comparisons, each based on the null hypothesis that the contrast is equal to zero. For example,

$$H: \mu_1 = \mu_2$$

or, equivalently,

$$H: \mu_1 - \mu_2 = 0$$

would be tested by using the contrast

$$L = \bar{x}_1 - \bar{x}_2$$

to form the test statistic. Or,

$$H: \frac{\mu_1 + \mu_2}{2} = \mu_3$$

or, equivalently,

$$H: \mu_1 + \mu_2 - 2\mu_3 = 0$$

would be tested by the contrast

$$L = \bar{x}_1 + \bar{x}_2 - 2\bar{x}_3$$

According to this latter contrast, the null hypothesis claims that the mean in Group 3 is equal to the average of Groups 1 and 2. In the example on various types of instruction, this null hypothesis would claim that a group receiving programmed instruction plus audiovisual instruction scores no better in achievement, on the average, than groups receiving either method of instruction alone.

The variance of a contrast $L$ is estimated by

$$MS_w \sum_{i=1}^{k} \frac{\lambda_i^2}{n_i}$$

and the null hypothesis that the contrast $L$ equals zero can be tested by a $t$ test of the form

$$t = \frac{L}{\sqrt{MS_w \sum_{i=1}^{k} \frac{\lambda_i^2}{n_i}}}$$

with $N - k$ degrees of freedom. A decision to accept or reject the null hypothesis can be made by using the usual $t$-test procedure. The problem with just repeating this test for every contrast of interest, as already mentioned, is that the probability of a Type I error increases with the number of tests performed. Various multiple comparison procedures have been designed to handle this problem. Prior to giving an overview of such procedures, we distinguish between comparisons that are planned or anticipated prior to data collection and ones that are based on inspection of the data.

A theoretical distinction is usually made between *a priori* comparisons, which are planned prior to data collection and based on the specific research questions to be answered, and *a posteriori* comparisons, which are made subsequent to the data collection and may be determined by inspection of the group means. A priori comparisons would be used in cases where specific hypotheses have been formulated about which groups should differ and which should not, based on the rationale behind the research. In the example on types of instruction, an obvious a priori comparison would be the three instruction groups with the control group, since one intent of the study is to determine whether instruction of any kind leads to higher achievement scores than none at all. A posteriori comparisons are ones that are unplanned, and the researcher usually picks out those means that appear to be dissimilar and tests them to see whether the differences are statistically significant. Logically, a priori comparisons are made regardless of whether the ANOVA $F$ is significant, and a posteriori comparisons only follow the finding of a significant $F$. This distinction is not always clear in practice.

There are several a posteriori (also called *post hoc*) multiple comparison procedures designed to allow for the comparison of all pairs of means following a significant $F$ from the ANOVA. The procedures vary according to the manner in which they control for Type I error. For the least-significant difference *(LSD)* method, developed by R. A. Fisher, the means are first ranked, and the largest compared with the smallest, by calculating the test statistic for the appropriate contrast and using the same specified error rate for each comparison. If the difference is found to be significant, the second largest is compared with the smallest, and so on. The result of this procedure is an analysis of which population means differ from which other population means. A similar procedure is the *studentized range*, developed by Tukey. The studentized range procedure is similar to the LSD method but requires that the sample sizes be equal or nearly equal and is designed to be more conservative than the LSD. In other words, fewer significant differences will be declared by Tukey's procedure than by the LSD. Another variant, called *Duncan's new multiple-range test*, tends to be more powerful than the other tests; thus there is a high probability of declaring a difference when there actually is a difference between the population means. Dunnett's test provides for the comparison of a control group with each of any number of experimental groups. Winer[46], Snedecor and Cochran[41], and Ferguson[14] all include fairly detailed discussions of many multiple comparison procedures, and all would be good references on this subject.

In addition to a posteriori comparisons developed for pairwise comparisons among means, there is a more general procedure, developed by Scheffé, which allows for all possible comparisons among means. This method is described in some detail in the next section of this book as an example of a method for making a posteriori comparisons. It has been included because it is general, easy to use, and commonly included in packaged computer programs. Next, use of a method called *orthogonal contrasts* for making a priori comparisons is described. Orthogonal contrasts allow the researcher to analyze the between groups sum of squares from ANOVA by dividing it into several independent parts representing differences between various group means. The last section of this chapter describes how orthogonal contrasts can be used for trend analysis.

# Analysis of Variance and Multiple Comparisons

## SCHEFFÉ TESTS

Scheffé tests are designed to allow for comparisons of all possible combinations of group means to determine which differ and which do not. The tests are designed in such a way that the probability of a Type I error is at most .01 or .05 (as set by the researcher) for any of the possible comparisons. This criterion makes it one of the most conservative multiple comparison procedures, so that it tends to yield fewer significant results than other methods. However, it is easy to use, can be used for making a posteriori comparisons (chosen after inspection of the data), and can be used for making any comparisons desired.

The procedure for Scheffé's test involves calculation of a test statistic that follows the $F$ distribution when the null hypothesis is true. As you will see, however, the fact that the Type I error is kept low means that the critical value with which the $F$ statistic is compared is determined in a slightly different way from the procedure for $F$ tests previously described. The $F$ ratio used to test the difference between two means, say, $\bar{x}_i$ and $\bar{x}_j$, is calculated as

$$F = \frac{(\bar{x}_i - \bar{x}_j)^2}{MS_w/n_i + MS_w/n_j}$$

where $n_i$ and $n_j$ are the number of subjects in groups $i$ and $j$, respectively, and $MS_w$ is the mean square within groups. An algebraically equivalent formula is

$$F = \frac{(\bar{x}_i - \bar{x}_j)^2}{MS_w \left[(n_i + n_j)/n_i n_j\right]}$$

To test the null hypothesis

$$H: \mu_i = \mu_j$$

one first consults the $F$ table to determine the $F$ required for significance at the desired level (e.g., .01 or .05), using $k - 1$ and $N - k$ degrees of freedom. Recall that $k$ is the number of groups and $N$ is the total number of subjects. Call this value $F_T$. Next, calculate

$$F' = (k - 1) \times F_T$$

The null hypothesis is rejected at the chosen level of significance whenever the $F$ statistic calculated for the comparison exceeds $F'$.

As an example, suppose that we wish to determine, for the example described in the previous two sections in this chapter, whether the mean posttest score for group 1 (programmed instruction) differs from the mean posttest score for group 2 (audiovisual instruction). The null hypothesis of no difference $H: \mu_1 = \mu_2$ is tested by calculating the test statistic

$$F = \frac{(\bar{x}_1 - \bar{x}_2)^2}{MS_w/n_1 + MS_w/n_2}$$

This $F$-test statistic, by substitution of the values for the example, is

$$F = \frac{(71.00 - 68.13)^2}{(77.274)/28 + (77.274)/30}$$
$$= 1.54$$

With $k - 1 = 4 - 1 = 3$ and $N - k = 100 - 4 = 96$ degrees of freedom, the $F$ required for significance at the .05 level (using 90 degrees of freedom for the denominator) is $F_T = 2.71$. Next,

$$F' = (k - 1) \times F_T$$
$$= (4 - 1) \times 2.71$$
$$= 8.13$$

The calculated $F$ statistic, $F = 1.54$, is less than 8.13, and so the null hypothesis of no difference between the means is retained. The analysis does not provide evidence that programmed instruction leads to better or worse achievement than audiovisual instruction. Similar comparisons could be carried out for any other pairs of means in this example.

The Scheffé method can be extended to any multiple comparison desired. For example,

$$H: \mu_1 + \mu_2 = \mu_3 + \mu_4$$

or

$$H: \mu_1 + \mu_2 + \mu_3 = 3\mu_4$$

and so on, can be tested by this method. Because of the fact that the procedure tends to be more conservative than others, a researcher will sometimes use a .10 level of significance instead of .01 or .05. Scheffé's method is a simple and straightforward procedure that allows for any comparisons of interest and that is available in several packaged programs (e.g., *Statistical Package for the Social Sciences*).

## ORTHOGONAL CONTRASTS

*Orthogonal contrasts* are a priori contrasts, which means that they are generally determined prior to data collection and based on the research questions posed by the study. They are chosen in such a way that they represent different, nonoverlapping sources of variation between the treatment groups. The procedure for orthogonal contrasts allows one to take the between-groups sum of squares and subdivide it into parts, each representing one of the contrasts. The word "orthogonal" simply refers to the independence among such contrasts, that is, the fact that they represent different pieces of the between-groups sum of squares. The researcher defines the contrasts in such a way as to make them orthogonal by following the mathematical rule described below. Mathematically, the requirement that insures orthogonality for two contrasts,

$$L_1 = \lambda_{11}\bar{x}_1 + \lambda_{12}\bar{x}_2 + \cdots + \lambda_{1k}\bar{x}_k$$

and

$$L_2 = \lambda_{21}\bar{x}_1 + \lambda_{22}\bar{x}_2 + \cdots + \lambda_{2k}\bar{x}_k$$

is the condition that

$$\sum_{i=1}^{k} \lambda_{1i} \lambda_{2i} = 0$$

In the example comparing the various types of instruction, the two contrasts suggested earlier,

$$L_1 = \bar{x}_1 - \bar{x}_2$$

and

$$L_2 = \bar{x}_1 + \bar{x}_2 - 2\bar{x}_3$$

are independent, because

$$\sum_{i=1}^{k} \lambda_{1i}\lambda_{2i} = \lambda_{11}\lambda_{21} + \lambda_{12}\lambda_{22} + \lambda_{13}\lambda_{23} + \lambda_{14}\lambda_{24}$$
$$= (1)(1) + (-1)(1) + (0)(-2) + (0)(0)$$
$$= 1 - 1 + 0 + 0$$
$$= 0$$

When two contrasts are orthogonal, as stated earlier, they represent different parts of the between-groups sum of squares, since this figure includes all the variation between groups. It turns out that each of the orthogonal contrasts represents a piece of the between-groups sum of squares with 1 degree of freedom. Just as the total sum of squares was partitioned into a between-groups sum of squares and a within-groups sum of squares, the between-groups sum of squares can be subdivided into contrasts. And since the between-groups sum of squares has $k - 1$ degrees of freedom, it can be divided into $k - 1$ orthogonal contrasts, each with 1 degree of freedom.

To describe a set of orthogonal contrasts, one sets up a table of the coefficients ($\lambda_{ij}$ values) to be used for each, as a way of checking on the orthogonality of the contrasts. As an example, consider the study we have discussed earlier in which various types of instruction are to be compared. The coefficients that would define the $3(k - 1)$ most logical orthogonal contrasts for this example are shown in Table 9-6a.

These coefficients define the contrasts

$$L_1 = \bar{x}_1 + \bar{x}_2 + \bar{x}_3 - 3\bar{x}_4$$
$$L_2 = \bar{x}_1 + \bar{x}_2 - 2\bar{x}_3$$
$$L_3 = \bar{x}_1 - \bar{x}_2$$

**Table 9-6a.** Coefficients Defining Orthogonal Contrasts for Comparison of Instructional Methods

|  | Group 1 (Programmed instruction) | Group 2 (Audiovisual instruction) | Group 3 (Programmed and audiovisual instruction) | Group 4 Control |
|---|---|---|---|---|
| $L_1$ | 1 | 1 | 1 | -3 |
| $L_2$ | 1 | 1 | -2 | 0 |
| $L_3$ | 1 | -1 | 0 | 0 |

# Analysis of Variance and Multiple Comparisons

and you can verify by the mathematical rule that these contrasts are indeed orthogonal.

Consider the intent of the contrasts we have just defined. They are designed to test the following three null hypotheses:

$$H_1: \frac{\mu_1 + \mu_2 + \mu_3}{3} = \mu_4$$

$$H_2: \frac{\mu_1 + \mu_2}{2} = \mu_3$$

$$H_3: \mu_1 = \mu_2$$

The corresponding research questions regarding the achievement scores are:

1. Is instruction on the average any better than no instruction?
2. Is a combination of both programmed and audiovisual instruction any better than either kind of instruction alone?
3. Is programmed instruction any better than audiovisual instruction?

These questions would be known prior to the study, since they are the obvious questions the researcher wants to answer.

After the orthogonal contrasts have been defined, the between-groups sum of squares can be partitioned into pieces corresponding to each contrast. For any contrast $L_i$,

$$SS_{L_i} = \frac{L_i^2}{\lambda_{i1}^2/n_1 + \lambda_{i2}^2/n_2 + \cdots + \lambda_{ik}^2/n_k}$$

represents that part of the between groups sum of squares associated with the contrast $L_i$. The sum of squares for each contrast is calculated in the same way. If the contrasts have been defined in such a way that they are orthogonal, the individual sums of squares will add to the between groups sum of squares from the original ANOVA. In the example with $L_1$, $L_2$, and $L_3$ defined as above, and the respective sums of squares calculated according to the formula just given, it will turn out that

$$SS_B = SS_{L_1} + SS_{L_2} + SS_{L_3}$$

where $SS_b$ is the between-groups sum of squares for the original ANOVA.

After the sum of squares associated with each contrast has been calculated, the data can be presented in a slightly modified ANOVA table, such as the one shown in Table 9-7.

Table 9-7. Mean Squares for ANOVA Using Orthogonal Contrasts

| Source of Variation | Sum of Squares | Degrees of Freedom | Mean Square | F |
|---|---|---|---|---|
| Between-groups | $SS_B$ | $k - 1$ | $MS_B$ | |
| Groups 1–3 vs group 4 | $SS_{L_1}$ | 1 | $MS_{L_1}$ | |
| Groups 1–2 vs group 3 | $SS_{L_2}$ | 1 | $MS_{L_2}$ | |
| Group 1 vs group 2 | $SS_{L_3}$ | 1 | $MS_{L_3}$ | |
| Within groups | $SS_W$ | $N - k$ | $MS_W$ | |
| Total | $SS_T$ | $N - 1$ | | |

As suggested by the table, the significance of each contrast is tested by the $F$ ratio

$$F = \frac{MS_{L_i}}{MS_w}$$
$$= \frac{SS_L/1}{SS_w/(N - k)},$$

which has an $F$ distribution with 1 and $N - k$ degrees of freedom, when the null hypothesis is true.

To illustrate how an orthogonal contrast is tested, we return to the example on differences in posttest scores by various types of instruction. Consider

$$L_1 = \bar{x}_1 + \bar{x}_2 + \bar{x}_3 - 3\bar{x}_4$$

which compares the three experimental groups with the control. Substitution of group means into the above formula gives

$$L_1 = 71.00 + 68.13 + 71.38 - 3(52.85)$$
$$= 51.96$$

as the numerical value of the contrast. The proportion of the between-groups sum of squares associated with this contrast is

Analysis of Variance and Multiple Comparisons

$$SS_{L_1} = \frac{L_1^2}{\lambda_{11}^2/n_1 + \lambda_{12}^2/n_2 + \lambda_{13}^2/n_3 + \lambda_{14}^2/n_4}$$

$$= \frac{(51.96)^2}{(1)^2/28 + (1)^2/30 + (1)^2/16 + (-3)^2/26}$$

$$= 5651.751$$

The $F$ ratio for testing the significance of this contrast is

$$F = \frac{MS_{L_1}}{MS_W}$$

$$= \frac{5651.751}{77.274}$$

$$= 73.14$$

which has an $F$ distribution with 1 and $N - k = 100 - 4 = 96$ degrees of freedom. The critical $F$ value at the .05 level with 1 and 90 degrees of freedom is $F = 3.95$, and the null hypothesis is clearly rejected. This analysis suggests that, on the average, any of the three forms of experimental instruction leads to higher achievement scores on the posttest than the control instruction. The remaining contrasts, of course, consider differences within the three experimental forms of instruction.

The partition of the between-groups sum of squares in orthogonal contrasts allows the investigator to describe in detail the nature of any differences among the group means. The between-groups sum of squares can also be divided into fewer than $k - 1$ parts. For example, since most of the between-groups sum of squares in the previous example is associated with the contrast $L_1$, the researcher could just as well leave the parts $SS_{L_2}$ and $SS_{L_3}$ lumped together, representing a sum of squares with 2 degrees of freedom. In this case the $F$ for the contrast $L_1$ is highly significant, and the $F$ for the contrasts $L_2$ and $L_3$ together,

$$F = \frac{MS_{L_2+L_3}}{MS_W} = \frac{(SS_{L_2} + SS_{L_3})/2}{MS_W}$$

(with 2 and 96 degrees of freedom) would be very low and nonsignificant. The researcher would conclude that any of the experimental forms of instruction is better than the control, in terms of achievement scores, but that the three experimental forms of instruction do not differ in their results. There are, of course, different sets of three orthogonal contrasts that could be defined for this example or for other similar kinds of data, and they should be chosen according to the research questions of interest to the investigator.

## TREND ANALYSIS

When the data come from an experiment in which the treatment groups represent equally spaced intervals along an underlying ordered continuum, there may be interest in determining whether a trend is present and what form it takes. For example, there are animal experiments in which the dose of a drug is increased by a constant amount across treatment groups, and the researcher wants to analyze the pattern of response to the varying doses, to determine at what dose the drug begins to be effective, and when the maximal effect is reached. In nursing research, the treatments may, for example, represent varying amounts of a particular nursing intervention.

Suppose that it is known that women who attend prepared childbirth education classes have lower levels of anxiety during labor and delivery than other women, as measured by a standard state anxiety scale, and it is believed that this effect is due to the knowledge and confidence gained as part of these classes. A hospital would prefer that all its prenatal patients attend such classes but they also would like to be cost-effective in running the classes. A nurse researcher has been hired to determine how much actual reduction in anxiety can be expected to result from various amounts of exposure to prepared childbirth education.

The researcher designs a study in which patients are randomized into three treatment groups. Each patient attends 4, 6, or 8 hours of classes, according to the assigned treatment. The resulting data consist of three means, representing each of the treatment groups, and, as expected, the anxiety score decreases as the number of hours of classes increases. Orthogonal contrasts can be used to test the significance of this trend and to determine whether the trend is linear (like a straight line), or whether the relationship is more complicated (curved).

You will recall from the preceding discussion of multiple comparisons that a contrast is simply a linear combination of treatment means, constructed in such a way that the sum of the coefficients is equal to zero. And orthogonal contrasts are contrasts constructed in such a way that they are independent; that is, they represent different parts of the between groups sum of squares. You will also recall that the number of orthogonal contrasts that can be tested for a given situation is equal to the number of treatment groups minus 1. For trend analysis, the number and types of trend that can be analyzed will depend on the number of treatment groups.

When there are just two treatment groups, there is only one comparison; thus

$$L = \bar{x}_1 - \bar{x}_2$$

Of course, in this case, a test for this contrast is equivalent to the $F$ test for the ANOVA, since there is only one contrast to be made. When there are three treatment groups, as in the childbirth education example, one can test for both linear and quadratic trends, by using these contrasts:

$$L_1 = \bar{x}_1 - \bar{x}_3$$
$$L_2 = \bar{x}_1 - 2\bar{x}_2 + \bar{x}_3$$

The contrast $L_1$ represents a linear trend, and $L_2$ represents a quadratic trend. For this example, you would calculate these two contrasts and test them for significance, as described in the preceding section.

Results of the analysis, combined with an inspection of the treatment means, would have implications for the design or modification of a prepared childbirth program. If the relationship is linear, the difference in means will be similar across the groups, and the contrast representing the linear trend will be significant. This would suggest that, across the range of class lengths used in the study, one could reduce anxiety during labor and delivery by a fixed amount per class hour added. If the anxiety level drops by a large amount for 6 hours compared with 4 hours but then decreases only slightly from 6 to 8 hours, the relationship is quadratic, and the test statistic for the quadratic contrast will be significant. These findings will suggest that one could not expect to gain much in reduced anxiety by offering more than 6 hours of class. If the anxiety is high for 4 hours of class, decreases only slightly for 6 hours, and then drops dramatically down for 8 hours of class, the quadratic trend will also be significant, and would suggest that one must offer at least 8 hours of class to have any substantial effect. It should be obvious that the interpretation of the results of a significant trend must be made in light of an examination of the group means.

The number of possible orthogonal contrasts continues to grow as the number of treatment groups increases. Tables of orthogonal polynomials are available that list the coefficients to be used, for each possible number of treatment means, to test each type of trend. Snedecor and Cochran[41] provide a discussion of how these coefficients are determined and also include a table which lists polynomials for experiments with up to 12 treatment groups. It is not necessary to carry out all of the possible tests allowed for by the degrees of freedom (number of treatment groups minus

1). For example, if the linear trend is highly significant, one might just leave the remainder of the between-groups sum of squares combined into an "other" term.

## SUMMARY

In this chapter, you have been introduced to the simple one-way ANOVA procedure, which can be used to test a hypothesis of no difference in group means. Various multiple comparison procedures which can be used to test specific patterns of differences between groups have also been described. In one-way ANOVA, the variable which defines the groups to be compared is considered the independent variable, and the variable for which the group means are calculated and compared is called the dependent variable. In Chapter 10, we will go on to discuss a more generalized form of ANOVA, in which there are two independent variables, so that the analysis becomes more complicated. The multiple comparison procedures already described in some detail in this chapter can be applied to the analysis of either of the independent ANOVA variables in the model to be described in Chapter 10.

## PROBLEMS

1. A researcher is interested in the effect of different teaching techniques on the length of time needed to perform a series of common nursing procedures and randomly assigns 24 student nurses to four groups, each of which is taught the procedures by a different technique. All the students are observed, and each is timed while carrying out the procedures. The mean length of time required is recorded for each group, and the results are shown in Table 9-8.

A one-way ANOVA is used to determine whether there is a significant difference in mean length of time among the four groups; the results are given in Table 9-9.

   (a) Complete the ANOVA table.
   (b) State the null hypothesis that can be tested by using the $F$-test statistic.
   (c) Test the null hypothesis, using the .05 level of significance.
   (d) Explain the results in substantive terms.

2. In Problem 6 of Chapter 3, a $t$ test for the difference between two means was carried out to compare mean pain scores for experimental and control group subjects classified as high on physical-danger trait anxiety. A second $t$ test was also done for the difference between two mean pain

Analysis of Variance and Multiple Comparisons

**Table 9-8.** Mean Length of Time Required to Perform Nursing Procedures

| Group | Mean Length of Time in Minutes |
|---|---|
| 1 | 5.38 |
| 2 | 8.40 |
| 3 | 6.14 |
| 4 | 3.00 |

scores for experimental and control group subjects classified as low on physical-danger trait anxiety. Now consider how the same analyses could be carried out by use of the ANOVA procedure described in this chapter.

(a) For the high physical-danger trait anxiety subjects, $\bar{x}$, the mean pain score for both experimental and control group subjects, is $\bar{x} = 0.3757$. Use this figure along with the two group means and sample sizes to calculate the mean square between groups required for ANOVA.

(b) As explained in this chapter, the mean square within groups is just the pooled estimate of variance across all the groups. In the case of two groups, this is the pooled estimate of variance used in the denominator of the $t$ test. What is the mean square within groups, according to your calculations for Problem 6 in Chapter 3?

(c) Use the answers to questions a and b to calcualte the $F$-test statistic for the ANOVA. Show that $F = t^2$, where $t$ is the $t$-test statistic obtained for the high physical-danger trait anxiety subjects in Problem 6 of Chapter 3; that is, show that the two procedures lead to equivalent test statistics.

(d) Repeat a, b, and c for the experimental and control group subjects classified as low on physical-danger trait anxiety. In this case, $\bar{x} = -0.6860$.

**Table 9-9.** Analysis of Variance for Group Differences in Length of Time Required to Perform Nursing Procedures

| Source of Variation | Sum of Squares | DF | Mean Square | F |
|---|---|---|---|---|
| Between groups | 82.22 | | | |
| Within groups | 85.93 | | | |
| Total | 168.15 | | | |

3. In Chapter 1, Problem 2, and in Chapter 3, Problem 7, a study of social and psychological influences on employment of married nurses was described. Among the factors identified in relation to employment status were career desirability, economic value of work, satisfaction with nursing, and conducive home situation. These factors are described in Problem 7 in Chapter 3. Part of the analysis included in this study was a comparison of mean scores on these four factors for nurses with different educational backgrounds. Tables 9-10 and 9-11 show the mean scores and ANOVA results for each of the four factors, for respondents classified by level of education.

(a) What null hypothesis is tested by the $F$-test statistic for career desirability?
(b) Test the null hypothesis stated in question a at the .05 level of significance.
(c) State your conclusion about how career desirability and level of education are related in substantive terms.
(d) Answer questions a, b, and c for the factors of economic value of work, satisfaction with nursing, and conducive home situation.
(e) Use the formula for within-groups mean square given in this chapter to calculate the mean square within groups for the ANOVA based on career desirability.
(f) Show how, using the mean square within groups, the $F$ value, and the degrees of freedom, you can work backward to reconstruct the complete ANOVA table for career desirability by level of education.

4. Referring back to the data in Problem 3:

(a) Calculate the $F$ ratio required for Scheffé's test for each of the six pairs of means of career desirability, using the formula given in this chapter.
(b) State and test the null hypothesis for each of the six $F$ ratios you have calculated in a, using the .10 level of significance.
(c) Repeat a and b for each of the other three factors analyzed by ANOVA in Problem 3.

5. For the study of the effect of different instructional methods on student achievement, which was used as an example in this chapter, a Scheffé test for the difference in means of groups 1 and 2 was calculated

**Table 9-10.** Differences in Employment Status Factors by Level of Education

| | | | | | Factor | | | | | | | |
|---|---|---|---|---|---|---|---|---|---|---|---|---|
| | Career Desirability | | | Economic Value of Work | | | Satisfaction with Nursing | | | Conducive Home Situation | | |
| Level of Education | $n$ | $\bar{x}$ | $s$ | $n$ | $\bar{x}$ | $s$ | $n$ | $\bar{x}$ | $s$ | $n$ | $\bar{x}$ | $s$ |
| Diploma only | 878 | 8.50 | 5.53 | 935 | 9.85 | 2.34 | 778 | 52.20 | 7.62 | 885 | 39.15 | 16.81 |
| Some college | 558 | 10.23 | 6.06 | 587 | 9.99 | 2.37 | 514 | 50.90 | 7.81 | 558 | 41.35 | 17.98 |
| Bachelor's degree | 281 | 9.51 | 5.91 | 290 | 9.74 | 2.36 | 251 | 51.39 | 7.80 | 281 | 38.34 | 17.68 |
| Graduate work | 137 | 11.66 | 6.32 | 142 | 9.78 | 2.33 | 121 | 51.33 | 8.43 | 139 | 46.33 | 19.83 |

**Table 9-11.** Analysis of Variance of Differences in Employment Status Factors by Level of Education

| Factor | F Value Calculated from ANOVA |
| --- | --- |
| Career desirability | 17.8474 |
| Economic value of work | 0.9057 |
| Satisfaction with nursing | 3.0419 |
| Conducive home situation | 8.6079 |

in the section on Scheffé tests. For each of the remaining pairs of means in this problem,

    (a) Calculate the Scheffé $F$-test statistic.
    (b) State the null hypothesis that can be tested by this $F$-test statistic.
    (c) Carry out the test and state your conclusion in substantive terms.

  6. For the study of the effect of different instructional methods on student achievement, three orthogonal contrasts were proposed in the section on orthogonal contrasts, and the first was calculated and tested for significance. For each of the remaining contrasts, $L_2$ and $L_3$,

    (a) Calculate the contrast.
    (b) Determine the sum of squares associated with the contrast.
    (c) Calculate the $F$-test statistic and test the contrast for significance, using the .05 level of significance.
    (d) State your conclusion in substantive terms.

  7. Referring back to Problem 3, consider the ANOVA carried out to test the null hypothesis that mean scores on the factor "conducive home situation" do not differ by level of education. Since there are four educational groups, the between-groups sum of squares has 3 degrees of freedom. Propose a set of three orthogonal contrasts that might be done, explaining the basis for your choice.

  8. Explain why multiple comparisons are not done when an ANOVA is performed to test for the difference in means between one experimental group and one control group.

# Chapter 10

## TWO-WAY ANALYSIS OF VARIANCE

The general intent of analysis of variance procedures is literally to analyze variance, that is, to break the total variation in the dependent variable into pieces, each representing a different part of the variation in individual observations. In its simplest form, *one-way ANOVA* (discussed in Chapter 9) the variation is divided into two parts, between-groups and within groups. In many research situations, the investigator wants to consider the simultaneous effect of several independent variables on the dependent variable of interest. The procedures to be described in this chapter allow for the incorporation of several categorical independent variables into one ANOVA procedure. The situation to be described in detail is two-way ANOVA, the case where two independent variables are present. The general method, however, can be extended to include any desired number of independent variables.

As an example, consider an investigation of the effects of the use of fetal monitors on fetal outcome, as measured by Apgar scores. A study to determine whether Apgar scores differ according to the presence or absence of fetal monitors would involve a comparison of two groups, those with fetal monitors and those without. (Assume randomization into two groups for this discussion.) The analysis could be done by a $t$ test for the difference in mean Apgar scores, or, equivalently, by one-way ANOVA. Suppose, however, that the researcher knows that Apgar scores might be affected by maternal stress during pregnancy, and has classified the study participants as high, medium, or low in stress, according to a questionnaire about experiences during pregnancy. The study subjects are, therefore, classified two ways: according to stress scores and to presence or absence of the fetal monitor. The subjects in such a study could be classified into six different groups, according to each possible combination of fetal monitor and stress level, that is,

|  | High | Medium | Low |
|---|---|---|---|
| Fetal monitor | 1 | 2 | 3 |
| No fetal monitor | 4 | 5 | 6 |

Two-way ANOVA would allow us to use such data to examine the effects of the two *factors,* stress and use of fetal monitor, on Apgar scores simultaneously.

The example we have just described is a clinical study, with subjects randomized into treatment groups and then classified on a second factor. Two-way ANOVA is also useful for other kinds of study, in which no experiment is done, but where the researcher wants to study the simultaneous effects of two independent categorical variables on a dependent variable. The data might come, for instance, from a survey or from records. For example, suppose that patient records were used to determine sex, type of insurance, and length of stay for all patients admitted with a particular diagnosis. A two-way ANOVA could be used to study the effects of sex and type of insurance (e.g., private, Medicare, no insurance) on length of stay.

In addition to providing for the simultaneous study of the effects of the two independent variables, the two-way ANOVA procedure allows for the investigation of interaction between the two factors. In the first example given above, if no interaction is present, the researcher can conclude that effects of the fetal monitor on Apgar scores are the same for each stress group. For example, use of the fetal monitor might result in higher Apgar scores within each of the stress groups. If, on the other hand, the fetal monitor resulted in higher Apgar scores in the high stress group and lower Apgar scores in the other two groups, the investigator would conclude that there is interaction between the two independent variables. Consider also the second example. If women have greater lengths of stay than men, regardless of type of insurance, there is no interaction, and the effects of sex and type of insurance are said to be additive. If, among those patients with private insurance, women stay longer than men, but among patients with Medicare or no coverage, there is no sex difference in length of stay, interaction is present. The ANOVA provides a separate sum of squares and significance test for the presence of an interaction effect. Before going on to a discussion of the model for two-way ANOVA, we will describe in more detail the kinds of effects to be measured by use of two-way ANOVA.

## MAIN EFFECTS AND INTERACTION EFFECTS

A *main effect* is the effect of one factor alone as opposed to the effect of its interaction with another factor. In our above examples, the effect of the fetal monitor on Apgar score, ignoring stress category, is a main effect, as in the effect of stress, ignoring the fetal monitor category. Similarly,

Analysis of Variance and Multiple Comparisons 227

the effect of sex on length of stay, ignoring type of insurance, is a main effect, as is the effect of type of insurance, disregarding sex. These main effects correspond to the effects of group differences described for one-way ANOVA, except that the situation is slightly more complicated for two-way ANOVA, because each individual is classified according to two variables (or factors) rather than one. The following example will illustrate the nature of and notation for main effects.

Refer again to the study using fetal monitors, and use the following notation for the unknown population values for the means:

|  | High | Medium | Low |  |
|---|---|---|---|---|
| Fetal monitor | $\mu_{11}$ | $\mu_{12}$ | $\mu_{13}$ | $\mu_{1\cdot}$ |
| No fetal monitor | $\mu_{21}$ | $\mu_{22}$ | $\mu_{23}$ | $\mu_{2\cdot}$ |
|  | $\mu_{\cdot 1}$ | $\mu_{\cdot 2}$ | $\mu_{\cdot 3}$ | $\mu$ |

For our discussion, we will assume an equal number of values in each *cell* (each row × column box in the table). In the usual ANOVA terminology, each independent variable is referred to as a *factor*, so that in our example, fetal monitor category is the *row factor* and stress category is the *column factor*. The individual rows or columns are referred to as *levels*, so that, for instance, the first level of the row factor is fetal monitor and the second level of the column factor is medium stress.

The quantity $\mu$ is the grand mean, that is, the mean of all the Apgar scores for the combined populations represented by all the cells. The $\mu_{i\cdot}$ are the row means, which in this instance are mean Apgar scores, respectively, for those with fetal monitor and those without fetal monitor, in these two hypothetical populations. The $\mu_{\cdot j}$ are the column means, here the mean Apgar scores for each of the three stress levels, again in these three hypothetical populations. The $\mu_{ij}$ are referred to as the *cell means* and are the population mean Apgar scores for those in each combination of fetal monitor category and stress category. So, for instance, $\mu_{23}$ is the mean Apgar score for low-stress patients with no fetal monitor, and so on. The analysis of main effects is concerned with the row and column means only.

The mean Apgar score for those with a fetal monitor, regardless of stress category, is denoted here by $\mu_{1\cdot}$, and the main effect of fetal monitor will be denoted by

$$\alpha_1 = \mu_{1\cdot} - \mu$$

In other words, the main effect of fetal monitor is the difference between the grand mean ($\mu$) and the mean for all those with fetal monitor. The value of $\alpha_1$ will be positive if use of the fetal monitor tends to increase the Apgar score, negative if it tends to lower the Apgar score, and zero if it makes no difference. Similarly, $\alpha_2$, the main effect of no fetal monitor, is

$$\alpha_2 = \mu_{2.} - \mu$$

The column effects are similarly defined and denoted as

$$\beta_1 = \mu_{.1} - \mu$$
$$\beta_2 = \mu_{.2} - \mu$$
$$\beta_3 = \mu_{.3} - \mu$$

In the general case, then,

$$\alpha_i = \mu_{i.} - \mu$$

is the main effect of level $i$ of the row factor and

$$\beta_j = \mu_{.j} - \mu$$

is the main effect of level $j$ of the column factor.

Consider the (concocted) means shown in Table 10-1.

In this example

$$\alpha_1 = \mu_{1.} - \mu$$
$$= 9 - 9$$
$$= 0$$

**Table 10-1.** Fictitious Mean Apgar Scores for Patients Classified by Use of Fetal Monitor and Stress Level, Additive Model

| Fetal Monitor | High Stress | Medium Stress | Low Stress | Total |
|---|---|---|---|---|
| Fetal monitor | $\mu_{11} = 8$ | $\mu_{12} = 9$ | $\mu_{13} = 10$ | $\mu_{1.} = 9$ |
| No fetal monitor | $\mu_{21} = 8$ | $\mu_{22} = 9$ | $\mu_{23} = 10$ | $\mu_{2.} = 9$ |
| Total | $\mu_{.1} = 8$ | $\mu_{.2} = 9$ | $\mu_{.3} = 10$ | $\mu = 9$ |

Stress Level

and, similarly, $\alpha_2 = 0$. The mean Apgar score for those with fetal monitor is equal to that for those without; in other words, the fetal monitor has no effect. Also,

$$\begin{aligned} \beta_1 &= \mu_{.1} - \mu \\ &= 8 - 9 \\ &= -1 \end{aligned}$$

which indicates that high stress has the effect of lowering the mean Apgar score by one unit. The corresponding effects for medium stress and low stress are $\beta_2 = 0$ and $\beta_3 = 1$, indicating that low stress is the most advantageous of the three groups, in terms of Apgar scores.

Each main effect depends on the other levels of the factor included and on the other factors specified for the hypothetical population under consideration. The main row effects sum to zero, as do the main column effects. If use of the fetal monitor tends to increase Apgar score, then nonuse of the fetal monitor must tend to decrease it. If high stress and medium stress tend to lower the Apgar score, then low stress must tend to increase the Apgar score enough that the sum of the effects is zero. If fetal monitors do not affect Apgar scores, the two means $\mu_{1.}$ and $\mu_{2.}$ will be equal (to each other and to $\mu$), and $\alpha_1$ and $\alpha_2$ will be zero, and the comparable result holds true for the column means. Of course, as usual, the sample estimates for means can differ as a result of sampling effects, even when the corresponding population means are equal to each other.

Now, still using this sample, let us discuss the meaning of *interaction effects*. To consider interaction effects, we move from the margins of the table of means (the row and column means) to the cell means. The degree of interaction is the extent to which the cell means cannot be predicted from the corresponding row and column means. Consider the cell that represents high-stress patients who receive the fetal monitor (the first row and first column). The mean Apgar score for this group, according to our notation, is $\mu_{11}$. If there is no interaction, the value of $\mu_{11}$ should be equal to the grand mean plus the sum of the row and column effects, that is,

$$\mu_{11} = \mu + \alpha_1 + \beta_1$$

If the above equation does not hold, then

$$(\alpha\beta)_{11} = \mu_{11} - (\mu + \alpha_1 + \beta_1)$$

measures the extent of deviation of the cell mean from the value predicted by the *additive* model. In general, the formula is

$$(\alpha\beta)_{ij} = \mu_{ij} - (\mu + \alpha_i + \beta_j)$$

Two illustrative examples follow.

First, return to the concocted means presented earlier, shown in Table 10-1.

In this example,

$$\mu + \alpha_1 + \beta_1 = 9 + 0 + (-1)$$
$$= 8$$
$$= \mu_{11}$$

so that

$$(\alpha\beta)_{11} = 0$$

and

$$\mu + \alpha_1 + \beta_2 = 9 + 0 + 0$$
$$= 9$$
$$= \mu_{12}$$

so that

$$(\alpha\beta)_{12} = 0$$

You can check by similar calculations for the remaining cells of the table that

$$(\alpha\beta)_{ij} = 0$$

in each case. This is an example where the effects are additive and no interaction is present. Looking at each column separately, we see that use of the fetal monitor has the same effect (i.e., none) regardless of stress level. Looking at the table across the rows, one can say that stress has the same effect, regardless of whether the fetal monitor is used (Apgar scores increase as stress decreases, within each row).

Now, consider another example where interaction is present, as indicated in Table 10-2. These values are again concocted.

Analysis of Variance and Multiple Comparisons 231

**Table 10-2.** Fictitious Mean Apgar Scores for Patients Classified by Use of Fetal Monitor and Stress Level, Interactive Model

|  | Stress Level |  |  |  |
|---|---|---|---|---|
| Fetal Monitor | High Stress | Medium Stress | Low Stress | Total |
| Fetal monitor | $\mu_{11} = 9$ | $\mu_{12} = 8$ | $\mu_{13} = 10$ | $\mu_{1\cdot} = 9$ |
| No fetal monitor | $\mu_{21} = 7$ | $\mu_{22} = 10$ | $\mu_{23} = 10$ | $\mu_{2\cdot} = 9$ |
| Total | $\mu_{\cdot 1} = 8$ | $\mu_{\cdot 2} = 9$ | $\mu_{\cdot 3} = 10$ | $\mu = 9$ |

In the above example,

$$\mu + \alpha_1 + \beta_1 = 9 + 0 + (-1)$$
$$= 8$$
$$\neq 9$$

so that

$$(\alpha\beta)_{11} = \mu_{11} - (\mu + \alpha_1 + \beta_1)$$
$$= 9 - 8$$
$$= 1$$

and there are several other cell means in the table for which

$$(\alpha\beta)_{ij} \neq 0$$

In this example the effects are not additive; that is, there is interaction. The interaction can be understood by inspection of each column. Use of the fetal monitor increases Apgar scores in the high-stress group, decreases Apgar scores in the medium-stress group, and has no effect in the low-stress group. The effect of the fetal monitor on Apgar scores differs according to the stress group, and interaction is present. The interaction can also be described by looking across each row. For those with fetal monitor, medium stress lowers the Apgar scores, high stress has no effect, and low stress increases the Apgar scores. For those without fetal monitor, high stress lowers the Apgar scores while medium and low stress increase the Apgar scores. The effect of stress is not the same for those with fetal monitor as for those without, and this is what we mean by interaction. In the next section we describe the mathematical model for two-way ANOVA and explain how the total sum of squares is partitioned to measure the main effects and interaction effects.

## THE GENERAL TWO-WAY ANOVA MODEL

For a two-way ANOVA situation, let us assume that we have observations on some continuous variable for individuals classified into groups according to two factors, which we will call the *row factor* and the *column factor*. Thus any combination of one level of the row factor with one level of the column factor defines a cell of the data table, that is, a group of individuals in the same classification on both independent variables. Although special procedures are available and many computer programs are designed to handle situations where the number of observations in each cell are unequal, the general model assumes an equal number in each cell, as we will assume in the following discussion. It is also assumed that the observations within each cell constitute a random sample from the corresponding population and that the observations in each cell are independent of those in the other cells.

To represent the observations, we will use the following notation shown in Figure 10-1.

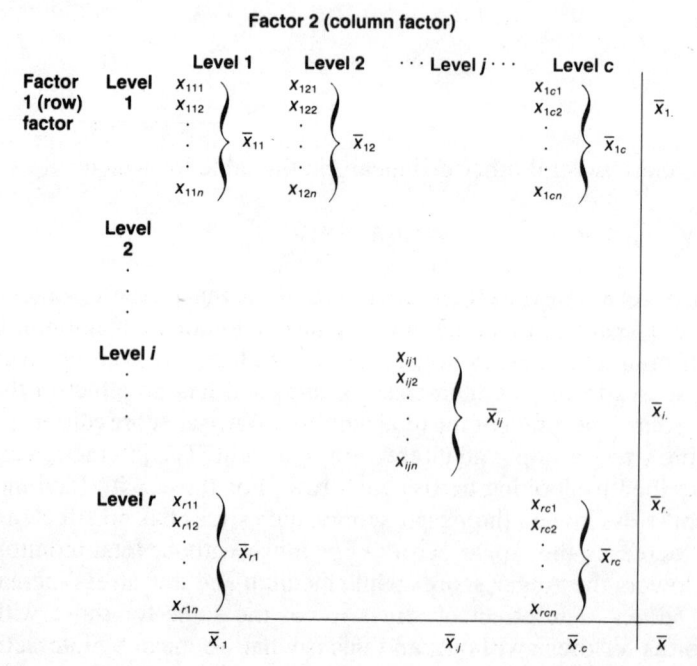

**Figure 10-1** Conventional notation system for two-way ANOVA with $r$ levels of the row factor and $c$ levels of the column factor.

Analysis of Variance and Multiple Comparisons

According to this notation,

$i$ = the row, $i = 1, \cdots, r$
$j$ = the column, $j = 1, \cdots, c$
$k$ = the observation number
$x_{ijk}$ = observation $k$ in row $i$ and column $j$
$n$ = number of observations in each cell
$\bar{x}_{ij}$ = mean of observations in row $i$, column $j$
$\bar{x}_{i.}$ = mean of observations in row $i$
$\bar{x}_{.j}$ = mean of observations in column $j$
$\bar{x}$ = mean of all the observations or the grand mean

For example, $x_{321}$ stands for the observation on the first individual in row 3 and column 2, $\bar{x}_{24}$ is the mean of all the observations in row 2 and column 4, $\bar{x}_{2.}$ is the mean of all the observations in row 2, and $\bar{x}_{.1}$ is the mean of all the observations in column 1.

For the study of Apgar scores described earlier, the treatment variable (fetal monitor vs no fetal monitor) can be arbitrarily designated as the row factor and the stress variable (high, medium, low) as the column factor. Thus factor 1 is treatment group, with $r = 2$ groups, and let us label level 1 as those patients with fetal monitor and level 2 as those patients without fetal monitor. And factor 2 is stress group, with $c = 3$ groups, and we will label level 1 as high stress, level 2 as medium stress, and level 3 as low stress. Thus, for example,

$$x_{211}, x_{212}, x_{213}, \cdots, x_{21n}$$

stand for the Apgar scores of the patients in row 2, column 1, that is, high-stress patients with no fetal monitor. In our notation, $\bar{x}_{21}$ is the mean Apgar score for these patients, where

$$\bar{x}_{21} = \frac{x_{211} + x_{212} + \cdots + x_{21n}}{n}$$

$$= \frac{\sum_{k=1}^{n} x_{21k}}{n}$$

In the following discussion of the model for two-way ANOVA, we consider the fixed effects model, as we did for one-way ANOVA. According to the fixed effects model, the observations ($x_{ijk}$) within each cell ($ij$)

are assumed normally distributed around a mean ($\mu_{ij}$) with variance $\sigma^2$, variance the same for each cell. Each observation is written as

$$x_{ijk} = \mu_{ik} + e_{ijk}$$

where $e_{ijk}$ stands for the deviation of the observation $x_{ijk}$ from its group mean $\mu_{ij}$. Using a formula given in the last section, we can write the two-way ANOVA model in a form that indicates the main effects and interaction effects.

Recall from the last section that the interaction effect is the degree to which the cell means deviate from the additive model. The interaction effect for each cell, therefore, was written as the difference between the cell mean and that predicted taking into account main effects only, that is,

$$(\alpha\beta)_{ij} = \mu_{ij} - (\mu + \alpha_i + \beta_j)$$

By simple algebraic transposition, this equation can be rewritten as

$$\mu_{ij} = \mu + \alpha_i + \beta_j + (\alpha\beta)_{ij}$$

In other words, the cell mean is equal to the grand mean plus main effects and interaction effects. Substituting the formula for $\mu_{ij}$ just obtained into the formula for $x_{ijk}$ shown above, we have

$$x_{ijk} = \mu + \alpha_i + \beta_j + (\alpha\beta)_{ij} + e_{ijk}$$

which is the mathematical model for two-way ANOVA.

As we noted for one-way ANOVA, the assumptions of normality and homogeneity of variance are seldom exactly achieved in practice. Although the ANOVA procedures are fairly robust to violations of these assumptions, you may again want to consult Snedecor and Cochran[41] on this issue. The assumption of an equal number of observations in each cell makes the main effects independent of each other and the interaction effects independent of the main effects and allows for partition of the total sum of squares into pieces representing these various effects. When there are unequal numbers of observations in each cell, as is often the case in nonexperimental research in nursing to which two-way ANOVA is applied, the different effects are not independent and the analysis become somewhat complicated. Nie et al.[34] explain the problem quite clearly, and many computer programs such as the ANOVA program in the *Statistical Package for the Social Sciences* are designed to handle data where the cell

# Two-Way Analysis of Variance

frequencies are unequal. The following discussion of partitioning the total sum of squares will provide a general idea of how to examine and interpret data handled by ANOVA, even though the partitioning, strictly speaking, holds only when the cell frequencies are equal.

## PARTITIONING THE SUM OF SQUARES IN TWO-WAY ANOVA

The total sum of squares for two-way ANOVA is the same total sum of squares as for one-way ANOVA. As you may recall, the total sum of squares is the numerator of the sample variance of the dependent variable, or in other words, it is the squared deviation of each observation from the grand mean, summed across all the observations. Using the notation for two-way ANOVA that we have introduced, we can write the total sum of squares as

$$\sum_{i=1}^{r} \sum_{j=1}^{c} \sum_{k=1}^{n} (x_{ijk} - \bar{x})^2$$

Just as the total sum of squares for one-way ANOVA is partitioned into parts representing different kinds of variation, the total sum of squares for two-way ANOVA can also be partitioned. Because we now have two independent factors instead of one, the total sum of squares can be broken into more than two parts. The algebra used to arrive at this partition is quite complicated and will not be given here. The final result is

$$\sum_{i=1}^{r} \sum_{j=1}^{c} \sum_{k=1}^{n} (x_{ijk} - \bar{x})^2 = \sum_{i=1}^{r} \sum_{j=1}^{c} \sum_{k=1}^{n} (x_{ijk} - \bar{x}_{ij})^2$$

$$+ nc \sum_{i=1}^{r} (\bar{x}_{i.} - \bar{x})^2 + nr \sum_{j=1}^{c} (\bar{x}_{.j} - \bar{x})^2$$

$$+ n \sum_{i=1}^{r} \sum_{j=1}^{c} (\bar{x}_{ij} - \bar{x}_{i.} - \bar{x}_{.j} + \bar{x})$$

According to this equation, the total sum of squares can be divided into four parts. It turns out that these parts are independent from each other and represent the different kinds of variation in the observations that are of interest in two-way ANOVA.

The first quantity,

$$\sum_{i=1}^{r} \sum_{j=1}^{c} \sum_{k=1}^{n} (x_{ijk} - \bar{x}_{ij})^2$$

is obtained by calculating the squared deviation of each observation from its cell mean, $\bar{x}_{ij}$, and then summing across all the observations. This quantity represents the variation of observations around their means within each cell. It is the measure for two-way ANOVA that corresponds to the within-groups sum of squares for one-way ANOVA and is referred to as the *within-groups sum of squares* or the *error sum of squares*, denoted by $SS_W$ or $SS_E$, respectively.

The expression of each observation as its group mean plus random deviation,

$$x_{ijk} = \mu_{ij} + e_{ijk}$$

becomes

$$x_{ijk} = \bar{x}_{ij} + e_{ijk}$$

when the sample mean $\bar{x}_{ij}$ is substituted for the population mean $\mu_{ij}$. Since the above equation is equivalent to

$$x_{ijk} - \bar{x}_{ij} = e_{ijk}$$

we can express the error sum of squares,

$$\sum_{i=1}^{r} \sum_{j=1}^{c} \sum_{k=1}^{n} (x_{ijk} - \bar{x}_{ij})^2$$

as

$$\sum_{i=1}^{r} \sum_{j=1}^{c} \sum_{k=1}^{n} e_{ijk}$$

This last formula shows algebraically that the error sum of squares represents variation of observations around their means within cells.

The second quantity in the partition

$$nc \sum_{i=1}^{r} (\bar{x}_{i.} - \bar{x})^2$$

is obtained by calculating the squared deviation of each row mean from the mean of all the observations and then summing the squared deviations across the rows. This quantity estimates the degree of difference between means of the row factor. It is the sum of squares between groups, where

# Two-Way Analysis of Variance

the groups are defined by the levels of the row factor in the design. It is called the *row sum of squares* or the *row treatment effect*, denoted by $SS_R$.

Now, recall that the row effect $\alpha_i$ is

$$\alpha_i = \mu_{i.} - \mu$$

that is, the difference between the row mean and the grand mean. The corresponding sample estimate is

$$\hat{\alpha}_i = \bar{x}_{i.} - \bar{x}$$

so that the row sum of squares

$$nc \sum_{i=1}^{r} (\bar{x}_{i.} - \bar{x})^2$$

can be written as

$$nc \sum_{i=1}^{r} \hat{\alpha}_i^2$$

In other words, the row sum of squares measures the main effect of the row factor.

The third quantity,

$$nr \sum_{j=1}^{c} (\bar{x}_{.j} - \bar{x})^2$$

is comparable to the row sum of squares, except that it is a sum of squared deviations of the column means from the mean of all the observations. This quantity estimates the degree of difference between means of the column factor. It is called the *column sum of squares* or the *column treatment effect*, denoted by $SS_C$. Again, recall that the column effect $\beta_j$ is the difference between the column mean and the grand-mean, so that

$$\beta_j = \mu_{.j} - \mu$$

The corresponding sample estimate is

$$\hat{\beta}_j = \bar{x}_{.j} - \bar{x}$$

so that the column sum of squares,

$$nr \sum_{j=1}^{c} (\bar{x}_{\cdot j} - \bar{x})^2$$

can be expressed as

$$nr \sum_{j=1}^{c} \hat{\beta}_j^2$$

Therefore, the column sum of squares measures the main effect of the column factor.

The fourth quantity in the partition of the total sum of squares,

$$n \sum_{i=1}^{r} \sum_{j=1}^{c} (\bar{x}_{ij} - \bar{x}_{i\cdot} - \bar{x}_{\cdot j} + \bar{x})^2$$

is a measure of interaction between the row and column factors. The amount by which this quantity deviates from zero is an estimate of the interaction between the row and column factors. It is called the *interaction sum of squares* or the *row × column interaction*, and will be denoted by $SS_I$. The fact that this sum of squares represents interaction is not obvious from the above formula, but can easily be demonstrated by algebraic manipulation of formulas used earlier in this chapter.

Remember that the formula for interaction is

$$(\alpha\beta)_{ij} = \mu_{ij} - (\mu + \alpha_i + \beta_j)$$

Substitution of sample values yields

$$\widehat{(\alpha\beta)}_{ij} = \bar{x}_{ij} - (\bar{x} + \alpha_i + \beta_j)$$
$$= \bar{x}_{ij} - [\bar{x} + (\bar{x}_{i\cdot} - \bar{x}) + (\bar{x}_{\cdot j} - \bar{x})]$$

so that

$$\bar{x}_{ij} = \widehat{(\alpha\beta)}_{ij} + \bar{x} + \bar{x}_{i\cdot} - \bar{x} + \bar{x}_{\cdot j} - \bar{x}$$

Using the above expression, we can rewrite the interaction sum of squares,

$$n \sum_{i=1}^{r} \sum_{j=1}^{c} (\bar{x}_{ij} - \bar{x}_{i\cdot} - \bar{x}_{\cdot j} + \bar{x})^2$$

# Two-Way Analysis of Variance

as

$$n \sum_{i=1}^{r} \sum_{j=1}^{c} \left[ \left\{ (\widehat{\alpha\beta})_{ij} + \bar{x} + \bar{x}_{i\cdot} - \bar{x} + \bar{x}_{\cdot j} - \bar{x} \right\} - \bar{x}_{i\cdot} - \bar{x}_{\cdot j} + \bar{x} \right]^2$$

$$= n \sum_{i=1}^{r} \sum_{j=1}^{c} (\widehat{\alpha\beta})_{ij}^2$$

since all the sample means cancel each other.

The degrees of freedom associated with the total sum of squares is $N - 1$, where $N$ is the total number of observations. In the two-way ANOVA described here, each cell has $n$ observations, so

$$N - 1 = rcn - 1$$

Remember that the between-groups sum of squares for one-way ANOVA has $k - 1$ degrees of freedom, where $k$ is the number of groups. Similarly, in two-way ANOVA, the degrees of freedom for the row sum of squares is $r - 1$, one less than the number of rows, and the degrees of freedom for the column sum of squares is $c - 1$. The within-groups sum of squares is a pooled estimate of variance across the cells, and one degree of freedom is lost for the variance estimate within each cell. The degrees of freedom associated with the variance estimate within each cell is thus $(n - 1)$, so that the degrees of freedom for the error sum of squares, pooled across all cells, is $rc(n - 1)$. In order for the degrees of freedom associated with the two main effects, the interaction effect, and the error to sum to the total degrees of freedom

$$rcn - 1$$

it turns out that the degrees of freedom associated with the interaction is

$$(r - 1) \times (c - 1)$$

The partition of the total sum of squares and total degrees of freedom that we have described here allows us to form $F$ ratios to test three null hypotheses of interest in two-way ANOVA. The three null hypotheses tested are

1. $H:$ $\alpha_1 = \alpha_2 = \cdots = \alpha_r = 0$ (or $\mu_{1\cdot} = \mu_{2\cdot} = \cdots = \mu_{r\cdot}$)
2. $H:$ $\beta_1 = \beta_2 = \cdots = \beta_c = 0$ (or $\mu_{\cdot 1} = \mu_{\cdot 2} = \cdots = \mu_{\cdot c}$)
3. $H:$ $(\alpha\beta)_{11} = \cdots = (\alpha\beta)_{rc} = 0$

These hypotheses correspond, of course, to null hypotheses of equivalence of row means (no row effect), equivalence of column means (no column effect), and no interaction. The procedure for testing these null hypotheses will be described in the next section and illustrated by application to an example.

## TESTING TWO-WAY ANOVA HYPOTHESES

For testing the null hypotheses in two-way ANOVA, one first calculates the mean square for each source of variation by dividing each sum of squares by its corresponding degrees of freedom, in the same fashion as for one-way ANOVA. For the fixed-effects model assumed here, $F$ ratios are calculated to test the null hypotheses as indicated in the chart shown in Table 10-3.

The $F$ ratio

$$F = \frac{MS_R}{MS_W}$$

is the test statistic for

$$H: \alpha_1 = \alpha_2 = \cdots = \alpha_r = 0$$

and can be shown to have an $F$ distribution with $r - 1$ and $rc(n - 1)$ degrees of freedom when the null hypothesis is true. The $F$ ratio

$$F = \frac{MS_C}{MS_W}$$

is the test statistic for

$$H: \beta_1 = \beta_2 = \cdots = \beta_c = 0$$

and is distributed as $F$ with $c - 1$ and $rc(n - 1)$ degrees of freedom when the null hypothesis is true. And

$$F = \frac{MS_I}{MS_W}$$

which tests

$$H: (\alpha\beta)_{11} = \cdots = (\alpha\beta)_{rc} = 0$$

**Table 10-3** Two-Way ANOVA

| Source of Variation | Sum of Squares | Degrees of Freedom | Mean Square | F |
|---|---|---|---|---|
| Between rows | $SS_R = nc\sum_{i=1}^{r}(\bar{x}_{i\cdot} - \bar{x})^2$ | $r - 1$ | $MS_R = SS_R/(r-1)$ | $MS_R/MS_W$ |
| Between columns | $SS_C = nr\sum_{j=1}^{c}(\bar{x}_{\cdot j} - \bar{x})^2$ | $c - 1$ | $MS_C = SS_C/(c-1)$ | $MS_C/MS_W$ |
| Row × column interaction | $SS_I = n\sum_{i=1}^{r}\sum_{j=1}^{c}(\bar{x}_{ij} - \bar{x}_{i\cdot} - \bar{x}_{\cdot j} + \bar{x})^2$ | $(r-1) \times (c-1)$ | $MS_I = SS_I/(r-1)\times(c-1)$ | $MS_I/MS_W$ |
| Error | $SS_W = \sum_{i=1}^{r}\sum_{j=1}^{c}\sum_{k=1}^{n}(x_{ijk} - \bar{x}_{ij})^2$ | $rc(n-1)$ | $MS_W = SS_W/rc(n-1)$ | |
| Total | $SS_T = \sum_{i=1}^{r}\sum_{j=1}^{c}\sum_{k=1}^{n}(x_{ijk} - \bar{x})^2$ | $rcn - 1$ | | |

has an $F$ distribution with $(r - 1) \times (c - 1)$ and $rc(n - 1)$ degrees of freedom when the null hypothesis is true.

In each case the null hypothesis is rejected when the calculated $F$ ratio exceeds the value given in the table of the $F$ distribution, with level of significance chosen by the researcher. Usually, computer programs for ANOVA include all these $F$ ratios on the printout, but, in fact, it is logical to perform the tests in a sequential fashion. If the interaction is significant, the effects of the row variable differ across categories of the column variable, and the main effects are not of interest. Rather, the cell means are studied to determine the nature of the interaction effect. If interaction effects are not significant but row or column effects are significant, the row or column means are useful in interpretation of the results of the study. The following example illustrates the use of two-way ANOVA and interpretation of the results.

In a study to determine factors in variation of knowledge about diabetes and general health, Lowery and DuCette[30] classified 90 diabetic patients into three groups according to length of time since diagnosis and into two groups according to their scores on Rotter's Internal–External Control Scale. On the basis of studies that have shown internally controlled persons to be more active information seekers than externally controlled persons, these researchers predicted that their group of internal diabetics would score higher on a test of diabetes and health information than their group of external diabetics. Scores on the information test were analyzed by ANOVA, using both length of illness and locus of control as independent variables, so that the main effects of these two factors as well as any interaction effects could be simultaneously investigated. These researchers divided the information test into four subtests and analyzed the differences in scores on the subtests. For our example, we have combined the subtest scores together into a total diabetic and health information score, so that the example is a simplified version of the analysis given in Lowery and DuCette's paper. We have also assumed equal cell frequencies in our calculations, although cell frequencies were not given in the article.

Cell means for the diabetic and health information scores, calculated according to the assumption of equal cell frequencies, are given in Table 10-4.

Inspection of the row means suggests that internals scored higher than externals, which would support the main hypothesis of the study. The column means indicate higher information scores for those with diabetes for 6 years than for the other two groups. No pattern of interaction is apparent in the data, since the internals have higher scores than externals for each category of length of illness. These impressions can be checked by the ANOVA tests for main effects and interaction effects.

The ANOVA shown in Table 10-5 indicates the sources of variation and values for the $F$ tests. Each effect is tested by calculation of an $F$

# Two-Way Analysis of Variance

**Table 10-4** Mean Diabetic and Health Information Scores by Length of Illness and Locus of Control ($N = 90$)

| Locus of Control | Length of Illness |  |  | Total |
|---|---|---|---|---|
|  | Newly Diagnosed | 3 Years | 6 Years |  |
| Internal | 34.99 | 34.50 | 36.55 | 35.35 |
| External | 32.37 | 30.78 | 34.26 | 32.47 |
| Total | 33.68 | 32.64 | 35.41 | 33.91 |

ratio, dividing the appropriate mean square by the mean square within groups, as explained earlier in this section. The $F$ value, with the corresponding degrees of freedom, from the tables of the $F$ distribution, determines the $F$ value required for significance at the chosen level.

The locus of control effect is tested by the $F$ statistic:

$$F = \frac{MS_R}{MS_W}$$
$$= \frac{49.14}{5.59}$$
$$= 8.79$$

The $F$ required for significance at the .05 level with 1 and 80 degrees of freedom is

$$F_{.05}(1,80) = 3.96$$

**Table 10-5** Analysis of Variance for Differences in Mean Diabetic and Health Information Scores by Length of Illness and Locus of Control ($N = 90$)

| Source of Variation | Sum of Squares | DF | Mean Square | F |
|---|---|---|---|---|
| Locus of control | 49.14 | 1 | 49.14 | 8.79* |
| Length of illness | 25.72 | 2 | 12.86 | 2.30 |
| Interaction | 1.54 | 2 | 0.77 | 0.14 |
| Within groups | 469.56 | 84 | 5.59 |  |

*$p < .05$.

and so the null hypothesis is rejected.

Similarly, the length of illness effect is tested by the $F$ statistic:

$$F = \frac{MS_C}{MS_W}$$

$$= \frac{12.86}{5.59}$$

$$= 2.30$$

Tested against the required $F$ with 2 and 80 degrees of freedom,

$$F_{.05}(2,80) = 3.11$$

this null hypothesis is not rejected.

The interaction effect is tested by the $F$ statistic:

$$F = \frac{MS_I}{MS_W}$$

$$= \frac{.77}{5.59}$$

$$= 0.14$$

Since this is lower than the required $F$ for significance at the .05 level with 2 and 80 degrees of freedom ($F = 3.11$), the null hypothesis of no interaction is accepted.

The analysis thus supported the contention of the researchers that diabetics classified as internals according to Rotter's scale would score significantly higher on a test of diabetes and health information than diabetics classified as externals. In addition, there was no significant difference in scores according to length of illness (although it looks as if those with diabetes for 6 years would score higher than the other two groups if tested by a multiple comparison procedure). And finally, there was no significant interaction between locus of control and illness, since internals scored higher than externals, regardless of length of illness.

## ANOVA WITH MULTIPLE FACTORS

Two-way ANOVA is the simplest form of what are generally referred to as *factorial designs*. Factorial designs incorporate the simultaneous analysis of the effects of several factors or independent variables on the

# Two-Way Analysis of Variance

dependent variable. These designs are more efficient than ones considering only one independent variable, since data from each person or subject in the study can be used to consider the effects of several factors as well as interaction effects among the factors. Studies with 3 or 4 factors are not unusual in nursing research. These studies are commonly referred to by a terminology that indicates the number of levels of each factor. The study on locus of control just described would be referred to as a 2 × 3 ANOVA, indicating two levels of the row factor (locus of control) and three levels of the column factor (length of illness). A 2 × 3 × 3 ANOVA would describe a three-way ANOVA with three levels of the third factor, and so on. The inclusion of several factors in ANOVA makes the possible types of interaction numerous and often difficult to interpret. Refer to an advanced text such as Winer[46] or Klugh[29] for further discussion of higher-order factorial experiments.

Given the advantage that a factorial design allows one to simultaneously study the effects of several independent variables, researchers are sometimes inclined to include a large number of factors in one study. This procedure has some limitations, as we will discuss here. When a one-way ANOVA is done, the difference between the groups is tested by the following $F$ test:

$$F = \frac{MS_B}{MS_W}$$

$$= \frac{SS_B / (k - 1)}{SS_W / (N - k - 1)}$$

The numerator of this $F$ value measures differences among the groups defined by the independent variable of interest. All other sources of variation in the dependent variable are represented in the denominator of this $F$ test, that is, the within-groups mean square. The within-groups sum of squares, therefore, includes variation due not only to sampling error, but also to other independent variables that have not been measured in the study.

When a second independent variable is included in the analysis, the portion of the within groups sum of squares due to the effect of the second variable, plus the portion due to interaction, split off from the error sum of squares to become separate sums of squares. The effect of this is to reduce the error (unexplained) sum of squares, compared to what it would have been with the second factor ignored. Since the effect of the first variable is tested by an $F$ statistic that has the error sum of squares in its denominator, the effect of adding factors is to reduce the denominator of the $F$ statistic for the first factor. This makes this $F$ statistic larger and rejection of the null hypothesis more likely than if the second factor had been ignored. This is why researchers sometimes add as second or third factors variables not of primary interest to the research, but rather variables already known to affect the dependent variable under study.

It is not to the researcher's advantage to include as factors in the analysis variables whose effect on the dependent variable are likely to be trivial. If the effect of a factor is trivial, the sum of squares associated with it will be very small, and the error sum of squares will be only slightly decreased by the addition of this factor. Note that the degrees of freedom also change when factors are added. The error sum of squares has fewer degrees of freedom when two factors are included compared with one factor, and so forth. The decrease in degrees of freedom due to adding factors has the opposite effect of the decrease in the error sum of squares, as you can see by inspection of the formulas. Thus the addition of factors means a loss of degrees of freedom for the denominator sum of squares, which tends to decrease the statistic $F$ and increases the required value for rejection. If factors are included that do not reduce the error sum of squares enough to compensate for this loss of degrees of freedom, it becomes more difficult to obtain significance on the first factor (presumably the primary factor of interest). Usually only two (or three at the most) factors of primary interest to the research should be included in the kinds of research common to nursing. Additional factors not of primary interest should be included only if they are known or strongly suspected to affect the dependent variable.

## SUMMARY

You will recall from Chapter 9 that the one-way ANOVA procedure provides for a partition of the total variation in the dependent variable into a part due to between-groups variation and a part due to within-groups variation. In this chapter, the ANOVA procedure has been extended to situations in which there are two independent variables, and you have seen how the addition of a second independent variable introduces new measurable sources of variation. In two-way ANOVA, the total variation, as represented by the total sum of squares, can be divided into four parts that represent two main effects, an interaction effect, and an error term. Each of the main effects as well as the interaction effect can then be tested for significance. The addition of factors that have an effect on the dependent variable means that the effects of more than one factor can be investigated simultaneously. It also means that the error term is likely to be reduced, which makes the $F$ ratios used for the significance tests more powerful than if only one factor is studied.

# Two-Way Analysis of Variance

The meaning of a significant interaction term has also been introduced. When there is a significant interaction effect, one can conclude that the effect of one of the independent variables on the dependent variable is not constant but, rather, varies across the categories of the other independent variable. When there is no significant interaction, one can conclude that the data can be adequately described by an additive model. You may remember from the discussion of interaction in terms of the multiple regression model (Chapter 8) that, when interaction is present, one can obtain better prediction of the dependent variable by incorporating the interactive effect into the model. The same is true for interaction in ANOVA, which, as we have said, is just a special case of regression. Interaction in ANOVA is measured by a sum of squares that represents a part of the total sum of squares. By incorporating interaction, the general two-way ANOVA allows the interaction part of the total sum of squares to be removed from the error term. The effect of this (when there is interaction) is that the tests for main effects are more likely to yield significant results, since their denominator (the error term) has been reduced to take account of the interaction effect.

Interaction can take different forms, indicating different types of relationship among the variables. For example, consider the example of the effects of stress level and fetal monitors on Apgar scores. Suppose that the use of fetal monitors tends to have a calming effect among patients with high stress. This would make the labor progress more smoothly and result in higher Apgar scores than would occur in the absence of fetal monitors. Suppose, on the other hand, that for low-stress patients, the presence of fetal monitors creates anxiety, resulting in lower Apgar scores than would be found if monitors were not used. Data analysis from such a situation would result in a significant interaction effect, reflecting the fact that the use of fetal monitors would have opposite effects on high- and low-stress patients.

Interaction can also be significant when the effects are not opposite in nature. As an example of this, consider the study by Lowery and DuCette[31] described earlier in this chapter. These researchers examined simultaneously the effects of locus of control and length of illness on diabetes and health information scores among diabetic patients. According to their results, internals scored higher than externals for each category of length of illness, and there was no significant interaction effect. By imagining a hypothetical alternative outcome of this study, we can illustrate a second form of interaction.

Suppose that the hypothesis that internally controlled individuals are more active information seekers than externally controlled individuals is correct and that the gains in knowledge resulting from information seeking take place over an extended period of time. In this case the mean diabetic and health information scores for internals and externals might be similar among newly diagnosed patients. If the mean scores among externals increased only slightly as a function of length of illness while the mean scores for internals increased dramatically with length of illness, the difference between the means for the dependent variable for internals versus externals would continue to increase as the length of illness increased. Such data would yield a significant interaction effect, since, although means for both groups would increase across the time categories, they would increase at different rates. One could say that diabetes and health information scores do not increase over time independently of type of patient, but rather that the scores increase at different rates for the two patient groups.

These cases illustrate that the $F$ test for interaction indicates whether there is a significant interaction effect, but doesn't specify the form of the interaction. Intepretation of the particular form a significant interaction takes requires a detailed inspection of the pattern of variation in cell means, as in the examples given previously.

## PROBLEMS

1. In Problem 6 in Chapter 3, a study was described in which the effect of experimental information on pain experienced by surgical patients was investigated. A $t$ test was done to test for the difference in pain scores between experimental and control groups of patients classified as high on physical-danger trait anxiety. A second $t$ test was also done to test for the difference in pain scores between experimental and control groups of patients classified as low on physical-danger trait anxiety. In Problem 3 of Chapter 9, the same data were reanalyzed, using two ANOVA procedures instead of two $t$ tests, with equivalent results. Since subjects in this study were classified according to two factors, a two-way ANOVA could be applied to the data.

   (a) Explain in substantive terms what main effects would be tested.
   (b) Explain in substantive terms what interaction effect would be tested.
   (c) Do you think the interaction effect would be significant? Explain your answer.

2. Johnson et al.[24], in a study of the effects of various kinds of information on distress experienced by children during orthopedic cast removal, randomly assigned 84 children who had had a cast applied as a result of injury to one of three groups. The groups were as follows:

# Two-Way Analysis of Variance

Group 1. Children were given no preparatory information.
Group 2. Children were given taped information prior to cast removal about the procedures that would be carried out.
Group 3. Children were given taped information prior to cast removal about the sensory experiences they might expect.

The researchers hypothesized that children in group 3 would display less distress during cast removal than children in groups 1 and 2. In addition, the children were asked prior to cast removal how afraid they were of having the cast removed and were classified according to their responses into one of two groups:

Group 1. Not fearful
Group 2. Fearful

An observer who was unaware of the group assignments observed each child during the cast removal and assigned a distress score to each based on behavior during the cast removal. Scoring was done in such a way that a high score represented more distress than a low score. Summary data and analysis of the effects of fear and type of information are given in Tables 10-6 and 10-7.

(a) Is it reasonable to assume that the three information groups are alike with respect to age, prior experience with cast removal, and other variables that might affect the distress scores?
(b) Is it reasonable to assume that the two fear groups are alike with respect to the variables mentioned in question a?
(c) What difference does it make that the observer who scored distress during cast removal was unaware of the group to which each child belonged?

**Table 10-6** Mean Distress Scores by Information and Fear Groups ($N = 84$)

| Fear Groups | Group 1 (Control) $\bar{x}$ | $n$ | Group 2 (Procedure) $\bar{x}$ | $n$ | Group 3 (Sensation) $\bar{x}$ | $n$ | Total $\bar{x}$ | $n$ |
|---|---|---|---|---|---|---|---|---|
| Group 1 (not fearful) | 0.83 | 12 | 0.38 | 18 | 0.44 | 18 | 0.52 | 48 |
| Group 2 (fearful) | 1.12 | 16 | 1.17 | 12 | 0.60 | 10 | 1.00 | 38 |
| Total | 1.00 | 28 | 0.71 | 30 | 0.50 | 28 | 0.74 | 84 |

**Table 10-7** Analysis of Variance for Differences in Mean Distress Scores by Information and Fear Groups ($N = 84$)

| Source of Variation | Sum of Squares | DF | Mean Square | F |
|---|---|---|---|---|
| Information | 3.524 | 2 | | |
| Fear | 3.527 | 1 | | |
| Information × fear | 1.510 | 2 | | |
| Error | 45.708 | 78 | | |

(d) State in substantive terms the null hypothesis tested by the "Information" line in the ANOVA table.
(e) Calculate the F-test statistic for "Information."
(f) Test the "Information" null hypothesis, using the .05 level of significance.
(g) State in substantive terms your interpretation of the "Information" effect.
(h) Repeat steps d through g with reference to the "Fear" line in the ANOVA.
(i) Repeat steps d through g with reference to the "Information × fear" line in the ANOVA.

3. Reconsider the study described in Problem 2. Suppose that the researchers had not classified the children into groups according to "Fear." In this case, the analysis would be in the form of a one-way ANOVA with three groups.

(a) Construct the ANOVA table that would result. ("Total" sum of squares and "Information" sum of squares would, of course, be the same as in the table given.)
(b) State and test the null hypothesis.
(c) Explain the difference in results between the one-way ANOVA and the two-way ANOVA; that is, explain what was gained by adding the second factor, "fear."

4. Return to Problem 2. Since three information groups were included in this study, the "Information" sum of squares has 2 degrees of freedom, and thus two orthogonal contrasts can be made.

(a) Define two a priori orthogonal contrasts that could be made for comparisons among the information groups, based on the researchers' hypothesis.
(b) For each contrast, state the null hypothesis that can be tested.
(c) Calculate the sum of squares associated with each contrast.

# Two-Way Analysis of Variance

(d) Test the null hypothesis for each contrast. For the denominator for each $F$ test, use the error term used in the two-way ANOVA for the information effect.

(e) State the conclusion of the analysis in substantive terms.

5. In a study to evaluate the impact of a one-month management concepts course on 80 senior baccalaureate nursing students, Brock[2] used the Solomon Four-Group Design. This design requires the randomization of subjects into four groups, two experimental groups and two control groups. Both experimental groups receive the experimental treatment and are measured on a posttest, and one of these groups is also given a pretest. Neither control group receives the treatment, both are given a posttest, and one is also given a pretest. The advantage of this design over an experimental study with only two groups is that it makes possible the evaluation of effects of the pretest and interaction between the pretest and the treatment, as well as effects of the treatment itself. In Brock's study, each group consisted of 20 students, and the 40 students in the two experimental groups were given a 1-month course in management concepts. Pretests and posttests were done on the appropriate groups to measure knowledge of management concepts. The design was as follows:

|  | Pretest | No Pretest |
|---|---|---|
| Experimental | I | II |
| Control | III | IV |

Comparison of pretest scores for groups I and III indicated no significant difference. The mean posttest score for the experimental groups (I and II) together was 28.9, and for the control groups (III and IV) together was 17.63. Separate cell means were not included in the article. A two-way ANOVA for analysis of the effects of the "management course" and the pretest on the posttest scores yielded the results indicated in Table 10-8.

Table 10-8 is presented in a slightly different form from the model presented in this chapter. The "main effects" line is just a measure of the combined main effects, "treatment" and "pretest," as you can tell by adding together the sum of squares for the two main effects. And the "explained" line is a measure of the combined main effects and interaction effects, as you can check by adding together the sums of squares for both main effects and interaction. Computer output often includes these extra, summary tests in the ANOVA table, although they aren't usually of central importance in interpretation of the results.

(a) Why, in this study, would it be reasonable to assume that all four groups are alike in their knowledge of management concepts at the onset of the study?

**Table 10-8** Analysis of Variance for Difference in Mean Posttest Scores on Knowledge of Management Concepts by Treatment and Pretest ($N = 80$)

| Source of Variation | Sum of Squares | DF | Mean Square | F |
|---|---|---|---|---|
| Main effects | 2598.63 | 2 | 1299.31 | 102.45 |
| Treatment | 2542.51 | 1 | 2542.51 | 200.48 |
| Pretest | 56.11 | 1 | 56.11 | 4.42 |
| Treatment × pretest | 1.01 | 1 | 1.01 | 0.08 |
| Explained | 2599.64 | 3 | 866.55 | 68.33 |
| Residual (error) | 963.85 | 76 | 12.68 | |
| Total | 3563.49 | 79 | 45.11 | |

(b) Is the assumption stated in question a borne out by the pretest scores for groups I and III?
(c) Would it be reasonable to assume that all four groups are alike in other variables (e.g., age, IQ)?
(d) State in substantive terms the null hypothesis tested by the "Treatment" $F$ in the ANOVA table.
(e) Explain what ratio was used to calculate the $F$-test statistic for the "Treatment" line in the ANOVA.
(f) Test the "Treatment" null hypothesis, using the .05 level of significance.
(g) State in substantive terms your interpretation of the "Treatment" effects.
(h) Repeat steps d through g above with reference to the "Pretest" line in the ANOVA.
(i) Repeat steps d through g above with reference to the "Treatment × pretest" line in the ANOVA.

6. In Brock's[2] study, described in Problem 5, a $t$ test for the difference in posttest means for the experimental groups (I and II) together versus the control groups (III and IV) together was made, with the results shown in Table 10-9.

As you recall from the discussion of one-way ANOVA in Chapter 9, this $t$-test is equivalent to a one-way ANOVA for the difference between two groups. Since $t = \sqrt{F}$, the corresponding $F$-test statistic would be

$$F = (13.939)^2$$
$$= 194.2957$$

Two-Way Analysis of Variance 253

**Table 10-9** Mean Post-test Scores on Knowledge of Management Concepts for Experimental versus Control Groups ($N = 80$)

| Groups | N | $\bar{x}$ | SD | t Value |
|---|---|---|---|---|
| Experimental (I,II) | 40 | 28.90 | 3.77 | |
| | | | | 13.939* |
| Control (III,IV) | 40 | 17.63 | 3.45 | |

*$p < .01$.

The $F$ for treatment in the ANOVA for these data is $F = 200.48$. It is higher than 194.2957 because the sum of squares due to the effect of the pretest and the treatment × pretest interaction have been identified and removed from the error sum of squares, reducing the denominator for the $F$ test for treatments (compared with a one-way ANOVA with the pretest classification ignored). If the pretest classification were ignored, the analysis would be one-way ANOVA. The treatment sum of squares, 2542.51, and the total sum of squares, 3563.49, would remain the same. The other sources of variation and remaining degrees of freedom which appear in Table 10-8 would be combined into one error term. Reconstruct the one-way ANOVA that would result, and verify that the $F$-test statistic would be $F = 194.2957$.

7. Lindeman and Stetzer[30], in a study of the effect of preoperative visits by operating room nurses, randomized adult patients admitted to the hospital for surgery into two groups. Patients in the experimental group received a preoperative visit designed to reduce anxiety and have a positive effect on general patient welfare in the postoperative period. Patients in the control group received no visit. Among the measures used as indicators of postopertaive anxiety was the Palmar Sweat Index (*PSI*). The PSI is scored so that a low score indicates a higher level of anxiety than a high score. Since the researchers thought that the patients' age and the degree of surgical trauma might also influence postoperative anxiety, each patient's age group and degree of surgical trauma were recorded and included in the analysis. For the analysis of variations in PSI, a 2 × 3 × 3 ANOVA was used. The factors were

A = Age (16–44, 45–59, 60+)
B = Preoperative visit (yes, no)
C = Surgical trauma (minor, moderate, extensive)

Table 10-10 gives the three-way ANOVA used to test the effects of these three factors on postoperative PSI.

**Table 10-10** Analysis of Variance of Differences in Mean PSI by Age, Treatment, and Degree of Surgical Trauma ($N = 176$)

| Source of Variation | DF | Mean Square | F Ratio |
|---|---|---|---|
| Age (A) | 2 | 10511.52 | 12.65* |
| Visit or no visit (B) | 1 | 3077.76 | 3.70 |
| Surgical trauma (C) | 2 | 9186.96 | 11.05* |
| A × B | 2 | 231.68 | 0.28 |
| A × C | 4 | 3135.20 | 3.77* |
| B × C | 2 | 5273.48 | 6.35* |
| A × B × C | 4 | 660.70 | 0.80 |
| Within cells | 158 | 831.03 | |
| Total | 175 | 1163.60 | |

*$p < .05$.

The article also contained a table of mean PSI scores by degree of trauma and preoperative visit, as shown in Table 10-11.

The PSI means for the three age groups were 51.81 (16–44 years), 26.21 (45–59 years), and 24.00 (60+ years). Mean PSIs for age groups were not reported separately by preoperative visit or degree of surgical trauma.

(a) What null hypothesis is tested by the F-test statistic for age?
(b) State the substantive conclusion of the F test for age.
(c) Repeat steps a and b for the visit or no-visit factor and for the surgical trauma factor.
(d) Repeat a for the interaction term B × C.

**Table 10-11** Mean Palmar Sweat Index by Treatment and Degree of Surgical Trauma ($N = 176$)

| Treatment | Degree of Trauma | | |
|---|---|---|---|
| | Minimum | Moderate | Extensive |
| Preoperative visit | 66.30 | 29.18 | 21.03 |
| No preoperative visit | 31.84 | 36.19 | 19.50 |

# Two-Way Analysis of Variance

(e) For the $B \times C$ interaction, explain the results in substantive terms, by referring to Table 10-11 above.

(f) Explain why the significant $A \times C$ interaction cannot be interpreted on the basis of the information given in Tables 10-10 and 10-11.

(g) If the researchers had not recorded age and degree of surgical trauma, they could have done a one-way ANOVA. The visit or not visit sum of squares and total sum of squares would have been the same as in Table 10-10, but the remaining variation would all be pooled into one error term. Explain what effect this would have on the $F$ test for visit or no visit.

# Chapter 11

## ANALYSIS OF VARIANCE, CONTINUED

**FIXED AND RANDOM EFFECTS**

In the previous two chapters one-way and two-way ANOVA designs have been discussed in some detail. In both of these chapters, ANOVA models referred to as *fixed-effects* models were presented. In fixed effects models, all of the levels of each factor included in the study are preselected by the investigator. For example, if sex is a factor, the two levels are male and female, and no other levels could be used. If type of treatment is a factor and the levels are surgical treatment versus medical treatment, the fixed-effects model would also be appropriate. If type of preparatory information given to patients is a factor, the specific levels of preparatory information are predetermined or fixed by the investigator. In all these examples, the conclusions of the study apply to only those levels of each factor included in the study. For sex as a factor, this is obvious, since there are only two levels. If type of treatment as described above is a factor, the researcher cannot generalize to other types of treatment (such as a combination of both medical and surgical procedures). In the third case, the researcher would not claim that the results of the study would necessarily hold for types of preparatory information not included in the actual study.

Contrast these situations with ones in which the researcher does want to generalize findings to levels of a factor other than those included in the study itself. For example, in a study of the effects of primary care on patient satisfaction among surgical patients, the researcher may include several hospitals in the study and use the factor hospitals as an independent variable because patient satisfaction varies by hospital. Or, several wards within one hospital may be used to constitute levels of a factor, if she has reason to think that patient satisfaction varies by wards. In these examples, the researcher is not interested in the specific hospitals or wards studied, but rather in the general effect of variation between hospitals or wards on patient satisfaction. The effects are no longer assumed to be fixed, as in the fixed-effects model, but are assumed to depend on the particular levels of the factor that are selected for inclusion in the study. These situations are appropriate for what is referred to as the *random-effects model* or the *components of variance model*.

In the fixed-effects model, the conclusions reached from the data analysis apply only to the specific levels of the factor that were included in the actual experiment. When the random-effects model is used, however, levels of a factor included in the study are assumed to be a random sample from a large population of levels. Although we will not discuss the theoretical details, the random-effects model can be shown to allow for generalization of the results to the population of all possible levels of a factor from which those levels included in the study were selected. Of course, variables such as hospitals or wards are not often selected at random, strictly speaking, so that the generalization to an appropriate population requires investigator judgment as to the representativeness of those hospitals or wards actually studied.

In ANOVA with more than one factor, it is possible to have all fixed factors, in which case the fixed-effects model is used. This is the most common situation in nursing research. On the other hand, if all the factors are random, the random-effects model is appropriate. If some factors are fixed and some are random, the situation is appropriate for a *mixed-effects model*. Fixed effects, random effects, and mixed effects are also referred to as *model I*, *model II*, and *model III*, respectively.

The significance of the difference in these models is in the way the $F$ tests for the various effects are constructed. For one-way ANOVA, the $F$ test for a significant difference between means is the same regardless of whether the factor is fixed or random. For more complicated designs, the ratio of mean squares to be used in calculating an $F$ test varies according to whether the factors are fixed or random. We will not discuss in detail the development of these tests here. However, Table 11-1 gives the appropriate $F$ ratios for each test for a two-way ANOVA, according to the nature of the factors.

In each case, the critical $F$ value is determined by using the numerator and denominator degrees of freedom of the corresponding $F$-test statistic. The appropriate tests when both factors are fixed, as shown above, are just those presented in the previous chapter, with each mean square tested against the within-groups mean square. As you can see, however, the denominator for the $F$ test varies in the other situations according to

**Table 11-1.** F-Test Ratios for Two-Way ANOVA by Type of Factor (Fixed vs. Random)

| Source of Variation | Mean Square | Row Factor Fixed, Column Factor Fixed (Fixed Effects) | Row Factor Random, Column Factor Random (Random Effects) | Row Factor Random, Column Factor Fixed (Mixed Effects) |
|---|---|---|---|---|
| Factor R | $MS_R$ | $F = MS_R/MS_W$ | $F = MS_R/MS_I$ | $F = MS_R/MS_W$ |
| Factor C | $MS_C$ | $F = MS_C/MS_W$ | $F = MS_C/MS_I$ | $F = MS_C/MS_I$ |
| R × C interaction | $MS_I$ | $F = MS_I/MS_W$ | $F = MS_I/MS_W$ | $F = MS_I/MS_W$ |
| Error | $MS_W$ | | | |

whether the factor tested is fixed or random. For ANOVA designs with more than two factors, the tests become increasingly complicated. Consult a text such as Winer[46] for procedures to determine the appropriate F ratios for any ANOVA designs.

As you may have begun to surmise, ANOVA is not a simple procedure, but actually a complicated area of statistical analysis that has almost endless possibilities for variations in design of studies and analysis of data. In the remainder of this chapter we will briefly discuss just a few of those ANOVA variations that are used or can easily be used in nursing research. You may want to consult an advanced experimental design book for detailed information about these or other ANOVA problems. Winer[46] is an excellent reference.

## RANDOMIZED BLOCKS

One technique commonly used to increase the precision in an experiment is called a *randomized blocks* design. In this design, subjects are first divided into homogeneous groups called *blocks,* and then treatments are assigned at random within the groups. As an example, consider the study of the effect of an antihypertensive drug on blood pressure. Subjects could be randomly assigned to experimental (drug) and control groups, and a one-way ANOVA used to test for a significant difference in blood pressure decrease during a given time period. In such an analysis, the between-groups sum of squares would represent the treatment effect, and all other sources of variation would be included in the within-groups sum of squares. However, we know there are age differences in blood pressure, and thus we could reduce the within-groups sum of squares by removing the effect of these age differences. We can do this by dividing the sample into several age groups and assigning individuals at random to the experimental and control groups within these age groups. Age is the *blocking factor* and becomes an identifiable source of variation in the analysis. Thus the age effect on blood pressure can be separated out from the within groups sum of squares, reducing the error or unexplained variation and thus increasing the precision of the $F$ test for a treatment effect. By increasing precision, we mean that the calculated $F$ ratio will be larger with the effect of age differences removed from the denominator (the within-groups sum of squares) than without, so that the $F$ test will be more likely to lead to rejection of the null hypothesis than if the effect of age diffeences had been ignored.

The randomized blocks procedure originated in agricultural experiments, where the blocks consisted of areas of land. Each area was subdivided into several plots called *sub-blocks*. Then within each area, treatments (e.g., different fertilizers) were randomly assigned to each sub-block into which each block or area of land was divided. Suppose, for example, that four fertilizers were to be tried, to provide a comparison of average yield of grain, and that three blocks of land were to be used for the study. Each of the three blocks would be divided into four equally sized areas, and then each of the four fertilizers would be assigned to one of the areas at random. Thus each type of fertilizer would be used once in each block. The intention was to randomize treatments within fairly homogeneous blocks. Each treatment group would thus contain measures on units of observation from each block, and this would tend to make the treatment groups similar at the outset of the study.

Randomized blocks designs are also commonly used in animal studies. Instead of just assigning rats to experimental treatments, an investigator will often randomly assign one littermate to the experimental group and the other to the control group. This procedure, which is a form of matching, tends to make the groups alike before the experiment, more so than they might be if all animals were simply assigned at random to treatment groups. The resulting data include individual observations and means for each experimental group, just like data that would result from simply assigning animals at random. However, each animal is identified with a particular block, that is, the litter from which it came. Thus the effect of the block can be separated out in the ANOVA, as you will see shortly.

The design for a simple randomized blocks study is like a two-way ANOVA; thus

|  |  | **Treatment** |  |  |  |
|---|---|---|---|---|---|
|  |  | 1 | 2 | ... | c |
|  | 1 | $x_{111}$ | $x_{121}$ |  |  |
|  |  | $x_{112}$ | $x_{122}$ |  |  |
|  |  | . | . |  |  |
|  |  | . | . |  |  |
|  |  | . | . |  |  |
| **Block** |  | $x_{11n}$ | $x_{12n}$ |  |  |
|  | 2 |  |  |  |  |
|  | . |  |  |  |  |
|  | . |  |  |  |  |
|  | . |  |  |  |  |
|  | r |  |  |  |  |

In this design, blocks are treated as a row factor and treatments as a column factor. In some situations, there may be only one observation per cell ($n = 1$), rather than the general model above. In this case, only a test for the treatment effect is made, as you will see in the following section on repeated measures.

The general design above is usually considered as a mixed-model ANOVA, with the blocks considered a random factor and the treatment a fixed factor. The appropriate $F$ tests for a two-way mixed-model ANOVA, as shown in the first section of this chapter, are illustrated in Table 11-2. According to this table, the random factor and the interaction are tested against the mean square within groups and the fixed factor against the interaction term. In the case of randomized blocks, the treatment is the fixed column factor and is thus tested against the interaction mean square, while the block is the random column factor and is tested against the within groups mean square.

**Table 11-2.** *F*-Test Ratios for Randomized Blocks Design

| Source of Variation | Mean Square | F Value |
|---|---|---|
| Row factor (random) | $MS_R$ | $MS_R/MS_W$ |
| Column factor (fixed) | $MS_C$ | $MS_C/MS_I$ |
| R × C interaction | $MS_I$ | $MS_I/MS_W$ |
| Error | $MS_W$ |  |

Note that if blocking had not been done, that is, if treatments were just randomly assigned to subjects, the analysis would be a one-way ANOVA, with the total sum of squares divided into between and within treatment sums of squares, that is

$$SS_T = SS_C + SS_W$$

and the $F$ test for treatment main effect would be

$$F = \frac{MS_C}{MS_W} = \frac{SS_C/(c-1)}{SS_W/(N-c)}$$

The assignment of treatments within blocks makes it possible to separate out the block main effect and block × treatment interaction from the within groups sum of squares, so that the partition of the total sum of squares now becomes

$$SS_T = SS_C + SS_R + SS_I + SS_W$$

where $SS_R$ represents the block effect, $SS_I$ the interaction, and $SS_W$ the reduced error term. In this case the $F$ test for treatment is

$$F = \frac{MS_C}{MS_I} = \frac{SS_C/(c-1)}{SS_I/[(r-1) \times (c-1)]}$$

If a successful blocking factor has been used, that is, a blocking factor that accounts for substantial variation in the dependent variable, then $SS_R$ will be relatively large. This means that $SS_I$ will be smaller than $SS_W$ from the one-way ANOVA, and so the denominator of the $F$ test when the block is used will tend to be smaller than with the block ignored, so that the precision or sensitivity of the experiment is increased.

Thus if a blocking factor is used that actually has a substantial influence on the dependent variable, the error term may be substantially reduced, increasing the chances of finding a significant treatment effect. If you see an analysis in which the mean square between blocks is very small relative to the treatment × block interaction, you may conclude that the investigator did not gain by using the randomized-blocks design and might as well have used a simple one-way ANOVA with all subjects randomized into treatment groups and the blocking factor ignored. Blocking may be used when the effect of the blocking factor itself is of major interest to the study, and suspected but not known to affect the dependent variable. It may also be used when it is known to affect the dependent variable but is not of particular interest to the researcher, just for the purpose of increasing precision of the experiment.

In nursing research, it is more common to measure extraneous variables known to affect the dependent variable and then to include them in the analysis than to actually use the blocking procedure just described. For example, in experiments to study the effect of preoperative instruction on postoperative outcome, a researcher may note patients' education and then use education and instruction group in a two-way ANOVA. The advantage of blocking on education, that is, randomizing to instruction groups within education levels, is that the chances of obtaining instruction groups similar in education are increased, and the number in each cell of the design can be made equal, thus greatly simplifying the analysis.

As an example of the sort of study in which randomized blocks might be used, consider the research by Johnson et al.[24] described in Problem 2 in Chapter 10. In this study, children were randomized into three groups prior to cast removal. One group received no preoperative information, one received procedural information, and one received sensory information. The children were also asked how afraid they were of having the cast removed and were classified according to their responses as either fearful or not fearful. A two-way ANOVA was used to study effects of information group and fear group on differences in mean distress scores. To use randomized blocks in such a situation, one would first classify the children into the fear–no-fear groups, which would be the blocking factor. Random assignment to information groups would then be made within the fear–no-fear groups.

It is sometimes difficult in terms of study methodology to use a randomized-blocks design. The procedure requires that subjects be classified into the appropriate blocks before the randomization into treatment groups is made. If the blocking factor is age group, education, and so on, this is easily accomplished. If the blocking factor is a more complicated variable, it may be more difficult. Consider the research by Kim[27], described in several problems in earlier chapters. Kim's research developed from several nursing research studies that suggested that preparatory information can be used to reduce anxiety and thereby reduce pain among surgical patients. She developed a contingency model that suggested that the effect of preparatory information on pain might be positive among patients low on a particular kind of trait anxiety (physical-danger) but negative in patients high on physical-danger trait anxiety. To use a randomized-blocks design for this study, one would first test patients on physical-danger trait anxiety, in order to classify them into the high or low group. There would be, therefore, two blocks, low anxiety and high anxiety. Within each of these blocks, then, patients would be randomized into experimental (preparatory information) or control (no preparatory information) groups. Such a blocking procedure would require calculation of the anxiety levels, so

Analysis of Variance, Continued

that it would not be possible to block, randomize within blocks, and carry out the experimental procedure within one contact with the subject. If possible to use, however, randomized blocks is a good design for reducing unexplained variation in the dependent variable and thus increasing sensitivity of the statistical test for the treatment effect.

## REPEATED MEASURES

Another design commonly used in nursing research is one in which the same subjects are observed at several different times, or under several different treatment conditions. This is called a *repeated-measures* design, since repeated observations are made on each individual. The fact that the same subjects are observed under each treatment condition means that there will be correlation between subjects' scores across treatments. Since the repeated-measures analysis is designed to take account of this correlation, the resulting statistical test is more powerful than the one that would result from observing a different group of subjects under each treatment condition, that is, an ordinary one-way ANOVA. Repeated use of the same subjects also makes it possible to use fewer subjects than required for a comparison of independent group means.

An example of a repeated-measures ANOVA is a study in which the temperatures of individuals are taken at several points during the day to determine whether temperatures tend to rise from morning to evening. Any before–after study, where some dependent variable is observed for all subjects before and after a treatment, is also an example of a repeated-measures ANOVA design. Repeatedly testing students at several points during a course provides data for a repeated-measures ANOVA. The trials do not necessarily have to represent time points. Measurement of blood pressure for the same subjects at different levels of activity would provide data for repeated-measures ANOVA, as would measurements of satisfaction among the same patients with different types of birth control.

The simplest sort of repeated measures design can be pictured as:

|          |   | Trials   |          |       |          |
|----------|---|----------|----------|-------|----------|
|          |   | 1        | 2        | ...   | c        |
|          | 1 | $x_{11}$ | $x_{12}$ | ...   | $x_{1c}$ |
| **Subjects** | 2 | $x_{21}$ | $x_{22}$ | ...   | $x_{2c}$ |
|          | . | .        | .        |       | .        |
|          | . | .        | .        |       | .        |
|          | . | .        | .        |       | .        |
|          | r | $x_{r1}$ | $x_{r2}$ | ...   | $x_{rc}$ |

In this design, subjects are the row factor and trials are the column factor. The columns represent different observations on the same subjects, which may be either observations at different time points or under different treatment conditions. If there are only two trials, such data can be handled by a paired $t$ test. With more than two trials, a *repeated-measures ANOVA* is appropriate. For this repeated-measures design, the subjects represent the row factor and the trials represent the column factor, so that the analysis is again a two-way ANOVA. The subjects are considered a random factor, since the researcher usually wants to generalize the results to subjects other than those included in the study. In other words, the same analysis is used as for a randomized-blocks design. This simple repeated measures design can in fact be regarded as a randomized-blocks design, with the subjects considered as blocks.

However, notice that in the repeated-measures design there is only one observation for each row × column combination, that is, only one observation per cell. This means that there is no within-cell variation (variation around cell means) and thus no within-cell sum of squares to be calculated. You can check on this by recalling that degrees of freedom for the within-cell sum of squares in two-way ANOVA is $rc(n - 1)$. When there is only one observation per cell, $n = 1$, so that

$$rc(n - 1) = rc(0)$$
$$= 0$$

indicating that there are no degrees of freedom available for within-cell variation.

Because there is no within-cell variation, the total sum of squares is partitioned as

$$SS_T = SS_R + SS_C + SS_I$$

The ANOVA table for this design is illustrated in Table 11-3.

The trial (or treatment effect) is tested by

$$F = \frac{MS_C}{MS_I}$$

just as in the randomized-blocks situation. In this case, no other tests are made, since there is no within-groups sum of squares with which to construct the other $F$ ratios.

With repeated-measures designs, the degrees of freedom are sometimes confusing. In earlier ANOVA designs, the total degrees of freedom was always $N - 1$, where $N$ stands for the number of subjects. In the

Analysis of Variance, Continued

**Table 11-3.** *F*-Test Ratio for Repeated Measures Design

| Source of Variation | Sum of Squares | Degrees of Freedom | Mean Square | F |
|---|---|---|---|---|
| Between subjects | $SS_R$ | $r - 1$ | $MS_R$ | |
| Between trials | $SS_C$ | $c - 1$ | $MS_C$ | $MS_C/MS_I$ |
| Trial × subject interaction | $SS_I$ | $(r - 1) \times (c - 1)$ | $MS_I$ | |
| Total | $SS_T$ | | | |

above design, the number of subjects is $r$ and the total degrees of freedom is $rc - 1$. This difference is, of course, due to the fact that repeated measures are being made on the same subjects.

An example of a repeated measures design comes from an investigation made by Derdiarian and Clough[11]. These researchers studied changes in levels of dependence and independence during the course of hospitalization among patients undergoing total hip or total knee replacement procedures. Tests measuring dependence and independence were obtained at five times: prehospitalization, presurgery, postsurgery, predischarge, and postdischarge. Such data can easily be handled by a repeated measures ANOVA, with subjects as rows and the five times of testing as columns. Although it is not discussed in this text, whenever there are more than two trials, it is possible to construct orthogonal comparisons of interest with respect to the trial factor. In the example, for instance, one could determine at which times, among the five measurement points, there were significant changes in the dependence and independence levels. Winer[46] includes an example of such an analysis.

## REPEATED MEASURES WITH RANDOM ASSIGNMENT

Another repeated-measures design that is used fairly frequently is one in which subjects are assigned randomly to treatment groups prior to repeated observation. In nursing research, the resulting measurements often consist of a pre-test and a post-test, so that change in an experimental group can be compared with change in a control group. This design is the one referred to by Campbell and Stanley[3] as the "pre-test–post-test control group design."

The design can be diagrammed as follows:

|  |  | **Trials** |  |  |  |
| --- | --- | --- | --- | --- | --- |
|  |  | 1 | 2 | ... | c |

**Subjects**

$\left.\begin{array}{c}1\\2\\3\\4\end{array}\right\}$ Treatment 1

$\left.\begin{array}{c}\cdot\\\cdot\\\cdot\end{array}\right\}$ Treatment 2

$\left.\begin{array}{c}\cdot\\\cdot\\\cdot\\\cdot\\r\end{array}\right\}$ Treatment $k$

The total number of subjects, $r$, are equally divided into the $k$ treatment groups, so that the number of subjects receiving each treatment is $r/k$.

In this design, subjects are again the row factor and trials the column factor. The total sum of squares can thus be partitioned into

$$SS_T = SS_R + SS_C + SS_I$$

the same partition as used for the repeated-measures design with no random assignment into groups. In this case, however, the row sum of squares, $SS_R$, includes not only variation among individual subjects, but also variation due to treatment. The row sum of squares, with $r - 1$ degrees of freedom, can thus be divided into two parts:

$$SS_R = SS_{\text{between treatments}} + SS_{\text{within treatments}}$$

with $(k - 1)$ and $(r - k)$ degrees of freedom, respectively. This is equivalent to considering the row sum of squares as a total sum of squares in a one-way ANOVA with just one observation per subject (the mean of all the trial scores for each subject).

The row × column interaction sum of squares, $SS_I$, can also be partitioned. This sum of squares, with $(r - 1) \times (c - 1)$ degrees of

# Analysis of Variance, Continued

freedom, includes both interaction between trials and treatment and interaction between trials and subjects within each treatment group. Thus

$$SS_I = SS_{\text{trials} \times \text{treatments}} + SS_{\text{trials} \times \text{subjects within treatments}}$$

with $(c - 1) \times (k - 1)$ and $(c - 1) \times (r/k - 1) \times (k)$ degrees of freedom, respectively, is the partition of the row × column interaction. Table 11-4 summarizes the partition of the total sum of squares for this analysis.

The analysis is similar to repeated measures analysis, except that there are two different types of error term. We will not discuss the theoretical basis for use of these error terms. Each $F$ test is interpreted according to the usual procedure, using the corresponding numerator and denominator degrees of freedom in each case to determine the critical value from the $F$ table. In a typical study with a control group and an experimental group, with a pretest and posttest on each, the $F$ test of greatest interest to the researcher is the interaction term. If the experiment is successful, the pre-tests should be similar for the groups because of the randomization, and the post-tests should differ because of the experimental treatment. This should be reflected in a significant trial × treatment interaction.

Research done by Rottkamp[38] illustrates the use of repeated measures with random assignment. The purpose of this research was to determine the effects on spinal cord-injured patients of behavior modification training in body positioning. Patients were randomly assigned to two groups. One group received the behavior modification training, and the other group received customary body positioning nursing care. One dependent variable of interest was frequency of daily changes of position, which was determined for all patients both before and after introduction of the experimental treatment. With subjects as rows divided into experimental and control subjects, and before and after behavior modification constituting the two trials (columns), the data fit a repeated measurements with random assignment design.

Although the model presented here assumes random assignment into treatment groups, many studies involve collection of data for two or more time points for two or more groups of subjects not formed by randomization. Such a study is illustrated by the research of Mims et al.[33]. These investigators analyzed changes in beliefs, attitudes, and behaviors of students following a 3-day human sexuality course. Three groups of students, medical, nursing, and graduate psychology students were included, so that the researchers could examine not only change over time, but differences in the degree of change for these three groups of students. The data from this study fit a repeated measurements with random assignment design, except that the groups were not formed by randomization. Many canned computer programs for analysis of repeated measures with subjects clas-

**Table 11-4.** *F*-Test for Repeated Measures With Random Assignment Design

| Source of Variation | Sum of Squares | Degrees of Freedom | Mean Square | F |
|---|---|---|---|---|
| *Between subjects* | $SS_R$ | $(r-1)$ | | |
| Between treatments | $SS_{RBTr}$ | $(k-1)$ | $MS_{RBTr}$ | $MS_{RBTr}/MS_{RWTr}$ |
| Between subjects within treatments | $SS_{RWTr}$ | $(r-k)$ | $MS_{RWTr}$ | |
| *Between trials* | $SS_C$ | $(c-1)$ | $MS_C$ | $MS_C/MS_{C \times RWTr}$ |
| *Trial × subject interaction* | $SS_I$ | $(r-1) \times (c-1)$ | | |
| Trials × treatments | $SS_{C \times Tr}$ | $(c-1) \times (k-1)$ | $MS_{C \times Tr}$ | $MS_{C \times Tr}/MS_{C \times RWTr}$ |
| Trials × subjects within treatments | $SS_{C \times RWTr}$ | $(c-1) \times (r/k-1) \times (k)$ | $MS_{C \times RWTr}$ | |
| Total | $SS_T$ | $(rc-1)$ | | |

sified into groups are designed to handle situations like this, where the groups are not formed by randomization, so that analysis of such data is seldom a problem.

## MULTIVARIATE ANOVA

The ANOVA situations we have discussed to this point are sometimes referred to as *univariate ANOVA*. In these situations, the effects of one or more factors on a single dependent variable are analyzed. There can be situations where more than one dependent variable may be of interest. For example, a drug might be expected to affect not only blood pressure, but also temperature and pulse rate. It is common to analyze such data by means of a series of ANOVA procedures, one for each dependent variable. If the observations on the dependent variables are obtained from the same subjects, however, they are correlated, and a measure of the simultaneous response to all the dependent variables is likely to be a better measure of treatment than each response considered separately. The procedure called *multivariate ANOVA* provides one overall test of significance for all the dependent variables taken together.

We will not go into derivation of tests for the multivariate ANOVA procedure. If you use a computer program to do multivariate ANOVA, you will obtain an overall $F$-test statistic for the null hypothesis of no treatment effects. The multivariate test takes account of the correlation among dependent variables, so that this test may result in statistical significance even when some or all of the corresponding univariate tests result in nonsignificant $F$ values. A multivariate ANOVA, with one independent variable and two or more dependent variables, which yields a significant $F$ ratio, indicates a significant overall treatment effect, taking into account the simultaneous response of the subjects to all the dependent variables. This may be a better indication of a total treatment effect than individual $F$ tests on each dependent variable. See Winer[46] for further discussion on this topic, as well as for many other complicated ANOVA topics not discussed in this text.

## SUMMARY

In the last several chapters, several ANOVA procedures have been described. The ones we have discussed include factorial designs, randomized blocks, and repeated measures designs. In some of the presentations, for simplicity of notation, we have assumed equal cell frequencies. When the cell frequencies are not equal, as is often the case in nursing research studies, the notation and analysis become more complicated. As we have pointed out along the way, many computer programs are designed to account for inequalities in frequencies, so this should not generally be a problem in data analysis. See Winer[46] for details of the mathematical development of many designs with unequal cell frequencies.

Analysis of variance as a statistical technique originated as a method for analyzing data that result from experiments. In the classical one-way ANOVA situation, the researcher randomizes individuals into the treatment groups. In a factorial design, an equal number of subjects are randomly assigned to each possible treatment combination, and the result of this is that the independent variables (the factors) are independent. As you have seen, many research problems in nursing and other behavioral sciences involve collection of data from intact groups, that is, groups not formed by randomization. Individuals are assigned to groups on the basis of characteristics they already possess, such as level of education. When group assignment is not based on randomization, the independent variables are intercorrelated.

Because computer programs have been designed to handle unequal cell frequencies, researchers sometimes partition continuous variables such as education into groups, such as high, medium, and low, so that ANOVA can be used. The effect of this procedure, as explained at the end of Chapter 4, is the loss of variability among the subjects and reduced sensitivity of the statistical tests. When the independent variables are both qualitative and quantitative, it is tempting to categorize the quantitative variables so that a fancy ANOVA procedure can be carried out, with each independent variable treated as a factor. A preferable procedure is multiple regression analysis. This is easily accomplished by the use of dummy coding for the qualitative independent variables and allows the quantitative independent variables to retain their original values.

This chapter has covered only a few of the many possible ANOVA designs. Specialized designs like Latin Squares have not been described. Neither have nested or hierarchical designs, in which not all possible treatment combinations are represented. These designs are very rarely used in nursing research. If necessary, you can refer to Snedecor and Cochran[41]; Winer[46], Klugh[29], or other references repeatedly cited in the ANOVA chapters for explanations of these topics. Computer programs are also available to handle many of the designs that have not been discussed in this text.

The use of multiple comparisons was discussed in detail only in relation to one-way ANOVA. Their use can be extended to more complicated ANOVA designs. In two-way ANOVA, for example, any main effect that has more than one degree of freedom (i.e., more than two levels of the factor) can be subdivided into orthogonal contrasts. Multiple comparison

# Analysis of Variance, Continued

procedures can also be applied to repeated measures designs, as well as to most other ANOVA designs. The references just cited in the above paragraph have examples of such procedures. Nie et al.[34], as well as Cohen and Cohen[8] also explain in more detail about the relationships between regression analysis and ANOVA that have frequently been alluded to in this text. In Chapter 12 we will discuss the use of analysis of covariance (ANOCOVA), usually conceptualized as a combination of regression and ANOVA procedures.

## PROBLEMS

1. In Problem 7 in Chapter 10, a study of the effect of preoperative visits by operating room nurses was described. In this study, patients were randomized into two groups. In the experimental group, each patient received a preoperative visit designed to reduce anxiety and have a positive effect on postoperative patient welfare. Age and degree of surgical trauma were also measured and included in an analysis of differences in the Palmar Sweat Index (PSI). Explain how this study could be redesigned, using randomized blocks. Explain what the blocks would be and how the randomized procedure would be carried out. For simplicity, you can omit age as a study variable.

2. Suppose that in a sample of 153 patients, systolic blood pressure is recorded for the first 3 days of hospitalization, so that change during the first 3 days can be evaluated. The blood pressure measures, as shown in Table 11-5, are taken for 3 days on the same subjects, so that a repeated-measures ANOVA can be used to analyze the data. The analysis is shown in Table 11-6.

   (a) Calculate the mean squares for the table.
   (b) What null hypothesis can be tested by this analysis?
   (c) Calculate the $F$ ratio required to test the null hypothesis.
   (d) Test the null hypothesis, using the .01 level of significance.
   (e) State your findings in substantive terms.
   (f) Why couldn't a paired $t$ test be used for this analysis?

**Table 11-5.** Systolic Blood Pressure for First 3 Days of Hospitalization ($N = 153$)

| Day 1 | | Day 2 | | Day 3 | |
|---|---|---|---|---|---|
| Mean | SD | Mean | SD | Mean | SD |
| 122.9 | 71.9 | 116.4 | 29.1 | 104.1 | 44.1 |

**Table 11-6.** Repeated-Measures Analysis of Variance of Change in Systolic Blood Pressure for First 3 Days of Hospitalization ($N = 153$)

| Source of Variation | Sum of Squares | DF | Mean Square | F |
|---|---|---|---|---|
| Between subjects | 510,531 | 152 | | |
| Between trials | 27,633 | 2 | | |
| Trial × subject | 700,170 | 304 | | |
| Total | 1,238,334 | 458 | | |

3. Isenberg[21] investigated the relationship between the experience of surgery and changes in the speed of time perception. She reasoned that, as a result of metabolic changes associated with the surgical experience, surgical patients should experience a speeding up of time perception following surgery and that there should be a greater speedup for patients having major surgery than for patients having minor surgery. Several measurements of time perception were obtained from 72 subjects (36 having major surgery and 36 having minor surgery) on the day before surgery and on each of several days after surgery. For one measure of time perception, a verbal estimation of a 20-second interval, the investigator asked each subject to estimate how many seconds passed between the time she said "start" and the time she said "stop" (the actual clock time was 20 seconds). According to the theoretical rationale on which the study was based, she hypothesized that subjects would estimate the 20-second interval as longer after surgery than before, and that the difference would be greater for patients having major surgery than for patients having minor surgery. Group means for the estimates for the two groups of patients, for the day before and the day after surgery, are shown in Table 11-7.

A repeated measures ANOVA was used for analysis of the difference between groups and change over time. Results are given in Table 11-8.

(a) Calcualte all the relevant mean squares for the above table.
(b) Calculate the relevant $F$ values for the ANOVA.
(c) State the null hypothesis tested by the $F$-test statistic for "between groups."
(d) Test the null hypothesis stated in step c, using the .001 level of significance.
(e) State in substantive terms the conclusion, based on your answers to c and d.
(f) Answer the questions in c, d, and e for the "between trials" and "trial × group" $F$-test statistics.

Analysis of Variance, Continued

**Table 11-7.** Mean Verbal Estimation of 20-Second Interval for the Day Before and the Day After Surgery, for Patients Having Major Surgery and Patients Having Minor Surgery ($N = 72$)

| Group | Trial: Day Before Surgery | Trial: Day After Surgery | Day Before Surgery–Day After Surgery |
|---|---|---|---|
| Minor Surgery ($N = 36$) | 32.67 | 37.25 | 4.58 |
| Major surgery ($N = 36$) | 45.50 | 108.19 | 62.69 |
| Total ($N = 72$) | 39.08 | 72.72 | 33.64 |

(g) Does the analysis support the relationships hypothesized by the researcher?

4. To study the effect of relaxation training on the frequency of intake of pro re nata (prn) medication for relief of tension, Tamex et al.[42] studied 60 patients on prn minor tranquilizers and sedatives in a psychiatric

**Table 11-8.** Repeated-Measure Analysis of Variance of Change in Mean Verbal Estimation of 20-second Interval from the Day Before Surgery to the Day After Surgery, for Patients Having Major Surgery and Patients Having Minor Surgery ($N = 72$)

| Source of Variation | Sum of Squares | DF | Mean Square | F |
|---|---|---|---|---|
| Between subjects | 198973.69 | 71 | | |
| Between groups | 63168.31 | 1 | | |
| Between subjects within groups | 135805.38 | 70 | | |
| Between trials | 40736.69 | 1 | | |
| Trial × subject interaction | 43014.32 | 71 | | |
| Trial × group | 30392.13 | 1 | | |
| Trial × subjects within groups | 12622.19 | 70 | | |

nursing unit of a veterans administration (VA) hospital. Subjects were randomly assigned to three groups, as follows:

Group A. Control, no training
Group B. Live instruction in relaxation training
Group C. Taped instruction in relaxation training

The researchers reported mean number of tranquilizers and hypnotics taken on day of admission and study day 1, by group, as indicated in Table 11-9.

This design fits that for repeated measures with random assignment.

(a) Describe the three null hypotheses that could be tested for the data.
(b) If the relaxation training were effective, which of the $F$ tests would you expect to be significant, and why?
(c) Although the relaxation training continued for 6 days, the data on number of tranquilizers and hypnotics were presented in the article only for the day of admission and study day 1. Can you guess why, based on the data shown in Table 11-9?

5. In Isenberg's study[21] (described in Problem 3) verbal estimates of a 20-second interval were obtained for 4 days following surgery for those patients in the major surgery group. The researcher hypothesized that the verbal estimates of a 20-second interval would speed up immediately following surgery and then gradually decline as the postsurgical period progressed. Means for the four postsurgical days are given in Table 11-10.

**Table 11-9.** Mean Number of Tranquilizers and Hypnotics Taken on Day of Admission and Study Day 1, by Treatment Group ($N = 60$)

| Drugs | Group | Day of Admission $\bar{x}$ | SD | Study Day 1 $\bar{x}$ | SD |
|---|---|---|---|---|---|
| Tranquilizers | A | 0.80 | 2.50 | 0.40 | 1.14 |
|  | B | 1.05 | 2.19 | 0.50 | 1.00 |
|  | C | 1.10 | 2.55 | 0.20 | 0.52 |
| Hypnotics | A | 1.80 | 3.55 | 0.30 | 0.57 |
|  | B | 2.15 | 2.39 | 0.15 | 0.37 |
|  | C | 1.60 | 2.58 | 0.15 | 0.37 |

Analysis of Variance, Continued

**Table 11-10.** Mean Verbal Estimation of 20-second Interval for 4 Days Following Surgery, for Patients Having Major Surgery ($N = 36$)

| Day 1 | Day 2 | Day 3 | Day 4 |
|---|---|---|---|
| 108.19 | 86.94 | 53.89 | 28.25 |

Repeated measures ANOVA yielded the results shown in Table 11-11. For this problem, ignore the subdivisions of the between trials and error sums of squares.

(a) State the null hypothesis tested by the "between trials" $F$-test statistic.
(b) Test the null hypothesis described in step a.
(c) State in substantive terms the conclusion that can be made, based on your answers to a and b.
(d) Given your answer to c, your answers to problem 3, and by inspection of the means for the four postsurgical days, would you say the results support the effects of surgery on time perception hypothesized by the researcher?

6. In Table 11-11, the between-trials sum of squares, with 3 degrees of freedom, has been subdivided into three orthogonal contrasts. The analysis takes the form of trend analysis, as described in Chapter 9, except

**Table 11-11.** Repeated-Measures Analysis of Variance of Change in Mean Verbal Estimation of 20-second Interval for 4 Days Following Surgery, for Patients Having Major Surgery ($N = 36$)

| Source of Variation | Sum of Squares | DF | Mean Square | F |
|---|---|---|---|---|
| Between Trials | 134881.38 | 3 | 44960.46 | 144.31 |
| Linear | 134042.94 | 1 | 134042.94 | 220.84 |
| Quadratic | 173.36 | 1 | 173.36 | 0.77 |
| Residual | 665.08 | 1 | 665.08 | |
| Between subjects | 94471.88 | 35 | 2699.20 | |
| Error | 32714.13 | 105 | 311.56 | |
| Linear | 21244.31 | 35 | 606.98 | |
| Quadratic | 7835.14 | 35 | 223.86 | |
| Residual | 3634.68 | 35 | 103.85 | |

that in this problem the analysis is adapted to account for the repeated measures. The contrasts represent linear and quadratic trends, plus residuals. The error term has also been subdivided in a corresponding fashion. The linear part of the between-trials sum of squares measures the degree to which the four trial means lie on a straight line (constant decrease in estimation from day 1 to day 4). The quadratic part is a measure of the degree to which the trend across days is curvilinear (change in rate of decrease of estimation from day 1 to day 4). The residual is the part left over, which cannot be explained by either a linear or quadratic trend. According to the analysis, almost all the between-trials sum of squares can be attributed to linear trend, and the $F$ for linear trend is highly significant. What do these results suggest about the pattern of change in verbal estimation during the postsurgical period for patients having major surgery? See Winer[46] and Snedecor and Cochran[41] for further explanation of interpretation of results of trend analyses.

# Chapter 12

## ANALYSIS OF COVARIANCE

### USES OF ANOCOVA

In previous chapters we have discussed procedures for reducing unexplained variation in the dependent variable of interest in a study by use of various designs. Factorial designs have been described that allow for the simultaneous study of the effects of two or more independent variables, thus reducing unexplained variation. Randomized block designs and repeated measures designs also help reduce unexplained variation. Procedures such as multiple regression reduce unexplained variation as well, but usually through analysis of the data rather than by study design. In the ANOCOVA procedure the statistical technique of regression is used to reduce unexplained variation, followed by ANOVA to examine group differences. Analysis of covariance is described in this chapter as it is usually conceptualized, as a combination of regression and ANOVA. Since ANOVA is a special form of regression, such situations can also be handled by use of multiple regression analysis.

The intent of ANOCOVA is to provide statistical control for one or more variables that have not been controlled by the design of the study itself. It is appropriate for situations where one would like to study differences among means on a dependent variable for several groups, but where there is reason to suspect that the groups differ at the outset of the study. The procedure is used to adjust for, or eliminate the effect of initial differences among the groups, so that the ANOVA of the differences in means will be free of the effects of these initial, uncontrolled differences. Therefore, ANOCOVA is commonly used to analyze group differences in nonrandomized studies.

An example of such a study is an investigation of effects on final examination scores in classes where different teaching techniques have been used. In this type of study the subjects are probably not randomized into classes, but rather existing classes are used. The investigator wishes to use analysis of variance to compare mean scores on final examinations for the different classes. However, there may be differences in intelligence among the classes, which might be expected to affect the final exam scores. Analysis of covariance allows the researcher to control for group differences in intelligence while looking for a difference in examination scores that is due to the different teaching procedures.

Analysis of covariance may also be used to improve precision in the comparison of means in randomized studies. For example, in a controlled, experimental study of weight gain of babies given different formulas, some heavier babies may be placed in one group more frequently than another, despite the randomization procedure. If the sample sizes are very small, this initial difference between the groups can affect the final results. Adjustment for this initial difference in weight among the groups can be used to improve the precision of the final comparisons of weight gain. Analysis of variance allows the investigator to compare weight gain in the various groups with weight at the onset of the study controlled, that is, removing the effect of the subjects' original weight on the study of weight gain.

In both of these examples, there is a possibility that the comparison groups differed in some way at the outset of the study and, moreover, that they differed with respect to variables that might have an effect on the results of the final comparison of the groups. The purpose of ANOCOVA is to take these initial differences into account in such a way that they do not influence the final comparison of the means. The most common situation in which ANOCOVA is used, and the one to be described in this text, is the one in which the COVARIATES (the variables to be controlled) are quantitative in nature. Control of the covariates is followed by ANOVA with one or more factors, which are the independent variables of interest to the researcher.

You should note that some research situations do not fit this model. If the variables to be controlled are both qualitative and quantitative (e.g., sex and age), the model to be presented here is not appropriate. Or, it may be that the independent variable of major interest to the researcher is quantitative, so that there are no group means to compare. In such situations, a good approach is multiple regression, with inclusion of qualitative variables by use of dummy variables. The order of entry of variables can then be constrained in such a way that those to be controlled are entered prior to the independent variable of interest. The SPSS package provides for such analysis, for example, and Nie et al.[34] include a good explanation of the use and interpretation of ANOCOVA with both quantitative and qualitative variables.

Analysis of Covariance

## THE GENERAL ANOCOVA PROCEDURE

Consider a study design in which the subjects have been classified into $k$ groups, and the researcher wishes to test the null hypothesis of equality of group means. Suppose that the investigator also has data for each subject on a variable (covariate) that is suspected of being correlated with the dependent variable and should thus be controlled in the analysis. Let the dependent variable be represented by $y_{ij}$ and the covariate by $x_{ij}$. The observations can then be denoted as shown in Table 12-1. In relation to the example given earlier, the $y_{ij}$ values could represent weight gains for infants on $k$ different formulas, and the $x_{ij}$ values would be the birth weights for these same individuals. Notice that the dependent variable in this analysis of variance in labeled $y_{ij}$ instead of the $x_{ij}$ used before. The choice of symbols is purely arbitrary. We have switched to $y_{ij}$ here because $y_{ij}$ is used as a symbol for the dependent variable in regression, and you will see shortly how regression of $y$ on $x$ is used in ANOCOVA.

Analysis of covariance, as mentioned before, consists of regression followed by ANOVA. In order to control for the effect of the covariate $x$ on the dependent variable $y$, we begin by looking at the relationship between $x$ and $y$ as just an ordinary regression problem. This approach assumes, of course, a linear relationship between $x$ and $y$. You will recall how the regression analysis of variance divides the total sum of squares into one part due to regression and a second part representing deviations from regression. The table is constructed as shown in Table 12-2.

**Table 12-1.** Conventional Notation System for ANOCOVA with One Covariate and $k$ groups

| Group 1 | Group 2 | | Group $k$ | |
|---|---|---|---|---|
| $y_{11}\ x_{11}$ | $y_{21}\ x_{21}$ | $\cdots$ | $y_{k1}$ | $x_{k1}$ |
| $y_{12}\ x_{12}$ | $y_{22}\ x_{22}$ | $\cdots$ | $y_{k2}$ | $x_{k2}$ |
| . . | . . | | . | . |
| . . | . . | | . | . |
| . . | . . | | . | . |
| $y_{1n_1}\ x_{1n_1}$ | $y_{2n_2}\ x_{2n_2}$ | | $y_{kn_k}$ | $x_{kn_k}$ |
| $\bar{y}_1\ \bar{x}_1$ | $\bar{y}_2\ \bar{x}_2$ | | $\bar{y}_k\ \bar{x}_k$ | $(\bar{y},\bar{x})$ |

$i$ = Group number; $j$ = Observation number; $x_{ij}$; = Covariate variable for observation $j$ in group $i$; $y_{ij}$ = Dependent variable for observation $j$ in group $i$; $n_i$ = Number of observations in group $i$; $\bar{x}_i$ = Mean of covariate in group $i$; $\bar{y}_i$ = Mean of dependent variable in group $i$; $\bar{x}$ = Mean of all observations of covariate; $\bar{y}$ = Mean of all observations of dependent variable

**Table 12-2.** *F*-Test Ratio for ANOCOVA Covariate

| Source of Variation | Sum of Squares | DF | Mean Square | F |
|---|---|---|---|---|
| Regression | $\sum_{i=1}^{k}\sum_{j=1}^{n_i}(y'_{ij} - \bar{y})^2$ | 1 | $MS_R = SS_R/1$ | $MS_R/MS_D$ |
| Deviations | $\sum_{i=1}^{k}\sum_{j=1}^{n_i}(y_{ij} - y'_{ij})^2$ | $N - 2$ | $MS_D = SS_D/(N - 2)$ | |
| Total | $\sum_{i=1}^{k}\sum_{j=1}^{n_i}(y_{ij} - \bar{y})^2$ | $N - 1$ | | |

The only difference between this notation and the one used earlier for regression analysis is that the observations are classified into groups, so that each observation is represented by a $y_{ij}$ instead of simply by $y_i$.

According to this regression ANOVA, part of the total variation in $y$ (the regression sum of squares, $SS_R$) is due to the relationship between $x$ and $y$, and the other part (the deviations sum of squares, $SS_D$) is due to the effects of all other variables. Analysis of covariance allows us to make a comparison of treatment means using ANOVA, with the effect of $x$ eliminated. To eliminate the effect of $x$, we eliminate $SS_R$ from the variation that is to be considered by ANOVA from the total variation in $y$. We base the ANOVA on $SS_D$, the deviations sum of squares from the above regression analysis, since $SS_D$ represents the variation in $y$ with the effect of $x$ removed. Analysis of variance is then made by dividing the deviations sum of squares into a between-groups sum of squares and a within-groups sum of squares, as you will see shortly. If this ANOVA leads to rejection of the null hypothesis of equality of the treatment means, we will know that the difference in means cannot be attributed to group differences in the covariate, since the effect of the covariate will have been removed.

Consider for a moment the deviations sum of squares from the regression. Using the regression procedure, we calculate a regression equation for all the $x$ and $y$ observations, ignoring the placement of individuals in groups. Thus for each observed $y_{ij}$ value, there is a predicted value:

$$y'_{ij} = a + b_t x_{ij}$$

The deviations sum of squares, as you may recall, is just the sum of squared deviations of each observed value from the value predicted by the regression equation. Therefore, using the above formula for the predicted value, we can write the deviations sum of squares as

# Analysis of Covariance

$$\sum_{i=1}^{k}\sum_{j=1}^{n_i}(y_{ij} - y'_{ij})^2 = \sum_{i=1}^{k}\sum_{j=1}^{n_i}(y_{ij} - a - b_t x_{ij})^2$$

It can be shown algebraically that this equation can be expressed as

$$\sum_{i=1}^{k}\sum_{j=1}^{n_i}(y_{ij} - y'_{ij})^2 = \sum_{i=1}^{k}\sum_{j=1}^{n_i}(y_{ij} - \bar{y})^2 - b_t \sum_{i=1}^{k}\sum_{j=1}^{n_i}(y_{ij} - \bar{y})(x_{ij} - \bar{x})$$

The deviations sum of squares is the original total sum of squares reduced by an amount dependent on the degree of success of the prediction from the regression. If the prediction is not very good, most of the variation will remain in the deviations sum of squares, and the deviations sum of squares will be similar to the original sum of squares. If the prediction is very successful, that is, if the covariate is strongly correlated with the dependent variable, the deviations sum of squares may be substantially less than the original total sum of squares. This deviation sum of squares, on which the ANOVA is based, is often called the *adjusted total sum of squares*.

After the adjusted total sum of squares is determined, it is partitioned into between- and within-groups sums of squares. This is done by using what is called *within-groups regression*. Instead of doing one regression analysis for all of the $x$ and $y$ observations together, we can do one regression analysis for all $x$ and $y$ pairs within each of the $k$ treatment groups. The slope for each of these regressions is denoted as $b_i$. Analysis of covariance makes the assumption that the regression coefficient is the same for all of the within-group regressions, that is, that

$$b_1 = b_2 = \cdots = b_k = b_w$$

The gist of the above statement is that the strength of the relationship between the covariate and the dependent variable is assumed to be the same within each treatment group.

The within-groups regression analysis results in prediction equations that are the same for all the groups, since the strength of the relationship is assumed to be the same for all the groups. Denoting $y''_{ij}$ as predicted values for within-group regression to distinguish them from $y'_{ij}$, the predicted values for the regression analysis for all subjects together, we can write the prediction equations as

$$y''_{ij} = a_w + b_w x_{ij}$$

The sum of squared deviations from the within-group regression values can be written as

$$\sum_{i=1}^{k}\sum_{j=1}^{n_i}(y_{ij} - y''_{ij})^2 = \sum_{i=1}^{k}\sum_{j=1}^{n_i}(y_{ij} - a_w - b_w x_{ij})^2$$

which reduces algebraically to

$$\sum_{i=1}^{k}\sum_{j=1}^{n_i}(y_{ij} - y''_{ij})^2 = \sum_{i=1}^{k}\sum_{j=1}^{n_i}(y_{ij} - \bar{y}_i)^2 - b_w \sum_{i=1}^{k}\sum_{j=1}^{n_i}(y_{ij} - \bar{y}_i)(x_{ij} - \bar{x}_i)$$

The quantity

$$\sum_{i=1}^{k}\sum_{j=1}^{n_i}(y_{ij} - \bar{y}_i)^2$$

in the above equation is the sum of squared deviations of observations from their group means. This quantity represents the within-groups sum of squares that would be obtained by a one-way ANOVA with the effect of the covariate ignored. To obtain an adjusted within-groups sum of squares which takes the effect of the covariate into account, we reduce this original within-groups sum of squares by the quantity on the far right in the above equation, which is a measure of regression within groups. The *adjusted within-groups sum of squares*,

$$\sum_{i=1}^{k}\sum_{j=1}^{n_i}(y_{ij} - y''_{ij})^2$$

becomes the error term for the ANOVA that follows the regression in ANOCOVA.

The final quantity to be determined in ANOCOVA is the *adjusted between-groups sum of squares*. The original between-groups sum of squares has to be adjusted to eliminate the effect of the relationship between the $y$ values and the covariate $x$. In this case, however, the adjusted value can be obtained by subtraction. Just as the usual between-groups and within-groups sums of squares must add to the total, the adjusted values must add to the adjusted total. The adjusted between groups sum of squares is thus just the adjusted total sum of squares minus the adjusted within-groups sum of squares, or

## Analysis of Covariance

$$\sum_{i=1}^{k}\sum_{j=1}^{n_i}(y_{ij} - y'_{ij})^2 - \sum_{i=1}^{k}\sum_{j=1}^{n_i}(y_{ij} - y''_{ij})^2$$

$$= \left\{\sum_{i=1}^{k}\sum_{j=1}^{n_i}(y_{ij} - \bar{y})^2 - b_t \sum_{i=1}^{k}\sum_{j=1}^{n_i}(y_{ij} - \bar{y})(x_{ij} - \bar{x})\right\}$$

$$- \left\{\sum_{i=1}^{k}\sum_{j=1}^{n_i}(y_{ij} - \bar{y}_i)^2 - b_W \sum_{i=1}^{k}\sum_{j=1}^{n_i}(y_{ij} - \bar{y}_i)(x_{ij} - \bar{x}_i)\right\}$$

$$= \sum_{i=1}^{k}\sum_{j=1}^{n_i}(\bar{y}_i - \bar{y})^2 + \left\{b_W \sum_{i=1}^{k}\sum_{j=1}^{n_i}(y_{ij} - \bar{y}_i)(x_{ij} - \bar{x}_i)\right.$$

$$\left. - b_t \sum_{i=1}^{k}\sum_{j=1}^{n_i}(y_{ij} - \bar{y})(x_{ij} - \bar{x})\right\}.$$

The quantity

$$\sum_{i=1}^{k}\sum_{j=1}^{n_i}(\bar{y}_i - \bar{y})^2$$

is the sum of squared deviations of treatment group means from the grand mean, that is, the between-groups sum of squares that would result from one-way ANOVA with the covariate ignored. The adjusted between-groups sum of squares, as indicated by the equation above, is calculated by reducing the original between-groups sum of squares to take into account the effect of the covariate $x$.

After the sums of squares have been adjusted, the mean squares are computed and significance tests done as for an ordinary analysis of variance, using the adjusted sums of squares. Since a degree of freedom is used in the regression analysis, the total degrees of freedom for the subsequent ANOVA is $N - 2$ rather than $N - 1$. The ANOVA table is shown in Table 12-3. If the $F$ is significant, the researcher will conclude that the groups differ and that the difference is not due to the covariate, since the effect of the covariate has been eliminated. If the $F$ is nonsignificant, the researcher concludes that the groups do not differ significantly. A simple one-way ANOVA with the covariate ignored would have to be done to determine whether the groups would differ if the covariate had been ignored, of course, but this is seldom of interest to the investigator.

The results from ANOCOVA ordinarily include not only the ANOVA table based on the adjusted sums of squares, but also group means that have been adjusted to eliminate the effect of the covariate. Adjusted means

**Table 12-3.** Adjusted $F$-Test Ratio for ANOCOVA

| Source of Variation | Sum of Squares | DF | Mean Square | F |
|---|---|---|---|---|
| Between groups | $SS_B = SS_T - SS_W$ | $k - 1$ | $MS_B = SS_B/(k-1)$ | $MS_B/MS_W$ |
| Within groups | $SS_W = \sum_{i=1}^{k} \sum_{j=1}^{n_i} (y_{ij} - y_{ij}'')^2$ | $N - k - 1$ | $MS_W = SS_W/(N-k-1)$ | |
| Total | $SS_T = \sum_{i=1}^{k} \sum_{j=1}^{n_i} (y_{ij} - y_{ij}')^2$ | $N - 2$ | | |

Analysis of Covariance

that are similar to the unadjusted means suggest that the covariate has little effect. Adjusted means that are closer together than the unadjusted means suggest that some of the difference apparent in the unadjusted means is due to the effect of the covariate. The ANOVA on the adjusted values shows whether the difference in the adjusted means is significant. In the next section, an example of an actual nursing research problem is used to illustrate the use of ANOCOVA.

## TESTING AN ANOCOVA HYPOTHESIS

In a study of relationships between cognitive variables and nursing achievement, Johnson[23] classified 53 full-time students in a school of practical nursing as either congruent or noncongruent, based on their scores on a test to measure interest patterns. He hypothesized that those with congruent interest patterns would score higher in nursing achievement, as indicated by academic grades, than those with noncongruent interest patterns. Because achievement could be affected by the student's basic aptitude for nursing as well as by congruence or noncongruence of interest patterns, this investigator obtained a measure of initial nursing aptitude for each student. Thus, for each student, data were collected on initial nursing aptitude, congruence of interest patterns, and nursing achievement. The effect of initial nursing aptitude on nursing achievement was to be controlled in the ANOCOVA, so that initial nursing aptitude was considered as a covariate.

The null hypothesis for ANOCOVA is

$$H: \mu_1' = \mu_2' = \cdots = \mu_k'$$

or in this case, since there are only two groups, congruent and noncongruent, the null hypothesis becomes

$$H: \mu_1' = \mu_2'$$

For ANOCOVA, the prime notation is added to indicate that the null hypothesis is made for the adjusted means, with the effect of the covariate eliminated. In the case of our example, the null hypothesis is that there is no difference in mean achievement scores for those with congruent interest patterns compared with those with noncongruent interest patterns, with the effect of initial nursing aptitude eliminated. If the null hypothesis is rejected, we will conclude that nursing achievement differs for those with congruent interest patterns compared with those with noncongruent interest patterns, and that this difference is not attributable to a difference in initial nursing aptitude between the two groups.

Group means for the covariate (initial nursing aptitude) and the dependent variable (nursing achievement), both unadjusted and adjusted, are given in Table 12-4. The unadjusted achievement means, which are simply the means for the achievement scores, indicate a slightly higher value for the congruent group than for the noncongruent group. Either a $t$ test or, equivalently, a one-way ANOVA, would determine whether this difference is sufficient to be significant and thus support the researcher's hypothesis. The researcher also has data on the initial nursing aptitude, however, which must be taken into account.

The unadjusted nursing achievement scores indicate a mean for the congruent groups that is actually smaller than the mean for the noncongruent group. If the higher achievement in the congruent group were due to higher initial nursing aptitude than in the noncongruent group, we would expect the mean aptitude score to be higher in the congruent group than in the noncongruent group. In this particular example, therefore, inspection of the means suggests that the adjustment for initial nursing aptitude made by the ANOCOVA would not reduce the difference in nursing achievement between the congruent and noncongruent groups. This is apparent on consideration of the adjusted achievement means, which are almost the same as the unadjusted means.

It is common to carry out the ANOCOVA procedure even when inspection of the means indicates, as in this instance, that either ANOCOVA or one-way ANOVA with the covariate ignored would give the same results. In fact, if the analysis is done by computer, the researcher might not even have the means available for preliminary inspection, but might obtain them from the computer run that carries out the ANOCOVA

Table 12-4. Means for Initial Nursing Aptitude, Unadjusted and Adjusted Means for Achievement, for Students with Congruent and Noncongruent Interest Patterns ($N = 53$)

| | Group Means | |
|---|---|---|
| Variable | Congruent ($N = 26$) | Noncongruent ($N = 27$) |
| Initial nursing aptitude | 101.27 | 102.11 |
| Achievement (unadjusted) | 89.58 | 87.67 |
| Achievement (adjusted) | 89.60 | 87.64 |

# Analysis of Covariance

itself. The adjusted means for the dependent variable require calculation of at least the regression part of the ANOCOVA, so that the adjusted means would normally result from the ANOCOVA procedure itself.

The ANOVA table for the example used here, using the adjusted sums of squares with the effect of initial nursing aptitude removed, is given in Table 12-5. Since 53 subjects were used, with the usual 1 degree of freedom lost from the total sum of squares and one lost by the regression procedure that preceded the ANOVA, there are 51 degrees of freedom in the analysis. The within-groups degrees of freedom, which would be $N - k$ (or 51) in an unadjusted ANOVA, also is reduced by 1 and thus becomes 50.

According to Table D in the Appendix, the value required for significance at the .05 level with 1 and 50 degrees of freedom is

$$F_{.05}(1,50) = 4.03$$

Since the calculated $F$ value of 4.16 exceeds the tabled critical value of 4.03, the researcher decides that the null hypothesis can be rejected. In other words, the researcher concludes that those with congruent interest patterns have significantly higher nursing achievement scores than those with noncongruent interest patterns, and that this difference cannot be attributed to a difference in initial nursing aptitude. The difference must either be a causal one; that is, congruent interest patterns actually lead to higher achievement than noncongruent interest patterns, or else the difference must be due to other factors not taken into account in the study.

## ANOCOVA WITH MULTIPLE COVARIATES

Analysis of covariance can be extended to situations in which there are two or more covariates. Such a situation is common when a researcher wants to compare means on several groups that were not formed by

**Table 12-5.** Analysis of Covariance for Differences in Mean Achievement, for Students with Congruent and Noncongruent Interest Patterns, Controlling for Initial Nursing Aptitude ($N = 53$)

| Source of Variation | Sum of Squares | DF | Mean Square | F |
|---|---|---|---|---|
| Between groups | 50.96 | 1 | 50.96 | 4.16 |
| Within groups | 613.15 | 50 | 12.26 | |
| Total | 664.11 | 51 | | |

randomization and has data on several variables that might differ between the comparison groups and might also be correlated with the dependent variable. For example, Volicer et al.[45], in their study of medical–surgical patient differences in hospital stress, considered several patient characteristics that might account for differences in hospital stress between medical and surgical patients. These included variables such as age, education, number of previous hospitalizations, and life stress prior to hospitalization. The use of ANOCOVA in this study allowed for the elimination of the effect of such background characteristics in the comparison of differences in hospital stress between medical and surgical patients.

When more than one covariate is to be considered, ANOCOVA requires the use of multiple regression analysis. The multiple regression procedure described in earlier chapters is used to develop a regression equation to predict the dependent variable of the study, using the covariates as predictor variables. Subsequently, ANOVA is done on the sums of squares adjusted to take account of the effect of the predictors indicated by the regression analysis. Results of a computer ANOCOVA (such as SPSS) often indicate which of the covariates were actually found to correlate significantly with the dependent variable.

The inclusion of several covariates in ANOCOVA results in loss of several degrees of freedom for the ANOVA part of the procedure, since a degree of freedom is lost for each covariate entered into the multiple regression procedure. If covariates that have no effect on the dependent variable are included, there will be little adjustment in the sums of squares, even though degrees of freedom are lost. This works against the researcher's intent to increase precision and may make it harder to detect treatment (group) differences. For very large samples, the loss of degrees of freedom will not be significant, but in other cases, the indiscriminate inclusion of many covariates can be to the researcher's disadvantage. In such situations, the decision about which variables will be used as covariates should be made carefully. For example, there may be previous research or theoretical information that indicates likely covariates, or preliminary inspection of the data can be made to indicate which potential covariates correlate with the dependent variable and differ between the groups.

Analysis of covariance can be extended to situations in which there is more than one factor to be considered in the analysis, such as factorial designs or repeated-measures designs. See either Winer[46] or Snedecor and Cochran[41] for further discussion of such procedures. If several predictors are of interest in the analysis but the intent of the research does not correspond to the model described in this chapter, some form of multiple regression can be used to handle the analysis. Multiple regression can also be used in situations where interaction has not been taken into account in the ANOCOVA presented. See Nie et al.[34] or Cohen and Cohen[8] for further discussion of these topics.

Analysis of Covariance

## PROBLEMS

1. In Chapter 9, a study[16] was described in which different instructional methods were used to teach hospital personnel about problems involved in contamination and decontamination of respiratory therapy equipment. The subjects were randomized into four groups, as follows:

   Group 1.  Programmed instruction
   Group 2.  Audiovisual instruction
   Group 3.  Programmed and audiovisual instruction
   Group 4.  Commercial programmed instruction

One-way ANOVA indicated significant group differences in achievement following the experimental intervention. Suggest a variable that might be used as a covariate in this study, and explain how its use might strengthen the study findings.

2. Refer back to the study by Cleland et al.[5], discussed in Chapter 1, Problem 2, Chapter 3, Problem 7, and Chapter 9, Problem 3. In this study, the researchers compared mean scores on four factors related to employment of nurses in different educational levels (see Chapter 9, Problem 3 for the data). Differences by educational level were found for the factors of career desirability, satisfaction with nursing, and conducive home situation. Explain why age might be a reasonable covariate to use for further investigation of these differences. How would the use of age as a covariate facilitate the interpretation of educational differences found in this study?

3. One type of data that fit a repeated measures ANOVA with (or without) random assignment is pre-test and post-test scores for two or more groups receiving different experimental interventions. Explain how such data can also be handled using ANOCOVA.

4. In a hypothetical study of the effect of four drugs on blood pressure, 24 patients are randomly assigned to four groups of six each. One-way ANOVA to test for group differences in blood pressure after administration of the drugs results in the analysis shown in Table 12-6. Due to the small number of patients in each group, the researcher is concerned that the groups might not have been alike in mean blood pressure at the outset of the study and thus uses ANOCOVA to test for differences in the groups with the effects of blood pressure at the start of the study controlled. Results are as indicated in Table 12-7.

   (a) What null hypothesis can be tested by the information given in Table 12-6?

**Table 12-6.** Analysis of Variance of Differences in Mean Blood Pressure After Drug Treatment, for Patients on Four Drugs ($N = 24$)

| Source of Variation | Sum of Squares | DF | Mean Square | F |
|---|---|---|---|---|
| Between groups | 1636 | 3 | | |
| Within groups | 2018 | 20 | | |
| Total | 3654 | 23 | | |

    (b) Calculate the mean squares and the $F$-test statistic for Table 12-6.
    (c) Test the null hypothesis for Table 12-6, using the .05 level of significance.
    (d) State the conclusion in substantive terms.
    (e) Considering that the treatment groups were formed by randomization, how could blood pressure at the outset of the study differ among the groups?
    (f) What is the covariate that is controlled by the ANOCOVA?
    (g) What does the difference between the total sum of squares in Tables 12-6 and 12-7 ($3654 - 3200 = 454$) represent?
    (h) Repeat steps a through d for the data shown in Table 12-7.

    5. In Problem 6 at the end of Chapter 3 as well as at other places in this text, an investigation of the relationship between preoperative information about sensation and pain was described. The researcher demonstrated by use of $t$ tests that, for patients low on physical-danger trait anxiety, the experimental group receiving preparatory information reported lower pain that the control group receiving no preparatory information. In addition, for patients high on physical-danger trait anxiety, the experimental group receiving preparatory information reported higher pain than

**Table 12-7.** Analysis of Covariance for Differences in Mean Blood Pressure After Drug Treatment for Patients on Four Drugs, Controlling for Blood Pressure at Beginning of Study ($N = 24$)

| Source of Variation | Adjusted Sum of Squares | DF | Mean Square | F |
|---|---|---|---|---|
| Between groups | 1400 | 3 | | |
| Within groups | 1800 | 19 | | |
| Total | 3200 | 22 | | |

Analysis of Covariance

**Table 12-8** Analysis of Covariance of Differences in Mean Pain Scores by Treatment, for Patients with High Physical-Danger Trait Anxiety, Controlling for Number of Years Since Last Surgery, Number of Children Delivered, Duration Between Last Pain Medication and Pain Measurement, and Number of Pain Medications ($N = 42$)

| Source of Variation (adjusted) | Mean Square | F |
|---|---|---|
| Explained | 2.153 | 3.477* |
| Residual | 0.619 | |
| Total | 0.838 | |

*$p < .05$.

the control group receiving no preparatory information. In an additional analysis, the researcher investigated the relationships between several extraneous variables and pain and found that pain scores were correlated with number of years since last surgery, number of children delivered, duration between last pain medication and pain measurement, and number of pain medications. The researcher then retested the major hypotheses of the study relating preparatory information and pain, using ANOCOVA to control for the effects of the four extraneous variables found to be associated with pain. The results of the ANOCOVA are reproduced separately in Tables 12-8 and 12-9, for patients with high physical-danger trait anxiety and patients with low physical-danger trait anxiety.

**Table 12-9** Analysis of Covariance for Differences in Mean Pain Scores by Treatment, for Patients with Low Physical-Danger Trait Anxiety, Controlling for Number of Years Since Last Surgery, Number of Children Delivered, Duration Between Last Pain Medication and Pain Measurement, and Number of Pain Medications ($N = 23$)

| Source of Variation (adjusted) | Mean Square | F |
|---|---|---|
| Explained | 1.643 | 4.781* |
| Residual | 0.344 | |
| Total | 0.686 | |

*$p < .05$.

(a) Why did the researcher decide to carry out this ANOCOVA procedure, when the $t$ tests comparing experimental groups had already been done and supported her hypotheses?
(b) Considering the ANOCOVA for patients with high physical-danger trait anxiety, how was the $F$-test statistic calculated?
(c) What null hypothesis can be tested by this $F$ statistic?
(d) Should the null hypothesis be accepted or rejected?
(e) State the conclusion in substantive terms.
(f) Repeat questions b through e for the ANOCOVA for patients with low physical-danger trait anxiety.

# Chapter 13
## FACTOR ANALYSIS AND DISCRIMINANT ANALYSIS

### FACTOR ANALYSIS

This section is intended to provide a brief introduction to the topic of factor analysis. This procedure is fairly controversial in statistics because interpretation of the results is thought to require more subjective judgment than is necessary for many other kinds of data analysis. The procedure is often used in situations where a large amount of data have been collected for each subject in a study, and the investigator wishes to reduce it to a more simplistic form.

*Factor analysis* is a way of looking at the structure of intercorrelations among a large number of variables, usually with the general intent of simplifying a large amount of data. The correlations among the variables may fall into some kind of pattern, so that there are clusters of variables that are highly correlated among themselves, and poorly correlated with variables in other clusters. This kind of clustering of variables according to their correlations with other variables makes it possible to identify "concepts," each measured by a cluster of several variables. These clusters may also be referred to as "dimensions" or "factors."

The measurement of concepts is of great importance to nursing research. Many, if not most, research projects in nursing involve an attempt to operationalize one or more concepts for which the investigator wants to obtain data in a quantitative form. For example, there are numerous studies in the literature dealing with concepts such as stress, anxiety, pain, aggression, adequacy of nursing care, satisfaction with nursing care, self-help ability, level of wellness, seriousness of illness, and so on. All the variables just named are *constructs;* they are hypothetical variables as distinguished from variables such as age, blood pressure, height, and weight. Researchers who plan to measure a hypothetical variable must invest considerable time in either finding instruments that have been developed and validated by previous studies, or in constructing their own measurement tools.

Construction of an instrument for measuring any particular concept may begin with a long list of questions or statements that the investigator believes are relevant for that concept. For example, one does not usually measure satisfaction with nursing care by asking patients "Are you satisfied with your nursing care? Please say yes or no." People are likely to give socially desirable answers to such global questions, particularly patients who think that their care might be affected by their response. It is more usual to use a checklist or set of questions, such as:

1. Did your nurse come right away when you pushed the call button?
2. Did your nurse answer your questions clearly and directly?
3. Was your nurse friendly to you?
4. Did you feel your nurse spent as much time with you as you needed?
5. Did your nurse seem to be interested in your progress?
6. Did your nurse check on your needs often enough?
7. Did your nurse do as much as possible to make you comfortable?

By talking with patients and nurses or other hospital personnel, the researcher can often construct a list of many questions that might be indicators of satisfaction with nursing care.

In the situation just described, it would be possible to consider the response to each of the questions as a variable in subsequent data analysis. More commonly, one hypothesizes that there are several factors involved in a concept such as satisfaction with nursing care, and that each specific question may be relevant as an indicator of one of the factors. In this case, the factors could be, for example, efficiency, compassion, and responsiveness. Factor analysis is a procedure that determines whether the responses to a set of specific questions such as those listed above can be categorized into groups that are then treated as factors. The researcher examines the clusters of variables suggested by the factor analysis procedure and determines whether conceptually meaningful names can be attached to them. The procedure then provides for calculation of factor scores that can be treated as variables in the data analysis.

As an actual example, consider research by Volicer et al.[45] on stress due to the experience of hospitalization. As part of this research, the authors devised the Hospital Stress Rating Scale (HSRS), which is based on 49 events related to the experience of hospitalization. The list of possible events was constructed by interviews with previously and presently hospitalized individuals and represents a wide variety of possible stresses related to hospitalization, from "having to sleep in a strange bed" to "not having friends visit you" to "not knowing for sure what illness you have."

The HSRS was constructed by asking a large sample of patients to rank all the events from the least stressful to most stressful. The question then arose as to whether these events might represent a small number of "stress factors" that could be measured, rather than 49 different types of stress. It was expected that perception of several events as measuring a common stress factor would result in similar ranks being given to those events, which would result in intercorrelations among ranks for that set of events. A factor analysis procedure was carried out to investigate this problem.

The factor analysis treated each of the 49 ranks as a separate variable. The results indicated that there were nine clusters of variables (events) apparent in the HSRS. These clusters were sets of events whose ranks tended to be intercorrelated with each other and that could then be named and referred to in subsequent analyses as "stress factors." The final set of nine stress factors yielded by this analysis were:

Factor 1. Unfamiliarity of surroundings
Factor 2. Loss of independence
Factor 3. Separation from spouse
Factor 4. Financial problems
Factor 5. Isolation from other people
Factor 6. Lack of information
Factor 7. Threat of severe illness
Factor 8. Separation from family
Factor 9. Problems with medications

Conceptualization of the HSRS events as a composite of factors allows one to measure and analyze the stress factors which represent nine hypothetical variables, instead of having to deal with an unwieldy set of 49 variables.

The basic factor analysis model can be written as follows:

$$x_1 = \lambda_{11}y_1 + \lambda_{12}y_2 + \cdots + \lambda_{1m}y_m + e_1$$
$$x_2 = \lambda_{21}y_1 + \lambda_{22}y_2 + \cdots + \lambda_{2m}y_m + e_2$$
$$\vdots$$
$$x_n = \lambda_{n1}y_1 + \lambda_{n2}y_2 + \cdots + \lambda_{nm}y_m + e_n$$

In the above equations,

$$x_1, x_2, \cdots, x_n$$

represent the $n$ observed random variables. The model assumes that all $n$ variables can be expressed as linear combinations of a set of $m$ variables,

$$y_1, y_2, \cdots, y_m$$

which are referred to as *factors*. Since the idea in factor analysis is to reduce a large amount of data to a simpler form, it is anticipated that $m$, the number of factors, will be substantially smaller than $n$, the original number of variables.

The $\lambda_{ij}$ values are referred to as *factor loadings*. For any variable $x_i$, the largest $\lambda_{ij}$ values (in standardized form) indicate which of the $y$ values are most important in determining the values of that variable. In addition, the largest $\lambda_{ij}$ values associated with any factor $y$, indicate the variables most related to that factor. The $e_i$ represent those parts of the $x_i$ that are not linear combinations of the $y$ values.

The $y$ values are assumed to be independently normally distributed with mean 0 and variance 1. It can be shown that $\lambda_{ij}$ is the covariance (or correlation, if standardized) of the $i$th response with the $j$th common factor, which is another way of saying that the factor loadings reflect the relative importance of each variable for a given factor.

Factor analysis provides a procedure for estimating the factor loadings based on sample data. A set of equations derived by the method of maximum likelihood must be solved to obtain these estimates. The correlation matrix for the original variables is used to determine factor loadings for each variable on each factor. There are actually several alternative procedures for carrying out a factor analysis. Consult a reference such as Harman[17] for an explanation of differences among the various procedures.

The model does not define a unique set of factor loadings, and procedures called *factor rotations* are carried out on the original factor matrix to change the loading values while still adhering to the factor analysis model. The rotations are manipulations involving orthogonal transformations of the originally estimated factor loading matrix. The results of a factor analysis will depend on the particular type of factor rotation used.

Characteristically, factor analysis is used as an attempt to describe data involving a large number of variates in a simplified manner. The intent is usually to describe the data contained in the original variables by a number of factors that is much smaller than the original number of variables. One procedure used is to make the factor loadings close to 0 or 1 by means of some rotation procedure. Ideally, the loading for any particular variable will be particularly high on one factor and low on all other factors. This makes it possible to identify each variable with the factor on which it loads most highly, that is, the factor most responsible for determining the value of the variable. We can then speak of factors as generally being represented by groups of variables, and it is these groups of variables that we hope to interpret as the main conceptual dimensions involved in the entire set of variables used originally. Substantive interpretations of the data can be greatly simplified by this kind of variable-factor identification.

Alternatively, one may use factor analysis to compute factor scores that can be analyzed in relation to other variables. Since the model assumes that each of the original variables can be written as a linear function of factors, this means that each factor can be expressed as a linear combination of variables. Given an observation on each variable for a sample of subjects, one can compute a factor score for each of the factors described by the factor analysis, and these scores can themselves be used as variables in further data analysis.

The actual procedures used in carrying out a factor analysis are quite complicated, and the brief introduction to the topic given here is not intended as an explanation that will equip readers to carry out factor analysis on their own. Nie et al.[34] describe the general ideas underlying various procedures used for factor analysis, the common types of factor rotation, and interpretation of the results. For a more mathematically sophisticated explanation of the topic, refer to Harman[17]. Kerlinger and Pedhazur[26] describe uses of factor analysis and factor scores in nonmathematical terms and also describe several research studies in which factor analysis was used.

## DISCRIMINANT ANALYSIS

The discussion of discriminant analysis to be included here, like the previous description of factor analysis, is intended to introduce the reader to the topic and suggest references for study. *Discriminant analysis* is a procedure for providing a statistical basis for distinguishing between two or more groups of people or other subjects. Using known characteristics of the individuals as well as their group membership, the researcher is able to determine whether the characteristics are useful in predicting the group to which each subject belongs.

Many examples can be given in nursing research in which it would be useful to be able to distinguish among two or more groups. For example, nurse educators might want to determine whether any characteristics of nursing students can be used to distinguish which individuals will actually join the profession of nursing following graduation and which will not. Or a researcher might want to know whether any characteristics of patients who attend prepared childbirth classes could be used to distinguish between those patients who eventually deliver without anesthesia and those who do not. Or another researcher might want to see whether any characteristics of diabetic patients given diet instruction can distinguish between those who follow the diet adequately, partly, and not at all.

In order to perform the discriminant analysis, the researcher must have a sample of subjects for which there are data on the characteristics or variables which are important discriminators as well as the group to which each individual belongs. Characteristics that might distinguish between nurses who practice and those who don't, for example, might include age at onset of study of nursing, marital status, IQ, high school grade-point average, and so on. Characteristics which might distinguish between patients who deliver with versus without anesthesia could include parity, age, previous delivery without anesthesia, education, and so on. A similar set of potentially relevant characteristics could be listed for the diabetic patients mentioned in the third example given above.

The first objective of a discriminant analysis is to see whether all or some of the selected characteristics can discriminate among the groups. The analysis provides a measure of the success with which such discrimination has been made. If the analysis indicates that the characteristics do indeed discriminate among the groups, the results may be useful for purposes of classification, a second objective. For new cases for which group membership is unknown, the researcher may use the information from the analysis to predict the group into which the case is most likely to fall. The cases can be classified on a probabilistic basis according to their known characteristics. Thus the analysis may be useful not just for understanding how groups differ, but for program planning for differential treatment of cases, according to their probability of belonging to each group.

The following discussion is limited to the case where a researcher wants to distinguish between two groups. References for more complicated situations are given at the end of the section. The procedure for two groups leads to the calculation of a quantity called a *discriminant function,* which is a linear combination of the selected characteristics or discriminating variables. The model for the discriminant function is

$$D = d_1 z_1 + d_2 z_2 + \cdots + d_n z_n$$

where the $z_i$ are the values of the discriminating variables, the $d_i$ are the weights determined by the procedure, and $D$ is the value of the function. If the discriminant function yields scores that tend to be similar for cases within each group (but different from cases in the other group), the function is useful in distinguishing between the two groups of cases.

As you may have noticed, this model looks very much like the model for multiple regression analysis. For a discriminant analysis with two groups, the analysis takes the form of a multiple regression analysis. The discriminating variables correspond to the independent variables in multiple regression analysis, and the group membership corresponds to the dependent variable. The groups can be designated by the codes 0 and 1, and then each individual is assigned a score of 0 or 1 on the dependent variable, according to the group to which the individual belongs.

The analysis is carried out exactly as a multiple regression, so a computer program that performs multiple regression analysis can be used for discriminant analysis with two groups. Simply assign each case the value 0 or 1 according to group membership, and designate this score as the dependent variable for the analysis. If the discriminating function is useful, the values predicted by the multiple regression equation will tend to be close to 0 for those cases in Group 0 and close to 1 for those cases in Group 1. Kerlinger and Pedhazur[26] give an example of such an analysis and explain how to assign cases to groups on the basis of the predicted score.

The usual $F$ test for significance of $R^2$ (the proportion of variance explained) can be used to determine whether significant prediction is achieved. A significant $F$ test indicates that assignment to groups using the equation is likely to be more accurate than chance alone. In other words, the discriminating variables do have some ability to distinguish between the groups. The data can also be treated in stepwise fashion, so that the researcher can determine which of the characteristics have significant discriminating power. For further examples and a discussion of interpretation of results of discriminant analysis, including situations where there are more than two groups, the reader is referred to Nie et al.[34] For additional reading, also with examples but taking a somewhat more mathematical approach, consult Overall and Klett[35]. Cohen and Cohen[8] also discuss discriminant analysis in the general context of multiple regression analysis.

## PROBLEMS

1. Everly and Falcione[13] used a factor analytic procedure to study dimensions of job satisfaction among staff registered nurses. They reported that earlier studies had conceptualized job satisfaction as a dichotomous variable consisting of intrinsic (psychological) rewards and extrinsic factors. The research by Everly and Falcione was done in an attempt to empirically establish factors related to job satisfaction. Nurses in the study were asked to indicate on a Likert-type scale the degree of importance for job satisfaction of each of several aspects of the working environment. Table 13-1 indicates factor loadings for each item that resulted from factor analysis with varimax rotation of the original 18 items. Factor loadings too low to be considered substantively meaningful were omitted from the article.

   (a) How would you describe the four dimensions of job satisfaction identified in this study?

**Table 13-1.** Retained Factor Loadings for Items Related to Job Satisfaction, Following Varimax Rotation of the Original 18 Items ($N = 144$)

|  | Factors |  |  |  |
|---|---|---|---|---|
| Item | I | II | III | IV |
| Adequacy of tools and equipment | | | | |
| Good working conditions | | .56 | | |
| Recognition of good work | | | | |
| Relations with fellow workers | .74 | | | |
| Hospital policy | | | | .83 |
| Job security | | | | |
| Relations with immediate supervisor | .62 | | | |
| Hospital's reputation | | | | |
| Respect for my suggestions | | | | |
| Enjoyment of my work | | .78 | | |
| Opportunity for advancement | | | .76 | |
| Salary | | | .64 | |
| Help from immediate supervisor | | | | |
| Employee benefits | | | .65 | |
| Opportunity to develop new skills and abilities | | .65 | | |
| Recognition of past service | | | | .62 |
| Relations with supervisory personnel | .74 | | | |
| Enjoyment in the opportunity to use my skills and abilities | | | | |

Reprinted from Everly, II, G.S., and Falcione, R.L. (1976). Perceived Dimensions of Job Satisfaction for Staff Registered Nurses. *Nursing Research,* 25: 346–348. American Journal of Nursing Company, New York, with permission.

(b) How might the factors be more useful for analysis of job absenteeism and turnover than the individual items?

2. Meleis and Farrell[32] used several standardized instruments to test 188 senior nursing students for intellectual characteristics, leadership, research orientation, and sociopsychological factors. One instrument used was the Registered Nurse Satisfactory Achievement Scale. Responses to the 18 items on this scale were factor analyzed to determine whether the items could be clustered into factors. Factor loadings for the rotated factor matrix are shown in Table 13-2. (Nonsignificant loadings were omitted from the article; for this example, they have been simulated.)

**Table 13-2** Factor Loadings for Rotated Factor Matrix for Responses to Items on Registered Nurse Satisfactory Achievement Scale ($N = 188$)

| Items | I | II | II | IV |
|---|---|---|---|---|
| 1. Speaking ability | .71 | .23 | .30 | .14 |
| 2. Reading ability | .82 | .07 | .36 | .40 |
| 3. Writing ability | .81 | .31 | .25 | .01 |
| 4. Manual dexterity | .61 | .31 | .32 | .08 |
| 5. Listening ability | .84 | .28 | .41 | .17 |
| 6. Communicating ability | .75 | .18 | .22 | .33 |
| 7. Well liked | .38 | .20 | .47 | .05 |
| 8. Well known at work | .54 | .06 | .47 | .13 |
| 9. Minimum quantity of work | .57 | .20 | .11 | .38 |
| 10. Theoretical orientation | .01 | .63 | .23 | .34 |
| 11. Time spent supervising | .23 | .26 | .81 | .41 |
| 12. Administrative advancement | .23 | .51 | .54 | .03 |
| 13. Contribution to teaching | .30 | .30 | .39 | .19 |
| 14. Work with patients | .24 | .32 | .12 | .84 |
| 15. Practice in profession | .31 | .05 | .29 | .72 |
| 16. Developmental contributions | .04 | .72 | .32 | .16 |
| 17. Publications | .15 | .75 | .21 | .38 |
| 18. Original work | .32 | .66 | .06 | .19 |

Reprinted from Meleis, A.I., and Farrell, K.M. (1974). Operation concern: A Study of Senior Nursing Students in Three Nursing Programs. *Nursing Research,* 23: 461–468. American Journal of Nursing Company, New York. With permission.

(a) By assigning each item to the factor on which it loads most highly, determine the factors or clusters of variables suggested by this analysis.
(b) Name each factor according to what you think it represents.
(c) Explain how these factors might be more useful in research on student achievement than the individual items.

3. In Problem 1 of Chapter 8, a study of factors that might affect smoking behavior among college students was described. In this study the researchers used multiple regression analysis to predict smoking behavior of the respondents, using the smoking behavior of father, mother, best

friend, and most friends as independent variables. Because the dependent variable, smoking behavior, is categorical, the multiple regression analyses carried out in this research are actually a form of discriminant analysis. For each of the following situations, explain which students would be studied, as well as what the nature of the dependent variable would be for the discriminant analysis, that is, how many groups there would be and how they would be defined.

(a) The researchers want to know whether parents' or peers' smoking behavior influences college students to take up smoking.
(b) The researchers want to know whether parents' or peers' smoking behavior affects how much smoking is done by those who do smoke.
(c) The researchers want to know whether parents' or peers' smoking behavior is related to whether those who do take up smoking have quit by the time they enter college.
(d) The researchers want to know whether information about parents' or peers' smoking behavior can be used to predict who will

**Table 13-3** Mean Scores of Cognitive and Noncognitive Characteristics for Students Entering a College of Nursing Program, by Subsequent Graduation Status ($N = 114$)

| Variables | Group 1 (Graduated) ($N = 72$) | Group 2 (Did Not Graduate) ($N = 42$) |
|---|---|---|
| IQ | 121 | 108 |
| SAT—Verbal | 341.19 | 168.67 |
| SAT—Mathematics | 347.29 | 168.52 |
| Gordon Personal Profile |  |  |
|   Ascendancy–leadership | 22.28 | 19.50 |
|   Responsibility | 25.07 | 23.43 |
|   Emotional maturity | 23.32 | 21.91 |
|   Sociability | 22.24 | 19.69 |
| Watson-Glaser Critical Thinking Examination | 73.82 | 59.60 |
| Kalisch Empathy Scale rating | 0.40 | 0.27 |

Reprinted from Richards, M.A. (1977). One Integrated Curriculum: An Empirical Evaluation. *Nursing Research*, 26: 90–95. American Journal of Nursing Company, New York. With permission.

# Factor Analysis and Discriminant Analysis

not smoke, who will smoke, and who will smoke but quit by college age.

4. Richards[37] studied both cognitive and noncognitive characteristics of 114 students entering a college of nursing program in 1972 to determine which characteristics might be predictive of successful completion of the program. Students were divided three years later into two groups, those who were graduating and those who had either failed or withdrawn. Mean scores for these two groups on the study characteristics are shown in Table 13-3.

(a) Explain why discriminant analysis would be an appropriate way to deal with the data.
(b) Explain what information would be gained by a discriminant analysis, over and above what would be gained by just comparing mean scores for the two groups on each variable.

# Chapter 14

# POWER AND SAMPLE SIZE

One of the most common questions asked of statisticians is "how large a sample should I take?" This question is often asked as if there should be a simple straightforward answer. In fact, there is no simple answer to this question, although there are some guidelines that can be useful in approximating an adequate sample size. The purpose of this chapter is to introduce the reader to some principles that can be used to make such approximations. Although the principal ideas are the same, the procedures differ according to the specific statistical tests that the researcher plans to apply to the data. Two specific situations will be described in detail, and further reading for other types of tests will be suggested.

The discussion of the issue of sample size presented here is dependent on an understanding of the concept of the *power* of a statistical test. The power of a statistical test of a null hypothesis is the probability of rejection of the null hypothesis when it is false. Power is related to the notions of Type I and Type II errors. Recall that Type I error is rejection of the null hypothesis when the null hypothesis is true. The probability of a Type I error is the significance level allowed for in testing the null hypothesis, commonly denoted by $\alpha$. Type II error is failure to reject the null hypothesis when it is false, and is denoted by $\beta$. Power, the probability of rejection of the null hypothesis when it is false, is by definition,

$$\text{Power} = 1 - \beta$$

Since most researchers state a null hypothesis that they think is false and that they hope to reject, it is clearly to the researcher's advantage to design a study in such a way as to make the power of the test relatively high.

Power of a test is very closely related to sample size. Throughout this book, the effect of sample size on the results of hypothesis tests has been discussed with reference to the formulas used to calculate the test statistics. Sample size parameters appear in formulas for calculation of test statistics in such a manner that large samples tend to make calculated test statistics larger than small samples. The effect of this is that a null hypothesis is more likely to be rejected when a large sample is used than when a small sample is used, other things being equal. As a result, power varies directly with sample size, that is, increases in sample size increase power. In published nursing research studies with very small samples and nonsignificant results, researchers commonly conclude that the null hypothesis is true. One intent of this chapter is to show that when very small samples are used, the power of the statistical test may be so low that the null hypothesis is unlikely to be rejected even when it is false. The conclusion in such cases should not be that the null hypothesis is supported, but rather that there is insufficient evidence to reject it, and the study should be redone with a larger sample.

Power is also related to $\alpha$, the significance level or the probability of a Type I error. The smaller the chosen $\alpha$ is the less likely it is that the null hypothesis will be rejected. Other things being equal, the significance level varies directly with power; therefore, the lower $\alpha$ is, the lower the power of the test. Since power varies inversely with the probability of a Type II error $\beta$, the practice of using a very small significance level tends to increase the probability of a Type II error while simultaneously decreasing power. The choice of $\alpha$ has an effect on the power of the test, and you will learn in this chapter how to determine how much the power of a test varies with different levels of $\alpha$ (e.g., .05 vs .01).

Considerations of the power of a statistical test are very often ignored in nursing research as well as in most other published research. Determination of the power of a test is a relatively complicated procedure that is different for each test. The power for a test of difference between means is determined differently than the power for a test of difference between two proportions, or for a correlation coefficient and so forth. In many statistics textbooks, particularly applied texts, the topic is either absent or just briefly mentioned. However, Cohen[7] offers a comprehensive and understandable explanation of the topic. The remainder of this chapter is based on extensive use of Cohen's book, and you are advised to consult this book for power analysis in your own research studies.

## COHEN'S APPROACH TO POWER ANALYSIS

In the beginning of this chapter, we discussed three parameters used in power analysis: power, sample size, and significance level. For carrying out power analysis, a fourth parameter is required that is somewhat more complicated than the other three and that differs for each type of statistical test. Cohen refers to this fourth parameter as *effect size*. The effect size, as stated by Cohen, is a measure of the "degree to which the null hypothesis is false." If, for example, one hypothesizes no difference in mean number of days of hospitalization for two groups of patients and the actual difference is 2 days, then the effect size is 2. Or if one hypothesizes no correlation between age and blood pressure and the actual correlation is .30, the effect size is .30. The tendency of large effects or differences to increase values of test statistics has been pointed out for several tests described in this text. The effect size is thus related to power in such a way that a large effect will result in a test with greater power compared with a small effect. In other words, the further the departure of parameters from values assumed by the null hypothesis, the greater the probability of rejection of the null hypothesis will be. Effect size is also related to sample size in such a way that a large effect is easier than a small effect to detect with a small sample (i.e., the null hypothesis is more likely to be rejected).

It is clear from these examples that the effect size is a number whose units can vary drastically, depending on the type of statistical test and the units of observation of the variables. For each of the statistical tests described in his book, Cohen has devised a procedure for calculating a standard effect size. This makes it possible to specify a metric-free index that can be used to determine power or sample size for any situation. If the researcher is able to estimate the difference between means or the expected correlation, or the difference she would consider nontrivial and that she would want to detect by rejection of the null hypothesis, the standard effect size can be calculated. Cohen also proposes guidelines for operationalizing the effect size as "small," "medium," or "large," based on the magnitude of various effects commonly observed in behavioral science research.

Cohen explains that power analysis is based on the interrelationships between the four parameters of sample size, significance level, effect size, and power. These four quantities are related in such a way that when any three are fixed, the fourth is determined. This makes four types of power analysis possible, two of which are discussed in great detail in Cohen's book and will be described in the examples given later in this chapter. Before going on to specific tests, we will briefly describe these two kinds of power analysis.

The first type of power analysis is the *determination of power,* given significance level, effect size, and sample size. If a researcher plans an experiment using a chosen significance level, effect size, and sample size, the power tables devised by Cohen can be used to determine the power of the test. In other words, the investigator can determine ahead of time how likely it is that the null hypothesis will be rejected. If the power turns out to be relatively small (e.g., a power of < .80, which is often conventionally considered "good"), the researcher may decide to redesign the study in such a way as to increase the power, most likely by increasing the sample size. This type of analysis can also be used on data from published studies to determine the power. That is, with the actual significance level, the reported effect, and the sample size, the power can be determined. For example, if the power is calculated as .10, one can conclude that with an actual effect size as large as that reported, the probability of obtaining significant results would be about .10. This low power suggests a new test of the same null hypothesis, but with data based on a larger sample.

The second type of power analysis is the determination of sample size, given the significance level, anticipated effect size, and desired power. Such an analysis can be used to answer the question posed at the outset of this chapter, "how large a sample should I take?" By setting the significance level, effect size anticipated, and power desired, the researcher can use the tables in Cohen's book to calculate the required sample size. This is the type of power analysis that is most likely to be useful to nurse researchers in the design of studies. If the tables indicate that the sample size necessary to obtain the desired power is a bit larger than the researcher had planned, the researcher might consider how to increase it, either by allowing more time for data collection so that more subjects can be included, or by considering additional study sites where subjects could be found. If the researcher is a doctoral student and the analysis suggests a sample size that would require 5 years for data collection, he or she should consider switching to another topic! It is not justifiable to proceed with a study using a sample size so small that the power will be very low. Such a situation indicates that the null hypothesis is very unlikely to be rejected even if it is false, and thus there is low probability of demonstrating any significant results.

Cohen's book has separate discussions of power analysis for each of many common test statistics. These include $F$ tests for analysis of variance and covariance and for multiple regression, as well as many tests for bivariate relationships. In each case, the discussion includes a detailed explanation of how to arrive at an effect size, followed by power tables and sample size tables, with explanations and illustrations of their use. It is not within the scope of this text to describe or even summarize all these situations individually, and the reader is referred to Cohen's book for detailed study. Included in the following two sections of this chapter are descriptions of the use of power analysis for two tests, the $t$ test for the difference between two means and the $F$ test for significance of the multiple correlation coefficient in multiple regression analysis. These two tests have been chosen because they are commonly encountered in nursing research (the $t$ test often presented as the equivalent analysis of variance with two groups), and determination of effect size can be more simply explained

## DIFFERENCE BETWEEN TWO MEANS

As you will recall, the null hypothesis tested by the $t$ test for the difference between two independent means is

$$H: \mu_1 - \mu_2 = 0$$

where $\mu_1$ and $\mu_2$ are the means of the two populations. The extent of departure from the null hypothesis is measured by the amount of difference between the means of the two populations. As the metric-free index of this effect size, Cohen uses the quantity

$$d = \frac{\mu_1 - \mu_2}{\sigma}$$

where $\sigma$ is the standard deviation of either population. He suggests that when prior information on which to estimate the value of $d$ is unavailable, one should select a small, medium, or large effect size according to the following criteria. A small effect size ($d = .2$) should be used in new areas of research, where the measurement of variables is not likely to be very precise, and where there is unlikely to be good experimental control. A medium effect size ($d = .5$) should be used to describe an effect likely to be visible to the naked eye. A large effect size ($d = .8$) would describe a gross perceptible difference, such as the difference in mean height between 13 and 18-year-old girls.

Cohen gives tables from which the sample size can be derived for this test, given the significance level, the effect size, and the desired power. Table 14-1 is an excerpt of some entries from the sample size table for $\alpha = .05$, using two-tailed tests. Entries in Table 14-1 are the sample size required for each of the two samples. So, for an anticipated effect size of $d = .50$, which Cohen refers to as medium, power of .50 would require 32 subjects in each sample, power of .80 would require 64 subjects in each sample, and so on. Notice that increase in power requires increase in sample size for any given effect size (look down any column), and that increase in effect size allows the researcher to decrease the number of subjects while maintaining the same power (look across any row). Cohen's tables clearly illustrate the nature of the relationships between the four parameters used in power analysis.

As an example, consider a researcher who wants to determine the effect of nurse preoperative teaching on postoperative anxiety, using an experimental design with a control group and an experimental group. Assume that the researcher has a theoretical basis for the belief that such teaching can affect anxiety, as well as an empirical basis that is founded on clinical experience. Although this might reasonably be considered a one-tailed situation, we will use a two-tailed significance level, since that will allow us to make use of the figures in Table 14-1 (Cohen also has tables for one-tailed tests). Let us also assume that the researcher will use a standardized anxiety test. It would be reasonable in this case to assume a medium effect size, or $d = .50$. If we assume that this investigator will use a significance level of .05, and would like to have a power of .80 (.20 allowance for the probability of a Type II error), we have specified all the parameters necessary to determine the required sample size.

According to the figures in Table 14-1, this researcher should have about 64 subjects in each of the two groups. If available resources allow for a maximum of 50 patients in each group, the researcher might go ahead, accepting a slightly lower power. Using Cohen's complete tables, the actual power that corresponds to 50 subjects per group could be determined. From our selected entries, we only know that it is larger than .50 and lower than .80. If the maximum number of patients to be studied is 10 or 15 in each group, due, for example, to the scarcity of the type of patients needed for the study or to the researcher's limited resources, this investigator might decide to forego the study as designed, since the power would be in the neighborhood of .20 to .25. If the researcher is in the fortunate and uncommon situation of having unlimited resources and an unlimited supply of patients, the power analysis suggests that 64 patients in each group will be adequate for the desired power, and an increase in sample sizes much beyond that is not worth the extra effort.

Table 14-1. Sample Size Required for Each of Two Samples for $t$ Test for Difference Between Means, for Selected Effect Sizes and Power, $\alpha = .05$, Two-Tailed Tests

| | | $d$ | |
|---|---|---|---|
| Power | .20 | .50 | .80 |
| .25 | 84 | 14 | 6 |
| .50 | 193 | 32 | 13 |
| .80 | 393 | 64 | 26 |

## MULTIPLE CORRELATION

As you may remember, the null hypothesis tested by the overall $F$ test for significance in multiple regression analysis is

$$H: \rho = 0$$

where $\rho$ stands for the population multiple correlation coefficient. This null hypothesis assumes that the observed values of the dependent variable are not correlated with those predicted by the regression equation based on the independent variables, or, equivalently, that no significant part of the variation in the dependent variable can be explained by the independent variables. The extent of departure from the null hypothesis can be measured by the size of $\rho$, the multiple correlation coefficient, which is equal to zero when the null hypothesis is true. As the metric-free index of this effect size, Cohen uses the quantity

$$L = \left\{\frac{R^2}{1-R^2}\right\} \times (N - u - 1)$$

In this formula, $R^2$ is the notation used by Cohen for the squared multiple correlation coefficient, $N$ is the sample size, and $u$ is the number of independent variables. As guidelines for small, medium, and large effects, when $R^2$ cannot be estimated from prior knowledge, Cohen uses the following values, which are stated in terms of $R^2$. A small effect size, $R^2 = .02$ ($R = .14$), would be anticipated in beginning research with unstandardized measures and considerable uncontrolled variation in the data. A medium effect size, $R^2 = .13$ ($R = .36$) would be of the magnitude commonly observed in correlational studies in behavioral research. A large effect size, $R^2 = .26$ ($R = .51$), is of the sort that would make nurse researchers' hearts beat faster and maybe cause them to throw their computer output around the room. The verbal descriptions of Cohen's effect sizes here are the present author's. As Cohen states, multiple regression analysis is somewhat more recent than the other procedures he describes, and the values he has suggested for small, medium, and large effects may have to be modified in the future, as more results of such forms of analysis become available.

In this case, we will illustrate the use of Cohen's power tables instead of sample size tables. The power tables provided by Cohen allow for determination of power, given the significance level, the effect size, and the sample size. One first calculates the quantity $L$, using the formula

Power and Sample Size

given above, since this is the index by which the values are located in the tables. Table 14-2 is an excerpt of some entries from the power table for $\alpha = .05$, as given by Cohen.

Each entry in Table 14-2 is the power resulting from the corresponding values chosen for the other parameters. For a value of $L$ of 12 with three independent variables, therefore, the power would be .84, with five independent variables the power would be .77, and so on. Notice that increases in $L$ (which result from either increases in $R^2$ or increases in $N$) increase the power of the test for a given number of independent variables (look across any row). The table also shows that for a given $L$, increases in the number of independent variables reduces power (look down any column). In other words, for a given $R^2$ and a given $N$, the test is more powerful if significant prediction can be obtained with fewer rather than more independent variables. This is, of course, related to the loss of degrees of freedom associated with the inclusion in a multiple regression of many irrelevant variables, as discussed in an earlier chapter.

Suppose, for example, we are considering a published research report in which the researcher considered five independent variables, including age, sex, life stress, number of previous hospitalizations, and seriousness of illness, as predictors of scores of patients on a hospital stress rating scale. The multiple regression analysis, let us assume, yielded a multiple correlation of

$$R = .40 \ (R^2 = .16)$$

between the observed stress scores and those predicted by the regression equation. The researcher reports that a total of 27 people were included in the study and that the analysis failed to lead to rejection of the null hypothesis and concludes that hospital stress is probably not associated with any of the five predictors used in the study.

**Table 14-2.** Power of Test of Null Hypothesis of No Prediction for Multiple Regression, for Selected Values of $L$ (Effect Size Index) and $u$ (Number of Independent Variables), $\alpha = .05$

| | | $L$ | |
|---|---|---|---|
| $u$ | 4.00 | 12.00 | 18.00 |
| 3 | 36 | 84 | 96 |
| 5 | 29 | 77 | 93 |
| 10 | 21 | 64 | 85 |

In order to consult Table 14-2, we must first calculate the index $L$ required for entry into the table. Substituting into the formula for $L$, we have

$$L = \left\{\frac{R^2}{1 - R^2}\right\} \times (N - u - 1)$$

$$= \left\{\frac{.16}{1 - .16}\right\} \times (27 - 5 - 1)$$

$$= 4$$

According to Table 14-2, for $L = 4$ and $u = 5$, the power is .29. In other words, the probability of detecting a value of $R^2 = .16$ as significant is about 29%. The researcher does not have evidence that the five predictors are unassociated with hospital stress, as was claimed. Such a small sample was used that the probability of failure to reject a false null hypothesis (Type II error) is .71 (1 − .29), that is, unreasonably large. The study should be repeated with a larger sample. You can check by substitution into the formula for $L$, for example, that with the same $R^2$, a sample of size $N = 69$ would result in $L = 12$ and a power of .77, as read from Table 14-2. In many such correlational studies it is often not difficult to make the sample large enough to ensure adequate power, since no randomization or experimental treatment is required. When a researcher has invested time and money into the development of a project, it should be worth the effort to check on the power that will result from the sample size being considered, and to attempt to increase it if necessary.

## PROBLEMS

1. Suppose that you are planning a study to determine whether there is any difference in patient satisfaction with nursing care received on the day shift as compared to the evening shift. You have devised your own scale for measuring satisfaction, and would like to ask a group of patients to rate their satisfaction with care received in the evening and a second group to rate their satisfaction with care received during the day, so that mean scores can be compared by a $t$ test. Suppose that this is a very preliminary study, no research has been done in the area, and you have no idea what the outcome is likely to be.

   (a) Suggest an appropriate effect size.
   (b) Determine the sample size for each group needed to attain a power of .80.

# Power and Sample Size

2. Suppose, for the research suggested in Problem 1, that you can obtain the hospital's permission for the study, provided you agree to interview no more than a total of 100 patients. Using the effect size you have chosen, decide whether you should go ahead with 100 patients, based on the power that the test is likely to have.

3. Suppose that, for the research suggested in Problem 1, you have a standard instrument available for measuring satisfaction with nursing care. Suppose that you also have made empirical observations which suggest to you that satisfaction with nursing care is higher in the evening than it is during the day.
   (a) Suggest an appropriate effect size.
   (b) Determine the sample size for each group needed to attain a power of .80.
   (c) Explain the difference between the sample sizes determined for this problem and for Problem 1.
   (d) Given a restriction of the total number of patients to 100, as described in Problem 2, should you go ahead with the study under the conditions described in Problem 3? Explain.

4. Suppose that you plan to interview obstetrical patients coming to a large outpatient facility that is run as a prepaid health care plan. You plan to obtain information which might be predictive of how long the patient will stay in the hospital. This information will be combined with other data about the labor and delivery in a study to determine significant predictors of length of hospital stay. For this study, assume a medium effect size ($R^2 = .13$) and also assume that 10 predictor variables will be used.
   (a) For a sample of $N = 40$, estimate the power of the test.
   (b) For a sample of $N = 100$, estimate the power of the test.
   (c) For a sample of $N = 150$, estimate the power of the test.
   (d) For a sample of $N = 200$, estimate the power of the test.
   (e) What would be a good sample size to provide adequate power for the analysis of data from this study?
   (f) Why would a sample of $N = 300$ or more not be necessary?

5. Suppose that a researcher has examined the difference in mean anxiety scores following surgery between an experimental group ($n_1 = 14$) of patients receiving preparatory information preoperatively and a control group ($n_2 = 14$) of patients receiving no preparatory information. The reported difference corresponds to an effect size of .50. The researcher

finds that the difference in means is not significant, according to the *t* test and concludes that preparatory information, at least of the type used, is not beneficial in terms of patient anxiety.

- (a) What was the power of the statistical test, according to Table 14-1?
- (b) Comment on the researcher's conclusion with reference to your answer to (a).

6. In a research methods class, students are required to jointly plan and carry out a research project. The project must include design of a study, data collection, computerization of the data, and analysis and interpretation of the findings. In such a situation, why might the instructor decide to forego a power analysis to help determine sample size?

7. Suppose that you plan a research project that will involve collection of a large amount of data. The analysis will require several statistical procedures, including chi-square and *t* tests and multiple regression analysis. What would be a reasonable way to use power analysis to determine an adequate sample size?

# REFERENCES

1. Bishop, Y. M. M., Fienberg, S. E., and Holland, P. W. (1975). *Discrete Multivariate Analysis: Theory and Practice*. MIT Press, Cambridge, Mass.
2. Brock, A. M. (1978). Impact of a Management-Oriented Course on Knowledge and Leadership Skills Exhibited by Baccalaureate Nursing Students. *Nursing Research,* 27:217–221.
3. Campbell, D. T., and Stanley, J. C. (1963). *Experimental and Quasi-experimental Designs for Research*. Rand McNally, Chicago.
4. Chang, B. L. (1978). Generalized Expectancy, Situational Perception, and Morale Among Institutionalized Aged. *Nursing Research,* 27:316–324.
5. Cleland, V., Bass, A. R., McHugh, N., and Montano, J. (1976). Social and Psychologic Influences on Employment of Married Nurses. *Nursing Research,* 25:90–97.
6. Cochran, W. G. (1963). *Sampling Techniques (2nd ed.)*. John Wiley and Sons, New York.
7. Cohen, J. (1977). *Statistical Power Analysis for the Behavioral Sciences* (revised ed.). Academic Press, New York.
8. Cohen, J., and Cohen, P. (1975). *Applied Multiple Regression/Correlation Analysis for the Behavioral Sciences*. Lawrence Erlbaum Associates, Hillsdale, New Jersey.
9. Corey, E. J. B., Miller, C. L., and Widlak, F. W. (1975). Factors Contributing to Child Abuse. *Nursing Research,* 24:293–295.
10. Denton, J. A., and Wisenbaker, Jr., V. B. (1977). Death Experience and Death Anxiety among Nurses and Nursing Students. *Nursing Research,* 26:61–64.
11. Derdiarian, A., and Clough, D. (1976). Patients' Dependence and Independence Levels on the Prehospitalization–Postdischarge Continuum. *Nursing Research,* 25:27–34.
12. Dittmar, S. S., and Dulski, T. (1977). Early Evening Administration of Sleep Medication to the Hospitalized Aged. A Consideration in Rehabilitation. *Nursing Research,* 26:299–303.
13. Everly II, G. S., and Falcione, R. L. (1976). Perceived Dimensions of Job Satisfaction for Staff Registered Nurses. *Nursing Research,* 25:346–348.
14. Ferguson, G. A. (1976). *Statistical Analysis in Psychology and Education* (4th ed.). McGraw-Hill, New York.
15. Friedman, M., and Rosenman, R. H. (1974). *Type A Behavior and Your Heart*. Fawcett, Greenwich, Connecticut.

16. Griggs, B. M. (1977). A Systems Approach to the Development and Evaluation of a Minicourse for Nurses. *Nursing Research,* **26:**34–41.
17. Harman, H. H. (1967). *Modern Factor Analysis* (2nd ed.). University of Chicago Press, Chicago.
18. Hegedus, K. S. (1978). *Use of Nursing Care Plans and Variations in Patient Outcomes.* Doctoral dissertation, Boston University.
19. Holmes, T. H., and Rahe, R. H. (1967). The Social Readjustment Rating Scale *Journal of Psychosomatic Research,* **11:**213–217.
20. Hong, E. K. (1978). *The Influence of Husband–Wife Compatibility Using FIRO-B and Sibling Complementarity on the Couple's Health.* Doctoral dissertation, Boston University.
21. Isenberg, M. A. (1978). *Relationship Between the Experience of Surgery and Perception of the Speed of Time.* Doctoral dissertation, Boston University.
22. Janis, I. J. (1958). *Psychological Stress,* John Wiley and Sons, New York.
23. Johnson, D. M. (1973). Relationships Between Selected Cognitive and Non-Cognitive Variables and Practical Nursing Achievement. *Nursing Research,* **22:**148–153.
24. Johnson, J. E., Kirchhoff, K. T., and Endress, M. P. (1975). Altering Children's Distress Behavior During Orthopedic Cast Removal. *Nursing Research,* **24:**404–410.
25. Keith, P. M., and Castles, M. (1976). Community Health Nurses' Preferences for Systems of Protection. *Nursing Research,* **25:**252–255.
26. Kerlinger, F. N., and Pedhazur, E. J. (1973). *Multiple Regression in Behavioral Research.* Holt, Rinehart, and Winston, New York.
27. Kim, S, (1978). *Preparatory Information, Anxiety, and Pain: A Contingency Model and Its Nursing Implications.* Doctoral dissertation, Boston Univesity.
28. Kirgis, C. A., Woolsey, D. B., and Sullivan, J. J. (1977). Predicting Infant Apgar Scores. *Nursing Research,* **26:**439–442.
29. Klugh, H. E. (1974). *Statistics: The Essentials for Research* (2nd ed.), John Wiley and Sons, New York.
30. Lindeman, C. A., and Stetzer, S. L. (1973). Effect of Preoperative Visits by Operating Room Nurses. *Nursing Research,* **22:**4–16.
31. Lowery, B. J., and DuCette, J. P. (1976). Disease-Related Learning and Disease Control in Diabetics as a Function of Locus of Control. *Nursing Research,* **25:**358–362.
32. Meleis, A. I., and Farrell, K. M. (1974). Operation Concern: A Study of Senior Nursing Students in Three Nursing Programs. *Nursing Research,* **23:**461–468.
33. Mims, F. H., Brown, L., and Lubow, R. (1976). Human Sexuality Course Evaluation. *Nursing Research,* **25:**187–191.
34. Nie, N. H., Hull, C. H., Jenkins, J. G., Steinbrenner, K., and Bent, D. H. (1975). *Statistical Package for the Social Sciences* (2nd ed.). McGraw-Hill, New York.
35. Overall, J. E., and Klett, C. J. (1972). *Applied Multivariate Analysis.* McGraw-Hill, New York.
36. Price, J. L., and Collins, J. R. (1973). Smoking among Baccalaureate Nursing Students. *Nursing Research,* **22:**347–350.

# References

37. Richards, M. A. (1977). One Integrated Curriculum: An Empirical Evaluation. *Nursing Research,* **26:**90–95.
38. Rottkamp, B. C. (1976). A Behavior Modification Approach to Nursing Therapeutics in Body Positioning of Spinal Cord-Injured Patients. *Nursing Research,* **25:**181–186.
39. Smith, H. W. (1975). *Strategies of Social Research: The Methodological Imagination.* Prentice-Hall, Englewood Cliffs, New Jersey.
40. Smyth, K., Call, J., Hansell, S., Sparacino, J., and Strodtbeck, F. L. (1978). Type A Behavior Pattern and Hypertension among Inner-City Black Women. *Nursing Research,* **27:**30–35.
41. Snedecor, G. W., and Cochran, W. G. (1967). *Statistical Methods* (6th ed.). Iowa State University Press, Ames, Iowa.
42. Tamez, E. G., Moore, M. J., and Brown, P. L. (1978). Relaxation Training as a Nursing Intervention Versus Pro Re Nata Medication. *Nursing Research,* **27:**160–165.
43. Turnbull, E. M. (1978). Effect of Basic Preventive Health Practices and Mass Media on the Practice of Breast Self-Examination. *Nursing Research,* **27:**98–102.
44. Volicer, B. J., and Burns, M. W. (1977). Preexisting Correlates of Hospital Stress. *Nursing Research,* **26:**408–415.
45. Volicer, B. J., Isenberg, M. A., and Burns, M. W. (1977). Medical–Surgical Differences in Hospital Stress Factors. *Journal of Human Stress,* **3:**3–13.
46. Winer, B. J. (1971). *Statistical Principles in Experimental Design* (2nd ed.). McGraw-Hill, New York.
47. Woods, N. F., and Earp, J. A. L. (1978). Women with Cured Breast Cancer: A Study of Mastectomy Patients in North Carolina. *Nursing Research,* **27:**279–285.

# APPENDIX

**Table A.** Proportions of Area Under the Standard Normal Curve

| $z$ | $1-P$* | $P$† | $z$ | $1-P$ | $P$ | $z$ | $1-P$ | $P$ | $z$ | $1-P$ | $P$ |
|---|---|---|---|---|---|---|---|---|---|---|---|
| 0.0 | .0000 | 1.0000 | 1.0 | .6827 | .3173 | 2.0 | .9545 | .0455 | 3.0 | .9973 | .0027 |
| 0.1 | .0797 | .9203 | 1.1 | .7287 | .2713 | 2.1 | .9643 | .0357 | 3.1 | .9981 | .0019 |
| 0.2 | .1585 | .8415 | 1.2 | .7699 | .2301 | 2.2 | .9722 | .0278 | 3.2 | .9986 | .0014 |
| 0.3 | .2358 | .7642 | 1.3 | .8064 | .1936 | 2.3 | .9786 | .0214 | 3.3 | .9990 | .0010 |
| 0.4 | .3108 | .6892 | 1.4 | .8385 | .1615 | 2.4 | .9836 | .0164 | 3.4 | .9993 | .0007 |
| 0.5 | .3829 | .6771 | 1.5 | .8664 | .1336 | 2.5 | .9876 | .0124 | 3.5 | .9995 | .0005 |
| 0.6 | .4515 | .5485 | 1.6 | .8904 | .1096 | 2.58 | .9901 | .0099 | 3.6 | .9997 | .0003 |
| 0.7 | .5161 | .4839 | 1.64 | .9000 | .1000 | 2.6 | .9907 | .0093 | 3.7 | .9998 | .0002 |
| 0.8 | .5763 | .4237 | 1.7 | .9109 | .0891 | 2.7 | .9931 | .0069 | 3.8 | .9999 | .0001 |
| 0.9 | .6319 | .3681 | 1.8 | .9281 | .0719 | 2.8 | .9949 | .0051 | 3.9 | .9999 | .0001 |
|  |  |  | 1.9 | .9426 | .0594 | 2.9 | .9963 | .0037 |  |  |  |
|  |  |  | 1.96 | .9500 | .0500 |  |  |  |  |  |  |

*$1-P$ = area between $\pm z$.
†$P$ = area beyond $\pm z$.

**Table B.** Percentage Points of the *t*-Distribution

| | Level of Significance for One-Tailed Test | | | | | |
|---|---|---|---|---|---|---|
| Degrees of Freedom, df | 0.10 | 0.05 | 0.025 | 0.01 | 0.005 | 0.0005 |
| | Level of Significance for Two-Tailed Test | | | | | |
| | 0.20 | 0.10 | 0.05 | 0.02 | 0.01 | 0.001 |
| 1 | 3.078 | 6.314 | 12.706 | 31.821 | 63.657 | 636.619 |
| 2 | 1.886 | 2.920 | 4.303 | 6.965 | 9.925 | 31.598 |
| 3 | 1.638 | 2.353 | 3.182 | 4.541 | 5.841 | 12.941 |
| 4 | 1.533 | 2.132 | 2.776 | 3.747 | 4.604 | 8.610 |
| 5 | 1.476 | 2.015 | 2.571 | 3.365 | 4.032 | 6.859 |
| 6 | 1.440 | 1.943 | 2.447 | 3.143 | 3.707 | 5.959 |
| 7 | 1.415 | 1.895 | 2.365 | 2.998 | 3.499 | 5.405 |
| 8 | 1.397 | 1.860 | 2.306 | 2.896 | 3.355 | 5.041 |
| 9 | 1.383 | 1.833 | 2.262 | 2.821 | 3.250 | 4.781 |
| 10 | 1.372 | 1.812 | 2.228 | 2.764 | 3.169 | 4.587 |
| 11 | 1.363 | 1.796 | 2.201 | 2.718 | 3.106 | 4.437 |
| 12 | 1.356 | 1.782 | 2.179 | 2.681 | 3.055 | 4.318 |
| 13 | 1.350 | 1.771 | 2.160 | 2.650 | 3.012 | 4.221 |
| 14 | 1.345 | 1.761 | 2.145 | 2.624 | 2.977 | 4.140 |
| 15 | 1.341 | 1.753 | 2.131 | 2.602 | 2.947 | 4.073 |
| 16 | 1.337 | 1.746 | 2.120 | 2.583 | 2.921 | 4.015 |
| 17 | 1.333 | 1.740 | 2.110 | 2.567 | 2.898 | 3.965 |
| 18 | 1.330 | 1.734 | 2.101 | 2.552 | 2.878 | 3.922 |
| 19 | 1.328 | 1.729 | 2.093 | 2.539 | 2.861 | 3.883 |
| 20 | 1.325 | 1.725 | 2.086 | 2.528 | 2.845 | 3.850 |
| 21 | 1.323 | 1.721 | 2.080 | 2.518 | 2.831 | 3.819 |
| 22 | 1.321 | 1.717 | 2.074 | 2.508 | 2.819 | 3.792 |
| 23 | 1.319 | 1.714 | 2.069 | 2.500 | 2.807 | 3.767 |
| 24 | 1.318 | 1.711 | 2.064 | 2.492 | 2.797 | 3.745 |
| 25 | 1.316 | 1.708 | 2.060 | 2.485 | 2.787 | 3.725 |
| 26 | 1.315 | 1.706 | 2.056 | 2.479 | 2.779 | 3.707 |
| 27 | 1.314 | 1.703 | 2.052 | 2.473 | 2.771 | 3.690 |
| 28 | 1.313 | 1.701 | 2.048 | 2.467 | 2.763 | 3.674 |
| 29 | 1.311 | 1.699 | 2.045 | 2.462 | 2.756 | 3.659 |
| 30 | 1.310 | 1.697 | 2.042 | 2.457 | 2.750 | 3.646 |
| 40 | 1.303 | 1.684 | 2.021 | 2.423 | 2.704 | 3.551 |
| 60 | 1.296 | 1.671 | 2.000 | 2.390 | 2.660 | 3.460 |
| 120 | 1.289 | 1.658 | 1.980 | 2.358 | 2.617 | 3.373 |
| ∞ | 1.282 | 1.645 | 1.960 | 2.326 | 2.576 | 3.291 |

Abridged from Fisher, R. A., and Yates, F. (Eds.). *Statistical Tables for Biological, Agricultural and Medical Research* (6th ed.), Oliver and Boyd Ltd., Edinburgh and London, 1963, Table III.

# Appendix

**Table C.** Percentage Points of Chi-Square Distribution

| Degrees of Freedom, $df$ | \.100 | \.050 | \.025 | \.010 | \.005 |
|---|---|---|---|---|---|
| 1 | 2.71 | 3.84 | 5.02 | 6.63 | 7.88 |
| 2 | 4.61 | 5.99 | 7.38 | 9.21 | 10.60 |
| 3 | 6.25 | 7.81 | 9.35 | 11.34 | 12.84 |
| 4 | 7.78 | 9.49 | 11.14 | 13.28 | 14.86 |
| 5 | 9.24 | 11.07 | 12.83 | 15.09 | 16.75 |
| 6 | 10.64 | 12.59 | 14.45 | 16.81 | 18.55 |
| 7 | 12.02 | 14.07 | 16.01 | 18.48 | 20.28 |
| 8 | 13.36 | 15.51 | 17.53 | 20.09 | 21.96 |
| 9 | 14.68 | 16.92 | 19.02 | 21.67 | 23.59 |
| 10 | 15.99 | 18.31 | 20.48 | 23.21 | 25.19 |
| 11 | 17.28 | 19.68 | 21.92 | 24.72 | 26.76 |
| 12 | 18.55 | 21.03 | 23.34 | 26.22 | 28.30 |
| 13 | 19.81 | 22.36 | 24.74 | 27.69 | 29.82 |
| 14 | 21.06 | 23.68 | 26.12 | 29.14 | 31.32 |
| 15 | 22.31 | 25.00 | 27.49 | 30.58 | 32.80 |
| 16 | 23.54 | 26.30 | 28.85 | 32.00 | 34.27 |
| 17 | 24.77 | 27.59 | 30.19 | 33.41 | 35.72 |
| 18 | 25.99 | 28.87 | 31.53 | 34.81 | 37.16 |
| 19 | 27.20 | 30.14 | 32.85 | 36.19 | 38.58 |
| 20 | 28.41 | 31.41 | 34.17 | 37.57 | 40.00 |
| 21 | 29.62 | 32.67 | 35.48 | 38.93 | 41.40 |
| 22 | 30.81 | 33.92 | 36.78 | 40.29 | 42.80 |
| 23 | 32.01 | 35.17 | 38.08 | 41.64 | 44.18 |
| 24 | 33.20 | 36.42 | 39.36 | 42.98 | 45.56 |
| 25 | 34.38 | 37.65 | 40.65 | 44.31 | 46.93 |
| 26 | 35.56 | 38.89 | 41.92 | 45.64 | 48.29 |
| 27 | 36.74 | 40.11 | 43.19 | 46.96 | 49.64 |
| 28 | 37.92 | 41.34 | 44.46 | 48.28 | 50.99 |
| 29 | 39.09 | 42.56 | 45.72 | 49.59 | 52.34 |
| 30 | 40.26 | 43.77 | 46.98 | 50.89 | 53.67 |
| 40 | 51.80 | 55.76 | 59.34 | 63.69 | 66.77 |
| 50 | 63.17 | 67.50 | 71.42 | 76.15 | 79.49 |
| 60 | 74.40 | 79.08 | 83.30 | 88.38 | 91.95 |
| 70 | 85.53 | 90.53 | 95.02 | 100.42 | 104.22 |
| 80 | 96.58 | 101.88 | 106.63 | 112.33 | 116.32 |
| 90 | 107.56 | 113.14 | 118.14 | 124.12 | 128.30 |
| 100 | 118.50 | 124.34 | 129.56 | 135.81 | 140.17 |

Abridged from Pearson, E. S., and Hartley, H. O. (Eds.). *Biometrika Tables for Statisticians*, Vol. I (3rd ed.). Cambridge University Press, London, 1966, Table 8.

**Table D.** Percentage Points of the $F$-Distribution, 5% Level of Significance

| $v_2$ \ $v_1$ | 1 | 2 | 3 | 4 | 5 | 6 | 7 | 8 | 9 | 10 | 12 | 15 | 20 | 24 | 30 | 40 | 60 | 120 | ∞ |
|---|---|---|---|---|---|---|---|---|---|---|---|---|---|---|---|---|---|---|---|
| 1 | 161.4 | 199.5 | 215.7 | 224.6 | 230.2 | 234.0 | 236.8 | 238.9 | 240.5 | 241.9 | 243.9 | 245.9 | 248.0 | 249.1 | 250.1 | 251.1 | 252.2 | 253.3 | 254.3 |
| 2 | 18.51 | 19.00 | 19.16 | 19.25 | 19.30 | 19.33 | 19.35 | 19.37 | 19.38 | 19.40 | 19.41 | 19.43 | 19.45 | 19.45 | 19.46 | 19.47 | 19.48 | 19.49 | 19.50 |
| 3 | 10.13 | 9.55 | 9.28 | 9.12 | 9.01 | 8.94 | 8.89 | 8.85 | 8.81 | 8.79 | 8.74 | 8.70 | 8.66 | 8.64 | 8.62 | 8.59 | 8.57 | 8.55 | 8.53 |
| 4 | 7.71 | 6.94 | 6.59 | 6.39 | 6.26 | 6.16 | 6.09 | 6.04 | 6.00 | 5.96 | 5.91 | 5.86 | 5.80 | 5.77 | 5.75 | 5.72 | 5.69 | 5.66 | 5.63 |
| 5 | 6.61 | 5.79 | 5.41 | 5.19 | 5.05 | 4.95 | 4.88 | 4.82 | 4.77 | 4.74 | 4.68 | 4.62 | 4.56 | 4.53 | 4.50 | 4.46 | 4.43 | 4.40 | 4.36 |
| 6 | 5.99 | 5.14 | 4.76 | 4.53 | 4.39 | 4.28 | 4.21 | 4.15 | 4.10 | 4.06 | 4.00 | 3.94 | 3.87 | 3.84 | 3.81 | 3.77 | 3.74 | 3.70 | 3.67 |
| 7 | 5.59 | 4.74 | 4.35 | 4.12 | 3.97 | 3.87 | 3.79 | 3.73 | 3.68 | 3.64 | 3.57 | 3.51 | 3.44 | 3.41 | 3.38 | 3.34 | 3.30 | 3.27 | 3.23 |
| 8 | 5.32 | 4.46 | 4.07 | 3.84 | 3.69 | 3.58 | 3.50 | 3.44 | 3.39 | 3.35 | 3.28 | 3.22 | 3.15 | 3.12 | 3.08 | 3.04 | 3.01 | 2.97 | 2.93 |
| 9 | 5.12 | 4.26 | 3.86 | 3.63 | 3.48 | 3.37 | 3.29 | 3.23 | 3.18 | 3.14 | 3.07 | 3.01 | 2.94 | 2.90 | 2.86 | 2.83 | 2.79 | 2.75 | 2.71 |
| 10 | 4.96 | 4.10 | 3.71 | 3.48 | 3.33 | 3.22 | 3.14 | 3.07 | 3.02 | 2.98 | 2.91 | 2.85 | 2.77 | 2.74 | 2.70 | 2.66 | 2.62 | 2.58 | 2.54 |
| 11 | 4.84 | 3.98 | 3.59 | 3.36 | 3.20 | 3.09 | 3.01 | 2.95 | 2.90 | 2.85 | 2.79 | 2.72 | 2.65 | 2.61 | 2.57 | 2.53 | 2.49 | 2.45 | 2.40 |
| 12 | 4.75 | 3.89 | 3.49 | 3.26 | 3.11 | 3.00 | 2.91 | 2.85 | 2.80 | 2.75 | 2.69 | 2.62 | 2.54 | 2.51 | 2.47 | 2.43 | 2.38 | 2.34 | 2.30 |
| 13 | 4.67 | 3.81 | 3.41 | 3.18 | 3.03 | 2.92 | 2.83 | 2.77 | 2.71 | 2.67 | 2.60 | 2.53 | 2.46 | 2.42 | 2.38 | 2.34 | 2.30 | 2.25 | 2.21 |
| 14 | 4.60 | 3.74 | 3.34 | 3.11 | 2.96 | 2.85 | 2.76 | 2.70 | 2.65 | 2.60 | 2.53 | 2.46 | 2.39 | 2.35 | 2.31 | 2.27 | 2.22 | 2.18 | 2.13 |
| 15 | 4.54 | 3.68 | 3.29 | 3.06 | 2.90 | 2.79 | 2.71 | 2.64 | 2.59 | 2.54 | 2.48 | 2.40 | 2.33 | 2.29 | 2.25 | 2.20 | 2.16 | 2.11 | 2.07 |
| 16 | 4.49 | 3.63 | 3.24 | 3.01 | 2.85 | 2.74 | 2.66 | 2.59 | 2.54 | 2.49 | 2.42 | 2.35 | 2.28 | 2.24 | 2.19 | 2.15 | 2.11 | 2.06 | 2.01 |
| 17 | 4.45 | 3.59 | 3.20 | 2.96 | 2.81 | 2.70 | 2.61 | 2.55 | 2.49 | 2.45 | 2.38 | 2.31 | 2.23 | 2.19 | 2.15 | 2.10 | 2.06 | 2.01 | 1.96 |

| | | | | | | | | | | | | | | | | | |
|---|---|---|---|---|---|---|---|---|---|---|---|---|---|---|---|---|---|
| 18 | 4.41 | 3.55 | 3.16 | 2.93 | 2.77 | 2.66 | 2.58 | 2.51 | 2.46 | 2.41 | 2.34 | 2.27 | 2.19 | 2.15 | 2.11 | 2.06 | 2.02 | 1.97 | 1.92 |
| 19 | 4.38 | 3.52 | 3.13 | 2.90 | 2.74 | 2.63 | 2.54 | 2.48 | 2.42 | 2.38 | 2.31 | 2.23 | 2.16 | 2.11 | 2.07 | 2.03 | 1.98 | 1.93 | 1.88 |
| 20 | 4.35 | 3.49 | 3.10 | 2.87 | 2.71 | 2.60 | 2.51 | 2.45 | 2.39 | 2.35 | 2.28 | 2.20 | 2.12 | 2.08 | 2.04 | 1.99 | 1.95 | 1.90 | 1.84 |
| 21 | 4.32 | 3.47 | 3.07 | 2.84 | 2.68 | 2.57 | 2.49 | 2.42 | 2.37 | 2.32 | 2.25 | 2.18 | 2.10 | 2.05 | 2.01 | 1.96 | 1.92 | 1.87 | 1.81 |
| 22 | 4.30 | 3.44 | 3.05 | 2.82 | 2.66 | 2.55 | 2.46 | 2.40 | 2.34 | 2.30 | 2.23 | 2.15 | 2.07 | 2.03 | 1.98 | 1.94 | 1.89 | 1.84 | 1.78 |
| 23 | 4.28 | 3.42 | 3.03 | 2.80 | 2.64 | 2.53 | 2.44 | 2.37 | 2.32 | 2.27 | 2.20 | 2.13 | 2.05 | 2.01 | 1.96 | 1.91 | 1.86 | 1.81 | 1.76 |
| 24 | 4.26 | 3.40 | 3.01 | 2.78 | 2.62 | 2.51 | 2.42 | 2.36 | 2.30 | 2.25 | 2.18 | 2.11 | 2.03 | 1.98 | 1.94 | 1.89 | 1.84 | 1.79 | 1.73 |
| 25 | 4.24 | 3.39 | 2.99 | 2.76 | 2.60 | 2.49 | 2.40 | 2.34 | 2.28 | 2.24 | 2.16 | 2.09 | 2.01 | 1.96 | 1.92 | 1.87 | 1.82 | 1.77 | 1.71 |
| 26 | 4.23 | 3.37 | 2.98 | 2.74 | 2.59 | 2.47 | 2.39 | 2.32 | 2.27 | 2.22 | 2.15 | 2.07 | 1.99 | 1.95 | 1.90 | 1.85 | 1.80 | 1.75 | 1.69 |
| 27 | 4.21 | 3.35 | 2.96 | 2.73 | 2.57 | 2.46 | 2.37 | 2.31 | 2.25 | 2.20 | 2.13 | 2.06 | 1.97 | 1.93 | 1.88 | 1.84 | 1.79 | 1.73 | 1.67 |
| 28 | 4.20 | 3.34 | 2.95 | 2.71 | 2.56 | 2.45 | 2.36 | 2.29 | 2.24 | 2.19 | 2.12 | 2.04 | 1.96 | 1.91 | 1.87 | 1.82 | 1.77 | 1.71 | 1.65 |
| 29 | 4.18 | 3.33 | 2.93 | 2.70 | 2.55 | 2.43 | 2.35 | 2.28 | 2.22 | 2.18 | 2.10 | 2.03 | 1.94 | 1.90 | 1.85 | 1.81 | 1.75 | 1.70 | 1.64 |
| 30 | 4.17 | 3.32 | 2.92 | 2.69 | 2.53 | 2.42 | 2.33 | 2.27 | 2.21 | 2.16 | 2.09 | 2.01 | 1.93 | 1.89 | 1.84 | 1.79 | 1.74 | 1.68 | 1.62 |
| 40 | 4.08 | 3.23 | 2.84 | 2.61 | 2.45 | 2.34 | 2.25 | 2.18 | 2.12 | 2.08 | 2.00 | 1.92 | 1.84 | 1.79 | 1.74 | 1.69 | 1.64 | 1.58 | 1.51 |
| 60 | 4.00 | 3.15 | 2.76 | 2.53 | 2.37 | 2.25 | 2.17 | 2.10 | 2.04 | 1.99 | 1.92 | 1.84 | 1.75 | 1.70 | 1.65 | 1.59 | 1.53 | 1.47 | 1.39 |
| 120 | 3.92 | 3.07 | 2.68 | 2.45 | 2.29 | 2.17 | 2.09 | 2.02 | 1.96 | 1.91 | 1.83 | 1.75 | 1.66 | 1.61 | 1.55 | 1.50 | 1.43 | 1.35 | 1.25 |
| ∞ | 3.84 | 3.00 | 2.60 | 2.37 | 2.21 | 2.10 | 2.01 | 1.94 | 1.88 | 1.83 | 1.75 | 1.67 | 1.57 | 1.52 | 1.46 | 1.39 | 1.32 | 1.22 | 1.00 |

$v_1$ = numerator degrees of freedom.
$v_2$ = denominator degrees of freedom.
Abridged from Pearson, E. S., and Hartley, H. O. (Eds.). *Biometrika Tables for Statisticians*, Vol. 1 (3rd ed.). Cambridge University Press, London, 1966, Table 18.

**Table D.** Percentage Points of the $F$-Distribution (Continued), 1% Level of Significance

| $v_2$ \ $v_1$ | 1 | 2 | 3 | 4 | 5 | 6 | 7 | 8 | 9 | 10 | 12 | 15 | 20 | 24 | 30 | 40 | 60 | 120 | ∞ |
|---|---|---|---|---|---|---|---|---|---|---|---|---|---|---|---|---|---|---|---|
| 1 | 4052 | 4999.5 | 5403 | 5625 | 5764 | 5859 | 5928 | 5981 | 6022 | 6056 | 6106 | 6157 | 6209 | 6235 | 6261 | 6287 | 6313 | 6339 | 6366 |
| 2 | 98.50 | 99.00 | 99.17 | 99.25 | 99.30 | 99.33 | 99.36 | 99.37 | 99.39 | 99.40 | 99.42 | 99.43 | 99.45 | 99.46 | 99.47 | 99.47 | 99.48 | 99.49 | 99.50 |
| 3 | 34.12 | 30.82 | 29.46 | 28.71 | 28.24 | 27.91 | 27.67 | 27.49 | 27.35 | 27.23 | 27.05 | 26.87 | 26.69 | 26.60 | 26.50 | 26.41 | 26.32 | 26.22 | 26.13 |
| 4 | 21.20 | 18.00 | 16.69 | 15.98 | 15.52 | 15.21 | 14.98 | 14.80 | 14.66 | 14.55 | 14.37 | 14.20 | 14.02 | 13.93 | 13.84 | 13.75 | 13.65 | 13.56 | 13.46 |
| 5 | 16.26 | 13.27 | 12.06 | 11.39 | 10.97 | 10.67 | 10.46 | 10.29 | 10.16 | 10.05 | 9.89 | 9.72 | 9.55 | 9.47 | 9.38 | 9.29 | 9.20 | 9.11 | 9.02 |
| 6 | 13.75 | 10.92 | 9.78 | 9.15 | 8.75 | 8.47 | 8.26 | 8.10 | 7.98 | 7.87 | 7.72 | 7.56 | 7.40 | 7.31 | 7.23 | 7.14 | 7.06 | 6.97 | 6.88 |
| 7 | 12.25 | 9.55 | 8.45 | 7.85 | 7.46 | 7.19 | 6.99 | 6.84 | 6.72 | 6.62 | 6.47 | 6.31 | 6.16 | 6.07 | 5.99 | 5.91 | 5.82 | 5.74 | 5.65 |
| 8 | 11.26 | 8.65 | 7.59 | 7.01 | 6.63 | 6.37 | 6.18 | 6.03 | 5.91 | 5.81 | 5.67 | 5.52 | 5.36 | 5.28 | 5.20 | 5.12 | 5.03 | 4.95 | 4.86 |
| 9 | 10.56 | 8.02 | 6.99 | 6.42 | 6.06 | 5.80 | 5.61 | 5.47 | 5.35 | 5.26 | 5.11 | 4.96 | 4.81 | 4.73 | 4.65 | 4.57 | 4.48 | 4.40 | 4.31 |
| 10 | 10.04 | 7.56 | 6.55 | 5.99 | 5.64 | 5.39 | 5.20 | 5.06 | 4.94 | 4.85 | 4.71 | 4.56 | 4.41 | 4.33 | 4.25 | 4.17 | 4.08 | 4.00 | 3.91 |
| 11 | 9.65 | 7.21 | 6.22 | 5.67 | 5.32 | 5.07 | 4.89 | 4.74 | 4.63 | 4.54 | 4.40 | 4.25 | 4.10 | 4.02 | 3.94 | 3.86 | 3.78 | 3.69 | 3.60 |
| 12 | 9.33 | 6.93 | 5.95 | 5.41 | 5.06 | 4.82 | 4.64 | 4.50 | 4.39 | 4.30 | 4.16 | 4.01 | 3.86 | 3.78 | 3.70 | 3.62 | 3.54 | 3.45 | 3.36 |
| 13 | 9.07 | 6.70 | 5.74 | 5.21 | 4.86 | 4.62 | 4.44 | 4.30 | 4.19 | 4.10 | 3.96 | 3.82 | 3.66 | 3.59 | 3.51 | 3.43 | 3.34 | 3.25 | 3.17 |
| 14 | 8.86 | 6.51 | 5.56 | 5.04 | 4.69 | 4.46 | 4.28 | 4.14 | 4.03 | 3.94 | 3.80 | 3.66 | 3.51 | 3.43 | 3.35 | 3.27 | 3.18 | 3.09 | 3.00 |
| 15 | 8.68 | 6.36 | 5.42 | 4.89 | 4.56 | 4.32 | 4.14 | 4.00 | 3.89 | 3.80 | 3.67 | 3.52 | 3.37 | 3.29 | 3.21 | 3.13 | 3.05 | 2.96 | 2.87 |
| 16 | 8.53 | 6.23 | 5.29 | 4.77 | 4.44 | 4.20 | 4.03 | 3.89 | 3.78 | 3.69 | 3.55 | 3.41 | 3.26 | 3.18 | 3.10 | 3.02 | 2.93 | 2.84 | 2.75 |
| 17 | 8.40 | 6.11 | 5.18 | 4.67 | 4.34 | 4.10 | 3.93 | 3.79 | 3.68 | 3.59 | 3.46 | 3.31 | 3.16 | 3.08 | 3.00 | 2.92 | 2.83 | 2.75 | 2.65 |

# Appendix

| $v_2$ | | | | | | | | | | | | | | | | | |
|---|---|---|---|---|---|---|---|---|---|---|---|---|---|---|---|---|---|
| 18 | 8.29 | 6.01 | 5.09 | 4.58 | 4.25 | 4.01 | 3.84 | 3.71 | 3.60 | 3.51 | 3.37 | 3.23 | 3.08 | 3.00 | 2.92 | 2.84 | 2.75 | 2.66 | 2.57 |
| 19 | 8.18 | 5.93 | 5.01 | 4.50 | 4.17 | 3.94 | 3.77 | 3.63 | 3.52 | 3.43 | 3.30 | 3.15 | 3.00 | 2.92 | 2.84 | 2.76 | 2.67 | 2.58 | 2.49 |
| 20 | 8.10 | 5.85 | 4.94 | 4.43 | 4.10 | 3.87 | 3.70 | 3.56 | 3.46 | 3.37 | 3.23 | 3.09 | 2.94 | 2.86 | 2.78 | 2.69 | 2.61 | 2.52 | 2.42 |
| 21 | 8.02 | 5.78 | 4.87 | 4.37 | 4.04 | 3.81 | 3.64 | 3.51 | 3.40 | 3.31 | 3.17 | 3.03 | 2.88 | 2.80 | 2.72 | 2.64 | 2.55 | 2.46 | 2.36 |
| 22 | 7.95 | 5.72 | 4.82 | 4.31 | 3.99 | 3.76 | 3.59 | 3.45 | 3.35 | 3.26 | 3.12 | 2.98 | 2.83 | 2.75 | 2.67 | 2.58 | 2.50 | 2.40 | 2.31 |
| 23 | 7.88 | 5.66 | 4.76 | 4.26 | 3.94 | 3.71 | 3.54 | 3.41 | 3.30 | 3.21 | 3.07 | 2.93 | 2.78 | 2.70 | 2.62 | 2.54 | 2.45 | 2.35 | 2.26 |
| 24 | 7.82 | 5.61 | 4.72 | 4.22 | 3.90 | 3.67 | 3.50 | 3.36 | 3.26 | 3.17 | 3.03 | 2.89 | 2.74 | 2.66 | 2.58 | 2.49 | 2.40 | 2.31 | 2.21 |
| 25 | 7.77 | 5.57 | 4.68 | 4.18 | 3.85 | 3.63 | 3.46 | 3.32 | 3.22 | 3.13 | 2.99 | 2.85 | 2.70 | 2.62 | 2.54 | 2.45 | 2.36 | 2.27 | 2.17 |
| 26 | 7.72 | 5.53 | 4.64 | 4.14 | 3.82 | 3.59 | 3.42 | 3.29 | 3.18 | 3.09 | 2.96 | 2.81 | 2.66 | 2.58 | 2.50 | 2.42 | 2.33 | 2.23 | 2.13 |
| 27 | 7.68 | 5.49 | 4.60 | 4.11 | 3.78 | 3.56 | 3.39 | 3.26 | 3.15 | 3.06 | 2.93 | 2.78 | 2.63 | 2.55 | 2.47 | 2.38 | 2.29 | 2.20 | 2.10 |
| 28 | 7.64 | 5.45 | 4.57 | 4.07 | 3.75 | 3.53 | 3.36 | 3.23 | 3.12 | 3.03 | 2.90 | 2.75 | 2.60 | 2.52 | 2.44 | 2.35 | 2.26 | 2.17 | 2.06 |
| 29 | 7.60 | 5.42 | 4.54 | 4.04 | 3.73 | 3.50 | 3.33 | 3.20 | 3.09 | 3.00 | 2.87 | 2.73 | 2.57 | 2.49 | 2.41 | 2.33 | 2.23 | 2.14 | 2.03 |
| 30 | 7.56 | 5.39 | 4.51 | 4.02 | 3.70 | 3.47 | 3.30 | 3.17 | 3.07 | 2.98 | 2.84 | 2.70 | 2.55 | 2.47 | 2.39 | 2.30 | 2.21 | 2.11 | 2.01 |
| 40 | 7.31 | 5.18 | 4.31 | 3.83 | 3.51 | 3.29 | 3.12 | 2.99 | 2.89 | 2.80 | 2.66 | 2.52 | 2.37 | 2.29 | 2.20 | 2.11 | 2.02 | 1.92 | 1.80 |
| 60 | 7.08 | 4.98 | 4.13 | 3.65 | 3.34 | 3.12 | 2.95 | 2.82 | 2.72 | 2.63 | 2.50 | 2.35 | 2.20 | 2.12 | 2.03 | 1.94 | 1.84 | 1.73 | 1.60 |
| 120 | 6.85 | 4.79 | 3.95 | 3.48 | 3.17 | 2.96 | 2.79 | 2.66 | 2.56 | 2.47 | 2.34 | 2.19 | 2.03 | 1.95 | 1.86 | 1.76 | 1.66 | 1.53 | 1.38 |
| $\infty$ | 6.63 | 4.61 | 3.78 | 3.32 | 3.02 | 2.80 | 2.64 | 2.51 | 2.41 | 2.32 | 2.18 | 2.04 | 1.88 | 1.79 | 1.70 | 1.59 | 1.47 | 1.32 | 1.00 |

$v_1$ = numerator degrees of freedom.
$v_2$ = denominator degrees of freedom.
Abridged from Pearson, E. S., and Hartley, H. O. (Eds.). *Biometrika Tables for Statisticians*, Vol. 1 (3rd 3d.). Cambridge University Press, London, 1966, Table 18.

# ANSWERS TO SELECTED PROBLEMS

## CHAPTER 2

1. (a) $17/20 = .85$
   (b) $3/20 = .15$
2. (a) $1200/2000 = .60$
   (b) $800/2000 = .40$
   (c) $5/5 = 1.00$
   (d) Pr (5 survivors) = .078
3. (a) $1.0000/2 = .50$
   (b) .9500
   (c) $.0500/2 = .025$
   (d) $1 - (.6892/2) = .6554$
   (e) $(.7699 - .0797)/2 = .3451$
   (f) $.50 + (.3829)/2 = .69145$
   (g) .9901
4. (a) $z = 0.0$
   (b) $z \cong 0.7$
   (c) $z = 1.96$
   (d) $z = 1.64$
   (e) $z \cong 1.3$
   (f) $z = 1.96$
   (g) $z = 2.58$
5. (a) $H: p_1 = p_2$, where $p_1$ equals the proportion among health oriented reporting more practice and $p_2$ equals the proportion among non-health-oriented reporting more practice.
   (b) $\hat{p}_1 = 16/90 = .1778$

327

(c) $\hat{p}_2 = 27/70 = .3857$
(d) $p = (16 + 27)/(90 + 70) = .2688$
(e) $z = -2.94$
(f) $-2.94 < -2.58$; reject
(g) $p = .0037$

6. (b) $H: p_1 = p_2$, where $p_1$ equals the proportion of full-term births among battered children and $p_2$ equals the proportion of full-term births among nonbattered children.
(c) $\hat{p}_1 = 28/34 = .8235$
(d) $\hat{p}_2 = 43/50 = .8600$
(e) $p = (28 + 43)/(34 + 50) = .8452$
(f) $z = -0.45$
(g) $0.45 < 1.96$; retain
(h) $p \cong .6892$

# CHAPTER 3

1. (a) $t = 2.262$
   (b) $t = 3.250$
   (c) $t = 2.093$
   (d) $t = 2.861$
   (e) $t = 2.101$
   (f) $t = 2.878$
   (g) $t \cong 2.042$
   (h) $t \cong 2.750$

2. (a) $t = 1.833$
   (b) $t = 2.821$
   (c) $t = 1.729$
   (d) $t = 2.539$
   (e) $t = 1.734$
   (f) $t = 2.552$
   (g) $t \cong 1.697$
   (h) $t \cong 2.457$

5. (a) $H: \mu = 7.2$
   (b) $t = -2.2$

Answers to Selected Problems

6. (b) $s_p^2 = 0.615$
   (d) $t = 3.24$
   (f) $s_p^2 = .394992$, $t = -4.46$
7. (b) $s_p^2 = 34.09$
   (c) $t = -6.68$
   (f) Economic value of work: $s_p^2 = 5.60$, $t = -0.92$
   Satisfaction with nursing: $s_p^2 = 60.42$, $t = -1.72$
   Conducive home situation: $s_p^2 = 311/51$, $t = -2.92$
8. (b) $\bar{d} = 9.43$
   (c) $s_d = 10.86$
   (d) $t = 3.98$

# CHAPTER 4

1. (a) Retain
   (b) Retain
   (c) Reject
   (d) Retain
   (e) Reject
   (f) Retain
4. (b) $90/160 = 56.25\%$
   (c) $43/160 = 26.88\%$
   (d) $26.88\%$
   (e) $26.88\%$
   (f) 
   | 24.19 | 65.81 |
   |---|---|
   | 18.82 | 51.18 |
   (g) $\chi^2 = 8.65$
   (i) $\sqrt{8.65} = 2.94$
5. (a)

|  |  | Alcohol |  |  |
|---|---|---|---|---|
|  |  | Yes | No |  |
| Nurse | Yes | 8 | 2 | 10 |
|  | No | 7 | 13 | 20 |
|  |  | 15 | 15 | 30 |

(c) $15/30 = 50\%$
(d) $8/10 = 80\%$
(e) $7/20 = 35\%$

(f) 
| 5 | 5 |
|---|---|
| 10 | 10 |

(g) $\chi^2 = 5.4$

6. (a) 
|  |  | Student | Staff |  |
|---|---|---|---|---|
| *Nurse* | Yes | 24 | 67 | 91 |
|  | No | 29 | 39 | 68 |
|  |  | 53 | 106 | 159 |

(b) $91/159 = 57.23\%$
(c) $24/53 = 45.28\%$
(d) $67/106 = 63.21\%$
(g) Expected values:

| 30.33 | 60.66 |
|---|---|
| 22.67 | 45.36 |

$\chi^2 = 4.64$

7. (b) $27/43 = 62.79\%$

(c) 
|  | Low | High |
|---|---|---|
| None | 11.30 | 6.70 |
| One | 5.02 | 2.98 |
| Two | 10.67 | 6.33 |

(d) $\chi^2 = 9.32$

# CHAPTER 5

5. (a) $x$ = science and health PACE subscale
   (b) $y$ = grade in nursing principles and skills course
   (c) $b_{y \cdot x} = .35$
   (d) positive
   (f) overall average: 88.99

Answers to Selected Problems                                                           331

6. (b) $y' = 167.87 - .86\,x$
   (c) $y' = 160.99$
   (d) $t = -4.89$

7. (a) Retain
   (b) Reject
   (c) Retain
   (d) Reject

8. (a) $F_{.01}(1,18) = 8.28$
   (b) $F_{.01}(1,28) = 7.64$
   (c) $F_{.01}(1,100) = 6.90$
   (d) $F_{.01}(1,1000) = 6.66$

9. (c) $b_{y \cdot x} = 0.89,\ a_{y \cdot x} = 91.46$
   (d) $y' = 127.06$
   (e) $s^2_{y \cdot x} = 308.469$
   (f) $s^2_x = 87.4$
   (h) $t = 1.83$

10. (a) Total SS = 5356.94
    Regression SS = 1038.3744
    Deviations SS = 4318.5656

    (b)
    Regression ANOVA

| Source of Variation | Sum of Squares | DF | Mean Square | F |
| --- | --- | --- | --- | --- |
| Regression | 1038.3744 | 1 | 1038.3744 | 3.366 |
| Deviations | 4318.5656 | 14 | 308.46897 | |
| Total | 5356.9400 | 15 | 357.12933 | |

   (d) $\sqrt{F} = \sqrt{3.366} = 1.83$


**CHAPTER 6**

2. (a) $s^2_x = 87.4$
   (b) $s^2_y = 357.29$
   (c) $r_{x \cdot y} = .44$
   (d) $r_{x \cdot y} = .89\,(\sqrt{87.4}/\sqrt{357.29}) = .44$
   (f) $t = 1.83$

3. (b) $t = -1.90$
4. (b) $t = -4.43$
   (g) $r^2_{x \cdot y} = (.20)^2 = 4\%$
   (h) $r_{x_2 x_3 \cdot x_1} = .07$
   (i) $t = 1.11$
5. (a) DE1 × death anxiety (zero order): $t = -1.04$
   DE1 × death anxiety (age controlled): $t = -0.58$
   DE1 × death anxiety (work experience controlled): $t = -0.95$
   DE1 × death anxiety (second order): $t = -0.14$
6. (a) $t = 0.54$
   (b) $t = 0.89$
   (c) $t = 1.33$
   (d) $t = 2.18$

# CHAPTER 7

1. (a)

Regression ANOVA

| Source of Variation | Sum of Squares | DF | Mean Square | F |
|---|---|---|---|---|
| Regression | 83.4 | 2 | 41.7 | 8.6875 |
| Deviations | 81.6 | 17 | 4.8 | |
| Total | 165.0 | 19 | | |

   (c) $F = [(.71)^2/2]/[\{1 - (.71)^2\}/17] = 8.64$
   (e) $\hat{R}^2 = .45$

2. $t = 1.71$

3. (f)

Regression ANOVA

| Source of variation | Sum of Squares | DF | Mean Square | F |
|---|---|---|---|---|
| Regression | 2910.54 | 2 | 1455.27 | 9.87 |
| Residual | 11056.14 | 75 | 147.42 | |
| Total | 13966.68 | 77 | | |

   (h) $F_{.01}(2,70) = 4.92$

Answers to Selected Problems

4. (a) Age
   (c) $R = .18$
   (d) $R^2 = 3.24\%$
   (j) $\hat{R}^2 = 12\%$
5. (a) $R^2 = 7\%$
   (b) $F = 1.91; F_{.05}(3,70) = 2.74$
   (e) $F = 3.37; F_{.05}(1,70) = 3.98$
   (f) $F = 5.35; F_{.05}(1,70) = 3.98$
6. (d) $F = 2.81; F_{.05}(3,70) = 2.74$
   (e) $F = 3.49; F_{.05}(1,70) = 3.98$

## CHAPTER 8

2. (b) e.g., $y$ = wife's health
   $x_1$ = socioeconomic status
   $x_2$ = years of education
   $x_1 x_2$ = socioeconomic status × years of education
   (c) $y = \alpha + \beta_1 x_1 + \beta_2 x_2 + \beta_3 x_1 x_2$
4. (a) Months since last delivery
   (c) 10.83%
   (e) Step 2: $F = 4.85; F_{.05}(1,48) = 4.04$
       Step 5: $F = 37.46; F_{.05}(1,44) = 4.06$
   (h) $\hat{R}^2 = 77\%$

## CHAPTER 9

1. (a)

ANOVA

| Source of Variation | Sum of Squares | DF | Mean Square | F |
|---|---|---|---|---|
| Between groups | 82.22 | 3 | 27.4067 | 6.38 |
| Within groups | 85.93 | 20 | 4.2965 | |
| Total | 168.15 | 23 | | |

(c) $F_{.05}(3,20) = 3.10$

2. (a) $MS_B = 6.4721$
   (b) $MS_W = 0.615$
   (c) $F = 10.5238$; $\sqrt{F} = 3.24$
   (d) $MS_B = 7.8701$; $MS_W = .394992$; $F = 19.9247$; $\sqrt{F} = 4.46$
3. (b) $F_{.05}(3,\infty) = 3.84$; $17.8474 > 3.84$
   (d) Economic value of work: $0.9057 < 3.84$
       Satisfaction with nursing: $3.0419 < 3.84$
       Conducive home situation: $8.6079 > 3.84$
   (e) $MS_W = 33.7765$
   (f) $MS_B = F \times MS_W = 602.8227$

ANOVA

| Source of Variation | Sum of Squares | DF | Mean Square | F |
|---|---|---|---|---|
| Between groups | 1808.4681 | 3 | 602.8227 | 17.8474 |
| Within groups | 62486.525 | 1850 | 33.7765 | |
| Total | 64294.9931 | 1853 | | |

4. (a) Diploma vs some college: $F = 30.23$
       Diploma vs bachelor's degree: $F = 6.43$
       Diploma vs graduate work: $F = 35.04$
       Some college vs bachelor's degree: $F = 2.87$
       Some college vs graduate work: $F = 6.66$
       Bachelor's degree vs graduate work: $F = 5.86$
   (b) $F_{.10}(3,\infty) = F_T = 2.08$; $F = 6.24$
       Diploma vs some college: $30.23 > 6.24$
       Diploma vs bachelor's degree: $6.43 > 6.24$
       Diploma vs graduate work: $35.04 > 6.24$
       Some college vs bachelor's degree: $2.87 < 6.24$
       Some college vs graduate work: $6.66 > 6.24$
       Bachelor's degree vs graduate work: $5.86 < 6.24$
5. (a) Group 1 vs group 3: $F = 0.02$
       Group 1 vs group 4: $F = 57.47$
   (c) $F_{.05}(3,90) = 2.71$; $F' = 8.13$
       Group 1 vs group 3: $0.02 < 8.13$
       Group 1 vs group 4: $57.47 > 8.13$

Answers to Selected Problems

6. (a) $L_2 = -3.63$
$L_3 = 2.87$
(b) $SS_{L_2} = 41.300746$
$SS_{L_3} = 119.29324$
(c) $F_{L_2} = 0.53$
$F_{L_3} = 1.54$

# CHAPTER 10

2. (e) $F = 3.01$
(f) $F_{.05}(2,70) = 3.13$
(h) $F = 6.02; F_{.05}(1,70) = 3.98$
(i) $F = 1.29; F_{.05}(2,70) = 3.13$

3. (a)

ANOVA

| Source of Variation | Sum of Squares | DF | Mean Square | F |
|---|---|---|---|---|
| Between groups | 3.524 | 2 | 1.762 | 2.81 |
| Within groups | 50.745 | 81 | 0.626 | |
| Total | 54.269 | 83 | | |

(b) $F_{.05}(2,80) = 3.11; 2.81 < 3.11$

4. (a)

| | Group 1 | Group 2 | Group 3 |
|---|---|---|---|
| $L_1$ | 1 | 1 | $-2$ |
| $L_2$ | 1 | $-1$ | 0 |

(c) $L_1 = .71; SS_{L_1} = 2.3790$
$L_2 = .29; SS_{L_2} = 1.2180$
(d) $F = 4.06; F = 2.08; F_{.05}(1,70) = 3.98$

5. (e) $F$ = Mean-square treatment/mean-square error = 2542.51/12.68
(f) $F_{.05}(1,70) = 3.98; 200.48 > 3.98$
(h) $F$ = Mean-square pretest/mean-square error
$= 56.11/12.68; F_{.05}(1,70) = 3.98; 4.42 > 3.98$
(i) $F$ = Mean-square treatment × pretest/mean-square error
$= 1.01/12.68; F_{.05}(1,70) = 3.98; 0.08 < 3.98$

6.

### ANOVA

| Source of Variation | Sum of Squares | DF | Mean Square | F |
|---|---|---|---|---|
| Between groups | 2542.51 | 1 | 2542.5100 | 194.24 |
| Within groups | 1020.98 | 78 | 13.0895 | |
| Total | 3563.49 | 79 | | |

7. (g)

### ANOVA

| Source of Variation | Sum of Squares | DF | Mean Square | F |
|---|---|---|---|---|
| Between groups | 3077.76 | 1 | 3077.76 | 2.67 |
| Within groups | 200552.24 | 174 | 1152.599 | |
| Total | 203630.00 | 175 | 1163.60 | |

# CHAPTER 11

2. (a) $MS_R$ (subjects) = 3358.757
   $MS_C$ (trials) = 13816.500
   $MS_{RC}$ (interaction) = 2303.191
   (c) $F = 6.00$
   (d) $F_{.01}(2,200) = 4.71$; $6.00 > 4.71$

3. (a) $MS_{RBTr} = 63168.31$
   $MS_{RWTr} = 1940.0768$
   $MS_C = 40736.69$
   $MS_{C \times Tr} = 30392.13$
   $MS_{C \times RWTr} = 180.317$
   (b) Between treatments (groups): $F = 32.56$
   Between trials (days): $F = 225.92$
   Trials (days) × treatments (groups): $F = 168.55$

5. (b) $F_{.05}(3,100) = 2.70$; $144.31 > 2.70$

6. Verbal estimation decreases from day 1 to day 4 in a linear fashion

Answers to Selected Problems

## CHAPTER 12

4. (b) $MS_B = 545.3333$
$MS_W = 100.9000$
$F = 5.40$
(c) $F_{.05}(3,20) = 3.10; 5.40 > 3.10$
(f) Blood pressure at beginning of the study
(h) $MS_B = 466.6667$
$MS_W = 94.7368$
$F = 4.93$
$F_{.05}(3,19) = 3.13; 4.93 > 3.13$

5. (b) $F = 2.153/0.619$
(f) $F = 1.643/0.344$

## CHAPTER 13

2. (a) Factor I:   items 1–6, 8, 9
Factor II:  items 10, 16–18
Factor III: items 7, 11–13
Factor IV:  items 14, 15

3. (a) Analysis would include all students in the sample; 2 groups: never smoked vs others.
(b) Analysis would include all current smokers in the sample; groups would be defined according to the amounts of smoking categorized by the data
(c) Analysis would include all who currently smoke or smoked but quit; 2 groups: current smokers vs past smokers.
(d) Analysis would include all students in the sample; 3 groups: never smoked, current smokers, smoked but quit.

## CHAPTER 14

1. (a) $d = .2$
(b) 393

2. No. Power would be slightly over .25.

3. (a) $d = .5$
   (b) 64
   (d) Yes. Power would be slightly less than .80.
4. (a) $L = 4.33$; power $> .21$
   (b) $L = 13.30$; power $> .64$
   (c) $L = 20.77$; power $> .85$
   (d) $L = 28.24$; power $> .85$
   (e) About 150
5. (a) .25

# Subject Index

## A

Acceptance region, 33
Additive effects, 179*ff*, 226
Alternative hypothesis, 11
Analysis of covariance, 227*ff*
   adjusted between groups sum of squares, 282
   adjusted total sum of squares, 281
   adjusted within groups sum of squares, 282
   covariates, 278*ff*
   model, 279*ff*
   multiple covariates, 287
   null hypothesis, 285
   test statistic, 283*ff*
   uses, 277*ff*
   within groups regression, 281
Analysis of variance, 186, 193*ff*
   components of variance, 257
   factorial designs, 244*ff*
   factors, 226, 245*ff*
   fixed effects, 195, 256
   interaction, 226*ff*
   main effects, 226*ff*
   mean square, 108
   mixed effects, 257
   model I, 195, 257
   model II, 257
   model III, 257
   multiple factors, 244
   multivariate, 269
   non-additivity, 226*ff*
   one-way, 193*ff*
      between groups sum of squares, 198
      cross-product, 197
      error mean square, 200
      error sum of squares, 197
      mean square between groups, 199
      mean square within groups, 200
      model, 194*ff*
      null hypothesis, 201
      partitioning degrees of freedom, 199
      partitioning sum of squares, 196*ff*
      test statistic, 201
      total sum of squares, 196
      treatment mean square, 200
      treatment sum of squares, 198
      uses, 193*ff*
      within groups sum of squares, 197
   proportion of variance, 205
   random effects, 257
   randomized blocks, 258*ff*
   and regression analysis, 105, 186, 204*ff*
   repeated measures, 194, 263*ff*
   treatment effect, 195
   two-way, 225*ff*
      additive effects, 229
      cell means, 227

---

Page numbers followed by *ff* indicate first page of discussion. Inclusive pages are not indicated.

Analysis of variance, two-way *(continued)*
    column factor, 227, 232
    column treatment effect, 237
    error sum of squares, 236
    interaction effects, 229*ff*
    interaction sum of squares, 238
    levels of factors, 227
    model, 232*ff*
    null hypotheses, 239*ff*
    partitioning degrees of freedom, 239
    partitioning sum of squares, 235*ff*
    row factor, 227, 232
    row treatment effect, 237
    row x column interaction, 238
    test statistics, 240*ff*
    uses, 225*ff*
    within groups sum of squares, 236
  univariate, 269
A posteriori comparisons, 209
A priori comparisons, 209
Association
  chi-square tests of, 68
  vs. causation, 126*ff*

## B

Bell curve, 25
Bias, 4*ff*
Binomial distribution, 19*ff*
  hypothesis test for a proportion, 22
  normal approximation, 28*ff*

## C

Categorizing data, 83*ff*
Causality, 127, 186
Cell frequencies, 72
Central limit theorem, 45
Chi-square, 66*ff*
  calculation, 70*ff*
  cell frequencies, 72
  degrees of freedom, 69*ff*
  distribution, 69*ff*
  expected values, 72
  goodness-of-fit tests, 68, 81*ff*
  and normal distribution, 73
  null hypothesis, 71
  observed values, 71
  partitioning of, 77*ff*
  R × C tables, 74*ff*
  tests of association, 68
  two by two tables, 66, 71*ff*
  uses, 66*ff*
Coding, 182*ff*
  dummy, 182*ff*
  effect, 184
  orthogonal, 184
Confidence intervals, 57*ff*
  for difference between two means, 58
  for population mean, 57
Confidence limits, 57*ff*
Continuous variable, 40
Correlation, 118*ff*
  coefficient, 119*ff*
    vs. regression coefficient, 118*ff*, 124
    calculation, 119
    multiple, 144
    null hypotheses, 122, 124
    point biserial correlation, 121
    rank correlation, 121
    test statistic, 122
    uses, 118*ff*
  first order, 131
  matrix, 120
  multiple, 144*ff*
  partial, 128*ff*, 153*ff*
  zero order, 131
Criterion variable, 59

## D

Degrees of freedom
  for analysis of variance, 199, 239
  for chi-square distribution, 69, 76
  for $F$ distribution, 110
  for $t$ distribution, 49
Dependent variable, 59
Descriptive statistics, 2
Difference between two means, 54*ff*
  estimate, 54
  null hypothesis, 46, 54

Subject Index

sampling distribution, 45
standard error of the difference, 46
test statistic, 46, 55
Difference between two proportions, 29*ff*
  estimate, 30
  mean, 30
  null hypothesis, 9, 29
  sampling distribution, 30
  standard error of difference, 30
  test statistic, 31
Discriminant analysis, 297*ff*
  discriminant function, 298
  and multiple regression, 298
  uses, 297*ff*
Dummy coding, 182*ff*
Duncan's new multiple range test, 210
Dunnett's test, 210

## E

Ethical concerns, 7
Estimates, 10
Expected values, 72

## F

*F* distribution, 108*ff*
  degrees of freedom, 108*ff*
  and *t* distribution, 110
*F* test
  in multiple regression, 148*ff*
  in one-way ANOVA, 201
  in two-way ANOVA, 240*ff*, 257*ff*
Factor analysis, 293*ff*
  factors, 296
  factor loading, 296
  factor rotations, 296
  model, 295
  uses, 294
Fisher's exact test, 71
Fisher's *z* transformation, 125

## G

Gaussian distribution, 25
Goodness-of-fit tests, 68, 81*ff*

## H

Hypothesis testing, 8
  for a correlation, 122
  for a mean, 50
  for a multiple correlation coefficient, 144
  for a proportion, 31
  for the difference between two means, 54
  for the difference between two proportions, 34

## I

Inference, 3, 7, 10
Inferential statistics, 2*ff*
Interaction, 172, 179, 226*ff*

## L

Least significant difference, 210
Level of significance, 24, 33, 305
Linear relationship, 93*ff*

## M

Main effect, 226*ff*
Matching, 59
Mean, 25, 43*ff*
  estimate, 50
  null hypothesis, 46, 50
  sampling distribution, 44
  standard error of the mean, 44
  test statistic, 45, 51
Mean square, 108
Method of least squares, 94
Multiple comparisons, 193, 206*ff*
  a posteriori, 209
  a priori, 209
  contrasts, 207
  null hypotheses, 208
  Scheffé tests for, 210*ff*
  test statistics, 209
  uses, 206*ff*
Multiple correlation, 144*ff*
  coefficient, 144*ff*

Multiple correlation *(continued)*
  power analysis for, 310
Multiple regression, 141 *(See also* Regression)
  dummy coding, 182*ff*
  estimated regression line, 145
  interaction in, 172, 179*ff*
  mean square, 147
  mean square deviation from, 147
  model, 143
  multiple regression coefficient, 144
  multiplicative terms, 181
  nonlinear relationships and, 171, 173*ff*
  null hypothesis, 145
  partitioning sum of squares, 146
  proportion of variance explained, 125*ff*, 149
  qualitative variables and, 172, 182*ff*
  shrinkage, 162
  standard partial regression coefficients, 161
  stepwise, 142, 150*ff*, 187
    backward solution, 151
    forward inclusion solution, 151
    null hypothesis, 158*ff*
    partial correlation in, 153*ff*
    test statistics, 158*ff*
    uses, 150*ff*, 187
  test statistic, 148
  uses, 141*ff*
Multivariate analysis, 141

## N

Nonlinear relationships, 93, 171, 173*ff*
Normal distribution, 24*ff*
  approximation to binomial distribution, 29
  area under normal curve, 26
  and chi-square distribution, 73
  mean, 25
  standard deviation, 25
  standard normal distribution, 27
  and *t* distribution, 49
  variance, 25
  *z* score, 27

Null hypothesis, 8
  rejecting, 10
  retaining, 10

## O

Observed values, 71
One-tailed tests, 53
Orthogonal contrasts, 210, 213*ff*
  formation, 213
  independence of, 214
  null hypothesis, 215
  tests, 216

## P

P value, 35
Paired data, 59*ff*
  reasons for pairing, 59
  repeated measures, ANOVA, 194, 263*ff*
  *t* test for paired data, 43, 59*ff*
Parameters, 25
Partial correlation, 128*ff*, 153*ff*
  calculation, 131
  coefficient, 130
  first order, 131
  null hypothesis, 132
  second order, 132
  in stepwise multiple regression, 153*ff*
  test statistic, 131
  uses, 128, 132
Partial regression coefficient, 143, 161
Partitioning of chi-square, 77*ff*
Pooled estimate of variance, 48, 200
Population, 3*ff*
Post hoc comparisons, 210
Power, 304*ff*
  analysis for difference between two means, 308
  analysis for multiple correlation, 310
  effect size, 305*ff*
  and Type I error
  and Type II error, 304
Pretest posttest control group design, 265

Probability distribution, 19
Product moment correlation coefficient, 119
Proportion, 28*ff*, 31*ff*
  estimate, 23
  mean, 29
  null hypothesis, 22
  sampling distribution, 28
  standard error, 29
  test statistic, 29
Proportion of variance, 125*ff*, 149, 205

# R

Random sample, 5
Randomization, 6
Randomized blocks, 258*ff*
  blocking factor, 259
  sub-blocks, 257
  test statistic, 261
  uses, 258*ff*
Regression, 91*ff* (*See also* Multiple regression)
  as analysis of variance, 105*ff*, 110, 186, 204*ff*
  coefficient, 100
  vs. correlation coefficient, 118*ff*
    estimate, 100
    null hypothesis, 103
    standard, 161
    test statistic, 104
  dependent variable, 92
  deviations from, 101*ff*
  fitted regression line, 97, 101*ff*
  independent variable, 92
  mean square, 109, 147
  mean square deviation from, 102, 109, 147
  method of least squares, 98
  model, 96
  multiple, 141*ff* (*See also* Multiple regression)
  null hypothesis, 103
  partitioning sum of squares, 105*ff*
  slope, 94
  test statistic, 104, 109
  total mean square, 109
  uses, 91
  y-intercept, 94
Rejection region, 34
Repeated measures ANOVA, 194, 263*ff*
Representative sample, 4
Research hypothesis, 8

# S

Sample, 3*ff*
  biased, 4*ff*
  hypothetical, 6
  vs. population, 3*ff*
  random, 5
  representative, 4
  simple random, 5
  stratified random, 5
  systematic random, 5
  variance, 47
Sample size
  in $t$ test for correlation coefficient, 123*ff*
  in $t$ test for difference between two means, 56
  in $F$ test in multiple regression, 150
  in $t$ test for a single mean, 52
  in $t$ test for regression coefficient, 104
  power and, 304*ff*
Sampling distribution, 28
  of a sample mean, 43
  of a sample proportion, 28
  of the difference between two sample means, 45
  of the difference between two sample proportions, 30
Scheffé tests, 210*ff*
Shrinkage, 162
Significant difference, 42
Slope of a straight line, 94
Standard deviation, 25, 27
Standard error
  of the difference, 46
  of the mean, 44
Sum of squares
  deviations, 108

Sum of squares *(continued)*
  regression, 108
Studentized range, 210

## T

$t$-distribution, 47*ff*
  degrees of freedom, 49
  and $F$ distribution, 110
  and normal distribution, 49
Test statistic, 36
Time series, 185
Trend analysis, 218*ff*
$t$-test
  in correlation, 122
  for difference between two means, 48, 55
  paired, 43, 59*ff*
  power of, 308
  in regression, 104
  for single mean, 48, 51
  as a special case of ANOVA, 194
  uses, 40*ff*
Two-by-two tables, 66, 71*ff*
Two-tailed tests, 53
Type I error, 23, 305
Type II error, 304

## V

Variable, 19
  binomial, 19
  categorical, 182
  constructs, 293
  continuous, 40
  criterion, 59
  dependent, 59, 92
  dichotomous, 182
  dummy, 182*ff*
  independent, 92
  predicted, 92
  predictor, 92
  range of values, 111
Variance
  pooled estimate of, 48
  proportion of variance explained, 125, 149, 205
  ratio, 109
  sample, 47

## Y

Yates' correction for continuity, 71
y-intercept, 94

## Z

$z$-score, 27*ff*
$z$ transformation, 125
zero order correlation, 131

# AUTHOR INDEX

## B

Bishop, Y.M.M., 81
Brock, A.M., 251–252
Burns, M.W., 135, 166, 176, 189

## C

Campbell, D.T., 12, 60, 265
Castles, M., 86
Chang, B.L., 15
Cleland, V., 13, 63, 222, 224, 289
Clough, D., 265
Cochran, W.G., 5, 48, 125, 179, 196, 210, 219, 234, 270, 276, 288
Cohen, J., 121, 125, 184, 186, 271, 288, 299, 305*ff*
Cohen, P., 121, 125, 184, 186, 271, 288, 299
Collins, J.R., 187, 301
Corey, E.J.B., 13, 38

## D

Denton, J.A., 136
Derdiarian, A., 265
Dittmar, S.S., 64
DuCette, J.P., 242, 247
Dulski, T., 64

## E

Earp, J.A.L., 14, 89
Everly, G.S., 299

## F

Falcione, R.L., 299
Farrell, K.M., 300
Ferguson, G.A., 71, 210
Friedman, M., 115, 133

## G

Griggs, B.M., 201*ff*, 289

## H

Harman, H.H., 296, 297
Hegedus, K.S., 134, 168, 169
Holmes, T.H., 180
Hong, E.K., 164, 189

## I

Isenberg, M.A., 272, 274–275

## J

Janis, I.J., 174
Johnson, D.M., 112, 132, 285
Johnson, J.E., 248, 250, 262

---

Page numbers followed by *ff* indicate the first page of discussion. Inclusive pages are not indicated.

## K

Keith, P.M., 86
Kerlinger, F.N., 143, 151, 178, 184, 297, 299
Kim, S., 62, 220, 248, 262, 290
Kirgis, C.A., 190
Klett, C.J., 143, 299
Klugh, H.E., 245, 270

## L

Lindeman, C.A., 253, 271
Lowery, B.J., 242, 247

## M

Meleis, A.I., 300
Mims, F.H., 267

## N

Nie, N.H., 160, 179, 185, 234, 271, 278, 288, 297, 299

## O

Overall, J.E., 143, 299

## P

Pedhazur, E.J., 143, 151, 178, 184, 297, 299
Price, J.L., 187, 301

## R

Rahe, R.H., 180
Richards, M.A., 303
Rosenman, R.H., 115, 133
Rottkamp, B.C., 267

## S

Smith, H.W., 8, 127
Smyth, K., 115, 133
Snedecor, G.W., 5, 48, 125, 179, 196, 210, 219, 234, 270, 276, 288
Stanley, J.C., 12, 60, 265
Stetzer, S.L., 253, 271

## T

Tamez, E.G., 273
Turnbull, E.M., 37, 85

## V

Volicer, B.J., 135, 166, 176, 189, 288, 294

## W

Winer, B.J., 181, 210, 245, 258, 265, 269, 270, 276, 288
Wisenbaker, V.B., 136
Woods, N.F., 14, 89

# NOTES